THE HSC
Handbook of Pediatrics

THE HSC
Handbook of
Pediatrics

The Hospital for Sick Children
Toronto, Canada

Editor

ANNE I. DIPCHAND, MD, FRCPC, FAAP
Formerly, Chief Resident, Department of Pediatrics
The Hospital for Sick Children, Toronto, Canada
Currently, Cardiology Fellow, Division of Cardiology,
Department of Pediatrics
The Hospital for Sick Children, Toronto, Canada

NINTH EDITION

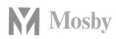

A Harcourt Health Sciences Company
St. Louis   London   Philadelphia   Sydney   Toronto

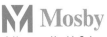
Mosby
A Harcourt Health Sciences Company

Vice President and Publisher, Medicine: Anne S. Patterson
Editor: Laura DeYoung
Associate Developmental Editor: Jennifer Byington Geistler
Project Manager: Patricia Tannian
Production Editor: Melissa Mraz Lastarria
Book Design Manager: Gail Morey Hudson
Manufacturing Manager: Dave Graybill
Cover Design: Teresa Breckwoldt

NINTH EDITION

Printed in the United States of America

Mosby, Inc.
11830 Westline Industrial Drive
St. Louis, Missouri 63146

Library of Congress Cataloging-in-Publication Data

The HSC handbook of pediatrics/the Hospital for Sick Children,
    Toronto, Canada. —9th ed./editor, Anne I. Dipchand.
        p.   cm.
    Includes bibliographical references and index.
    ISBN 0-8151-4664-7
    1. Pediatrics—Handbooks, manuals, etc.   I. Dipchand, Anne I.
II. Hospital for Sick Children.
    [DNLM: 1. Pediatrics—handbooks.   WS 39 H873 1997]
RJ48.H78   1997
618.92—dc21
DNLM/DLC   97-10

        00 01 / 9 8 7 6 5 4 3 2

CONTRIBUTORS

SANDRA ARNOLD, MD, FRCPC
Associate Chief Resident,
Department of Pediatrics,
The Hospital for Sick Children,
Toronto, Ontario, Canada
Dermatology

**MARIA P. SANDE-LEMOS
AZCUE, MD, PhD, FRCPC**
Staff Physician,
Department of Pediatrics (GI),
Hospital Fernando Fonseca,
Amadora, Portugal;
Formerly: Fellow,
Department of Gastroenterology
    and Nutrition,
The Hospital for Sick Children,
Toronto, Ontario, Canada
Gastroenterology

DARIUS J. BÄGLI, MDCM
Assistant Professor,
Department of Surgery,
Division of Urology,
The Hospital for Sick Children,
University of Toronto,
Toronto, Ontario, Canada
Urology

HANSA BHARGAVA, MD
Resident,
Department of Pediatrics,
The Hospital for Sick Children,
Toronto, Ontario, Canada
Nutrition

**SUSAN M.C. CAMPBELL, BSc,
MSc, MD**
Resident,
Department of Pediatrics,
The Hospital for Sick Children,
Toronto, Ontario, Canada
Adolescent Medicine

**SHARON MIELKE DELL, B.Eng.,
MD, FRCPC**
Consultant Pediatrician,
Toronto, Ontario, Canada;
Formerly:
    Associate Chief Resident,
Department of Pediatrics,
The Hospital for Sick Children,
Toronto, Ontario, Canada
Neurology/Neurosurgery

**ANNE I. DIPCHAND, MD, FRCPC,
FAAP**
Cardiology Fellow,
Division of Cardiology;
Formerly: Chief Resident,
Department of Pediatrics,
The Hospital for Sick Children,
Toronto, Ontario, Canada
*Editor, Emergencies, Lab Reference
Values, and Procedures*

ANH PHUONG DO, MD
Resident,
Department of Pediatrics,
The Hospital for Sick Children,
Toronto, Ontario, Canada
Metabolic Disease

WENDY H. EDWARDS, BScN, MD
Chief Resident,
Department of Pediatrics,
The Hospital for Sick Children,
Toronto, Ontario, Canada
Fluids and Electrolytes

GRAHAM ELLIS, PhD, FCACB, FRCPath, DABCC

Formerly:
Assistant Biochemist,
Department of Pediatric
  Laboratory Medicine,
The Hospital for Sick Children,
Toronto, Ontario, Canada
Laboratory Reference Values

DAVID WALLACE FEAR, MD, FRCPC

Chair, Pain Management
  Committee,
Department of Anaesthesia,
The Hospital for Sick Children,
Toronto, Ontario, Canada
Pain

VITO FORTE, MD, FRCSC

Department of Otolaryngology,
The Hospital for Sick Children,
Toronto, Ontario, Canada
Otalaryngology

MARYAM FOULADI, MD, FRCPC, FAAP

Fellow,
Department of Hematology and
  Oncology,
The Hospital for Sick Children,
Toronto, Ontario, Canada
Oncology

BETH DEBORAH GAMULKA, MDCM

Chief Resident
Department of Pediatrics,
The Hospital for Sick Children,
Toronto, Ontario, Canada
Rheumatology

SEAN GODFREY, MBChB, FRCPC

Consulting Pediatrician,
Toronto, Ontario, Canada;
Formerly: Resident,
Department of Pediatrics,
The Hospital for Sick Children,
Toronto, Ontario, Canada
Dentistry

ASTRID GUTTMANN, AB, BA, MSc, MDCM

Resident,
Department of Pediatrics,
The Hospital for Sick Children,
Toronto, Ontario, Canada
Surgery

JILL HAMILTON, MD, FRCPC

Fellow,
Department of Endocrinology;
Formerly: Chief Resident,
Department of Pediatrics,
The Hospital for Sick Children,
Toronto, Ontario, Canada
Endocrinology

GIANNOULA KLEMENT, BSc, MD, FRCPC

Fellow,
Department of Hematology and
  Oncology,
The Hospital for Sick Children,
Toronto, Ontario, Canada
Hematology

TOMMY KWOK LEUNG HO, MD

Resident,
Department of Pediatrics,
The Hospital for Sick Children,
Toronto, Ontario, Canada
Plastic Surgery

SHEILA J. JACOBSON, MBBCh, FRCPC

Staff Pediatrician,
Department of Pediatrics,
The Hospital for Sick Children,
Toronto, Ontario, Canada
Pain

FATIMA ROSHANALI KAMALIA, MD

Resident,
Department of Pediatrics,
The Hospital for Sick Children,
Toronto, Ontario, Canada
Orthopedics

JANE J-H KIM, MD FRCPC

Fellow,
Developmental Endocrinology,
National Institute of Child Health
and Human Development,
National Institutes of Health,
Bethesda, Maryland;
Formerly: Associate Chief
Resident,
Department of Pediatrics,
The Hospital for Sick Children,
Toronto, Ontario, Canada
Infectious Diseases

**JOEL A. KIRSH, BASc, MSc, MD,
FRCPC**

Fellow,
Division of Cardiology;
Formerly: Associate Chief
Resident,
Department of Pediatrics,
The Hospital for Sick Children,
Toronto, Ontario, Canada
Cardiology

STEPHEN P. KRAFT, MD, FRCSC

Staff Ophthalmologist,
Department of Ophthalmology,
The Hospital for Sick Children,
Toronto, Ontario, Canada
Ophthalmology

VICKY LEE, MD

Resident,
Department of Pediatrics
The Hospital for Sick Children,
Toronto, Ontario, Canada
Growth and Development

**ALEX VAN LEVIN, MD, FAAP,
FAAO, FRCSC**

Staff Ophthalmologist,
Department of Ophthalmology,
The Hospital for Sick Children,
Toronto, Ontario, Canada
Ophthalmology

**BARBARA L. MARINAC, BScPhm,
PharmD**

Coordinator, Therapeutic Drug
Monitoring,
Department of Pharmacy,
The Hospital for Sick Children,
Toronto, Ontario, Canada
Formulary

**MARCELLINA MIAN, MDCM,
FRCPC, FAAP**

Medical Director
Suspected Child Abuse and
Neglect (SCAN) Program
The Hospital for Sick Children;
Associate Professor of Paediatrics
and Behavioural Science
Faculty of Medicine
University of Toronto
Toronto, Ontario, Canada
Sexual Assault, Child Abuse

GAVIN MORRISON, MCRP, DCH

Consultant, Pediatric Intensive
Care Unit,
Guys Hospital,
London, Great Britain;
Formerly: Chief Fellow,
Department of Pediatric
Critical Care,
The Hospital for Sick Children,
Toronto, Ontario, Canada
Procedures

**SUMATHI NADARAJAH, BSc,
MSc, MD, FRCPC**

Pediatrician,
Mississauga, Ontario, Canada;
Formerly: Fellow,
Division of Immunology and
Allergy,
The Hospital for Sick Children,
Toronto, Ontario, Canada
Allergy and Immunology

GILLIAN D. OLIVER, MD, FRCSC, FACOG

Head, Division of Gynecology,
Department of Pediatrics,
The Hospital for Sick Children;
Assistant Professor,
Department of Obstetrics and
    Gynecology,
University of Toronto,
Toronto, Ontario, Canada
Gynecology

MARTIN PETRIC, PhD, SCM(CCM)

Staff Virologist,
Department of Microbiology,
The Hospital for Sick Children;
Associate Professor,
University of Toronto
Toronto, Ontario, Canada
Laboratory Reference Values

FRANCY PILLO-BLOCKA, RD, BSc, BA(A)

Clinical Dietician,
Division of Cardiology,
The Hospital for Sick Children,
Toronto, Ontario, Canada
Nutrition

ANNETTE O. POON, MB, BCh, FRCPC

Associate Chief, Department of
    Pediatric Laboratory Medicine,
Director, Clinical Biochemistry,
    Haematology Diagnostic
    Laboratory/Blood Bank,
The Hospital for Sick Children,
Toronto, Ontario, Canada
Laboratory Reference Values

CANDICE N. ROWE, MD, FRCPC

Pediatrician,
    Clinical Pharmacologist;
Formerly,
    Clinical Pharmacology Fellow,
Department of Clinical
    Pharmacology,
The Hospital for Sick Children,
Toronto, Ontario, Canada
*Adolescent Medicine and
Poisoning*

ASHER DANIEL SCHACHTER, MD, FRCPC

Nephrology Fellow,
Children's Hospital,
Boston, Massachusetts;
Formerly:
    Associate Chief Resident,
Department of Pediatrics,
The Hospital for Sick Children,
Toronto, Ontario, Canada
Nephrology

JOANNE L. SMITH, BScPhm

Coordinator, Drug Information
    Service,
Department of Pharmacy,
The Hospital for Sick Children,
Toronto, Ontario, Canada
Formulary

MELINDA SOLOMON, MD

Resident,
Department of Pediatrics,
The Hospital for Sick Children,
Toronto, Ontario, Canada
Respirology

JENNIFER STINSON, RN, BScN, MSc(W)

Clinical Nurse Specialist—
    Sedation,
Department of Anaesthesia,
The Hospital for Sick Children;
Clinical Associate,
Faculty of Nursing,
University of Toronto,
Toronto, Ontario, Canada
Pain

DAT J. TRAN, MD

Resident,
Department of Pediatrics,
The Hospital for Sick Children,
Toronto, Ontario, Canada
Hepatology

SHEILA UNGER, BSc, MD
Resident,
Department of Genetics,
The Hospital for Sick Children,
Toronto, Ontario, Canada
Genetics

GUY V. WIDRICH, MBBCH, FRCPC
NICU Fellow,
Department of Pediatrics,
The Hospital for Sick Children,
Toronto, Ontario, Canada
Neonatology

REVIEWERS

J.T.R. Clarke, MD, PhD, FRCPC
Professor,
Department of Pediatrics,
The Hospital for Sick Children,
Toronto, Ontario, Canada
Metabolic Disease

M. Teresa Costa, MD, MSc, FCCMG, FRCPC
Division of Clinical Genetics,
Departments of Pediatrics and
    Genetics,
The Hospital for Sick Children;
Assistant Professor,
Departments of Pediatrics and
    Medical Genetics,
University of Toronto,
Toronto, Ontario, Canada
Genetics

Peter N. Cox, MBChB, FFARCS, FRCPC
Clinical Director,
Department of Critical Care,
The Hospital for Sick Children;
Programme Director, Pediatric
    Critical Care,
University of Toronto,
Toronto, Ontario, Canada
Procedures

Denis Daneman, MB, BCh, FRCPC
Professor,
Department of Pediatrics,
University of Toronto;
Chief, Division of Endocrinology,
The Hospital for Sick Children,
Toronto, Ontario, Canada
Endocrinology

John J. Doyle, MD, FRCPC, FAAP
Assistant Professor,
Department of Pediatrics,
Division of Hematology/Oncology,
The Hospital for Sick Children,
Toronto, Ontario, Canada
Hematology

John F. Edmonds, MD
Staff Physician,
Department of Critical Care,
The Hospital for Sick Children,
Toronto, Ontario, Canada
Emergencies

Robert W. Enzenauer, MD, MPH, FAAP, FAAO, FACS
Ophthalmologist,
Children's Eye Physicians,
Denver, Colorado
Ophthalmology

E. Lee Ford-Jones, MD, FRCPC
Associate Professor,
Department of Pediatrics,
Division of Infectious Diseases,
The Hospital for Sick Children,
Toronto, Ontario, Canada
Infectious Disease

Mark L. Greenberg, MBChB, FRCPC, FAAP
Professor, Departments of
    Pediatrics and Surgery,
University of Toronto;
Director,
Department of Pediatrics,
    Division of Oncology,
The Hospital for Sick Children,
Toronto, Ontario, Canada
Oncology

Anne Marie Griffiths, MD, FRCPC

Associate Professor,
Department of Pediatrics,
University of Toronto,
Toronto, Ontario, Canada
Gastroenterology

Elizabeth Harvey, MD, FRCPC

Assistant Professor,
Department of Pediatrics,
University of Toronto;
Staff Nephrologist,
The Hospital for Sick Children,
Toronto, Ontario, Canada
Fluids and Electrolytes

D. Anna Jarvis, MD, MB, BS, FRCPC, FAAP

Medical Director,
Department of Pediatrics,
    Division of Emergency Services
The Hospital for Sick Children,
Toronto, Ontario, Canada
Emergencies

Douglas H. Johnston, MD

Head,
Division of Pediatric Dentistry,
The Hospital for Sick Children,
Toronto, Ontario, Canada
Dentistry

Daina Kalnins, RD, CNSD

Clinical Dietitian,
Departments of Critical Care and
    Respirology,
The Hospital for Sick Children,
Toronto, Ontario, Canada
Nutrition

Bernice R. Krafchik, MB, ChB, FRCPC

Head,
Department of Pediatrics,
    Division of Dermatology,
The Hospital for Sick Children,
Toronto, Ontario, Canada
Dermatology

Sang-Whay Kooh, MD, PhD, FRCPC

Associate Professor,
Department of Pediatrics,
The Hospital for Sick Children,
Toronto, Ontario, Canada
Endocrinology

Ronald Laxer, MD, FRCPC

Professor,
Department of Pediatrics,
University of Toronto;
Head, Division of Rheumatology,
The Hospital for Sick Children,
Toronto, Ontario, Canada
Rheumatology

Karen M. Leslie, MD, FRCPC

Staff Pediatrician,
Department of Pediatrics,
The Hospital for Sick Children;
Assistant Professor,
Division of Adolescent Medicine,
University of Toronto,
Toronto, Ontario, Canada
Adolescent Medicine

Daune L. MacGregor, MD, FRCPC

Professor,
Department of Pediatrics,
    Division of Neurology
The Hospital for Sick Children,
Toronto, Ontario, Canada
Neurology/Neurosurgery

Michael A. McGuigan, MD, MBA

Medical Director,
Ontario Regional Poison
    Control Centre,
The Hospital for Sick Children,
Toronto, Ontario, Canada
*Adolescent Medicine and
Poisoning*

Christine Newman, MD, FRCPC

Clinical Director,
Neonatal Intensive Care Unit,
Department of Pediatrics,
Division of Neonatology,
The Hospital for Sick Children,
Toronto, Ontario, Canada
Neonatology

David G. Nykanen, MD, FRCPC

Assistant Professor,
Department of Pediatrics,
The Hospital for Sick Children,
Toronto, Ontario, Canada
Cardiology

Mercer Rang, MBBS, FRCSC

Professor,
Department of Surgery,
University of Toronto;
Staff Orthopedic Surgeon,
The Hospital for Sick Children,
Toronto, Ontario, Canada
Orthopedics

J. Reisman, MD, FRCPC

Associate Professor,
Department of Pediatrics,
University of Toronto;
Department of Pediatrics,
  Division of Respirology,
The Hospital for Sick Children,
Toronto, Ontario, Canada
Respirology

Eve A. Roberts, MD, FRCPC

Associate Professor,
Department of Pediatrics,
  Medicine, and Pharmacology,
University of Toronto;
Staff Physician,
Departments of Gastroenterology
  and Nutrition,
The Hospital for Sick Children,
Toronto, Ontario, Canada
Hepatology

S. Wendy Roberts, MD, FRCPC

Associate Professor,
Department of Pediatrics,
University of Toronto;
Developmental Pediatrician,
Department of Pediatrics;
Director,
Child Development Centre,
The Hospital for Sick Children,
Toronto, Ontario, Canada
Growth and Development

Chaim M. Roifman, MD, FRCPC, FCACB

Head,
Department of Pediatrics,
Division of Immunology/Allergy,
The Hospital for Sick Children,
Toronto, Ontario, Canada
Allergy/Immunology

Norman D. Rosenblum, MD

Assistant Professor,
Department of Pediatrics,
University of Toronto;
Staff Nephrologist,
The Hospital for Sick Children,
Toronto, Ontario, Canada
Nephrology

Anthony D. Sandler, MD

Staff Surgeon,
Department of Surgery,
University of Iowa Hospitals and
  Clinics,
Iowa City, Iowa;
Formerly: Chief Surgical
  Resident,
Department of Pediatric Surgery,
The Hospital for Sick Children,
Toronto, Ontario, Canada
Surgery

Stanley H. Zlotkin, MD, PhD, FRCPC

Professor,
Departments of Pediatrics,
   Nutritional Sciences, and
   Gastroenterology/Nutrition,
University of Toronto,
Toronto, Ontario, Canada
Nutrition

Ronald M. Zuker, MD, FRCSC, FACS, FAAP

Professor,
Department of Surgery,
University of Toronto;
Head,
Division of Plastic Surgery,
The Hospital for Sick Children,
Toronto, Ontario, Canada
Plastic Surgery

FOREWORD

The Hospital for Sick Children Handbook of Pediatrics was initiated 41 years ago to provide essential information for the medical student, house-officer, and physician committed to the care of infants and children. The *HSC Handbook* does not purport to replace contemporary textbooks of Pediatrics or relevant information in the current scientific literature. Rather, *The HSC Handbook of Pediatrics* is organized in a compact, user-friendly design with the primary purpose to present a condensed and practical guide to the diagnosis and management of a wide array of pediatric disorders. The pocket-sized *Handbook* is always available to the care-giver while the library remains a necessary resource to augment information and learning.

The handbook has undergone extensive revision every 3 to 4 years to remain abreast of the development of new technology and the changing approaches to the diagnosis and management of complex and acute pediatric conditions. The ninth edition of the handbook is no exception. It is organized into 30 system-based chapters including new sections on pain management, gynecology, hematology and oncology, and genitourinary disorders in children. Acute emergencies are highlighted at the beginning of the handbook. Diagnostic procedures including new molecular techniques, laboratory reference values, and an updated formulary are also prominently presented.

The HSC Handbook of Pediatrics is a unique text in that each chapter is written by a pediatric house-officer or fellow who receives guidance and advice from a designated faculty member. The ninth edition of the handbook was edited by the chief resident, Dr. Anne Dipchand. Anne's dedication and hard work are clearly evident in the design and organization of the handbook. Finally, the ninth edition of *The HSC Handbook of Pediatrics* has become incorporated into the Mosby series of handbooks, which will enable this fine text to be circulated around the world.

Robert H.A. Haslam, MD, FRCPC

Formerly,
Professor and Chairman
Department of Pediatrics
The Hospital for Sick Children
Toronto, Canada

PREFACE

It is incredible how much new information can accumulate in five years. With that thought in mind, the exciting challenge of editing the ninth edition of *The HSC Handbook of Pediatrics* was undertaken. The eighth edition had achieved its goal of streamlining the text. With this foundation and three and a half years of "hands on use," the primary goal of the ninth edition has been to update and to improve access to the vast amount of information contained within. A secondary goal has been to have the ninth edition written "by pediatric trainees, for pediatric trainees." The final product clearly achieves this and represents the collective effort of many pediatric trainees and subspecialty fellows with tremendous support from faculty.

Each chapter has been revised and updated in keeping with advances in the practice of pediatrics and to ensure its accuracy. New features include a chapter devoted to Pain, the division of the Genitourinary chapter into independent chapters on Gynecology and Urology, and the establishment of separate chapters on Hematology and Oncology, emphasizing the uniqueness of the disorders within each of these subspecialties.

The section on Emergencies has been expanded extensively and outlines the acute management of common pediatric emergencies. It has been relocated to the front of the book and has an independent index for quick access to all emergency situations covered in the handbook. It is nicely complemented by the revised section on Procedures, which has a number of new diagrams to aid the user.

Comprehensive cross-referencing between chapters has been included to facilitate information retrieval. In addition, the chapters on Allergy and Immunology, Cardiology, Endocrinology, Fluids and Electrolytes, Gastroenterology, Growth and Development, Hepatology, Metabolic Diseases, Nephrology, and Neurology have been reorganized into more user-friendly formats.

Finally, the Formulary and Laboratory Reference Values sections have been thoroughly revised with the most up-to-date information available, making them tremendous resources for anyone involved in the diagnosis and management of pediatric diseases.

The ninth edition of *The HSC Handbook of Pediatrics* covers many major topics in the field of pediatrics spanning primary to quaternary care medicine. The exciting incorporation into the Mosby series of handbooks will facilitate its use by an even greater number of medical personnel around the world. It should continue to serve as a practical reference and a guide for all who participate in the care of infants and children. To four more years of reliable "hands on use!"

Anne I. Dipchand, MD, FRCPC, FAAP

ACKNOWLEDGMENTS

I would like to extend my heartfelt thanks to all of the people (too numerous to mention!) who helped to make the ninth edition of *The HSC Handbook of Pediatrics* a reality. I would especially like to thank the following people: Dr. Alan Goldbloom, Dr. Patricia Parkin, Alex Wright, and Neil Walker for helping me to get this project "off the ground" in the spring of 1995; Sharon Nancekivall, Claudia Anderson, Laurel Craven, and Bill Carter for helping me wade through the legal world of publishing contracts; Jennifer Byington Geistler for all of her help and advice in preparing the final manuscript for submission; and Melissa Lastarria for guiding me through the steps to publication.

Special thanks to Cheryl Wilson for the innumerable, tedious hours of word processing and editing; to Jan White and Krista Barnes, my "office buddies," for the laughs and for always being there when I needed help with *anything;* to Shawna, my friend and perpetual "release valve;" and to "the Associates" for their constant friendship and support.

Thank you to Dr. Robert Haslam, who provided me with special words of encouragement on a regular basis, especially over the last year and a half.

A very special thank you to my husband, Dr. Jake Kempenaar, who has supported me unselfishly and unwaveringly in fulfilling this goal.

Finally, thank you to my mentor and friend, Dr. Susan Tallett, for giving me the opportunity to edit the handbook, for giving me free reign in doing so, for being an endless source of wisdom and advice, and for the continuous support and encouragement in "getting the job done."

Anne I. Dipchand, MD, FRCPC, FAAP

To my parents
Betty Dipchand

and the late
Professor Cecil R. Dipchand

CONTENTS

ANNE DIPCHAND

CARDIOPULMONARY RESUSCITATION

- *See inside cover for quick guide to resuscitation drugs.*
- Precipitating factor in majority of pediatric cardiac arrests is not cardiac event but hypoxia secondary to respiratory failure or hypovolemia
- Arrhythmias in arrests: asystole following bradycardia (80%) or brady-

arrhythmias (10%); ventricular arrhythmias (10%) predominantly in underlying congenital heart disease or direct cardiac trauma
- Preceding history critical to definitive management

Basic Life Support (BLS)

- Determine unresponsiveness
- Call for help (trained pediatric rescuers should perform approximately 1 min of BLS before calling for help)
- Open airway
  1. Head extension to neutral position
  2. Chin lift
  3. Jaw thrust
- Check breathing
  1. Look, listen, and feel
  2. If patient is breathing, check for cause of coma (p. 9)
- Ventilate (if no or ineffective respirations)
  1. Mouth to mouth
  2. Mouth to mouth and nose
- Assess for chest movement; if chest not moving, consider airway obstruction (p. 458)
- If central pulse is slow (<80/min neonate; <60/min older infant and child), start cardiac compressions. (5 compressions : 1 ventilation); depress chest at least ⅓ of anteroposterior diameter of chest
  1. Infant: on sternum just below intermammary line, 100/min; depress 1.5-2.5 cm using two or three fingers
  2. Child: lower sternum, 80-100/min; depress 2.5-4 cm using heel of hand

Advanced Life Support (ALS, ABCs)

Airway, Breathing

- Initial assessment (respiratory effort, air entry, cyanosis, respiratory distress)
- Establish airway
  1. Position (head tilt, jaw thrust, "sniffing" position)
  2. Clear airway of any foreign bodies and/or suction secretions
  3. Bag and mask ventilation with 100% O_2; if ineffective, reassess positioning, mask size, seal, airway patency; consider oral airway
  4. Endotracheal intubation (p. 498)
- Provide 100% O_2 if possible. Nonrebreathing bag provides 70%-90% O_2; anesthetic bag delivers 100% O_2

Circulation

- Output
  1. Assess cardiac output (femoral, brachial, or radial pulse); if bradycardic, pulseless, or asystolic, start compressions as outlined above Check effectiveness of compressions by palpating femoral pulse
  2. Check blood pressure
  3. Check rhythm on cardiac monitor or with "quick look" paddles (see p. 60)
- Parenteral Access
  1. Attempt peripheral IV once or twice, then try intraosseous (p. 490) or central vein

2. Potential central sites include femoral, internal jugular, or external jugular veins (p. 490); should be accessed by most experienced personnel present
3. Consider venous cutdown (p. 494); should only be attempted by experienced personnel
4. When access secured, obtain blood for laboratory investigations as appropriate
5. Obtain rapid blood glucose measurement (e.g., Chemstrip)
6. For intravascular volume expansion, start with isotonic crystalloid (normal saline or Ringer's lactate) at initial dose of 20 ml/kg, then assess response by looking at changes in heart rate (HR), peripheral perfusion, capillary refill, and blood pressure; repeat bolus as necessary; consider other volume expanders, including colloid (5% albumin), packed red blood cells, whole blood, or fresh frozen plasma (FFP)

Drugs

- *See inside cover for quick guide to resuscitation drugs*
- See Table I-1 for recommended therapy
- If IV access not yet established, endotracheal route (ETT) can be used for epinephrine, atropine, or lidocaine
- **Oxygen:** 100% or as close to 100% as able to be delivered effectively
- **Epinephrine:** indicated for pulseless arrest, asystole, bradycardia, hypotension (poor cardiac output)
  - 1:10,000 strength at dose of 1 ml + 0.1 ml/kg (min 1 ml) via IV/IO (0.1 mg + 0.01 mg/kg)
  - Second and subsequent doses use 1:1,000 strength at dose of 0.1 ml/kg q 3-5 min (0.1 mg/kg)
  - ETT dose: 1:1,000 strength, 0.1 ml/kg
  - Infusion: 0.05-1.0 µg/kg/min (Fig. I-1)
- **Sodium Bicarbonate:** indicated for prolonged arrest or documented metabolic acidosis
  - 8.4% strength (1 mmol/ml) at dose of 1-2 mmol/kg IV initially (1-2 ml/kg)
  - Subsequent doses q10-20 min empirically or based on blood gas monitoring
  - Use 4.2% strength (0.5 mmol/ml) for neonates
  - Infusion: mix 8.4% strength 1:1 with D5W; 1 ml = 0.5 mmol, run at 1 ml/kg/hr

Table I-1 Drug Therapy in Cardiopulmonary Resuscitation

Diagnosis	First-line therapy	Secondary therapy
Asystole, bradycardia, or normal rate with no pulse	O_2, $NaHCO_3$, epinephrine, fluid bolus	Atropine, dextrose, ± calcium
Ventricular fibrillation	O_2, defibrillation	Lidocaine, $NaHCO_3$, epinephrine, ± bretylium
Sinus tachycardia	O_2, fluid bolus	
Tachyarrhythmias	See p. 60	

Drug dose ranges (µg/kg/min):

- Epinephrine, Morphine: 0.1 — 1.0
- Nitroglycerin, Salbutamol: 0.5 — 10
- Isoproterenol: 0.05 — 1.0
- Dopamine: 1.0 / 2.0 — 25

Amount (mg) to Put into 50 ml Syringe

Infusion rate values are in ml/hr.

µg/kg/min	0.15 × wt	0.3 × wt	0.6 × wt	1.5 × wt	3 × wt	6 × wt	15 × wt	30 × wt	60 × wt
0.05	1								
0.075	1.5								
0.1	2	1							
0.2	4	2	1						
0.3	6	3	1.5						
0.4	8	4	2						
0.5	10	5	2.5	1					
0.6	12	6	3						
0.7	14	7	3.5						
0.8	16	8	4						
0.9	18	9	4.5						
1	20	10	5	2	1				
1.5		15	7.5	3	1.5				
2		20	10	4	2	1			
2.5				5	2.5				
3			15	6	3	1.5			
3.5				7	3.5				
4			20	8	4	2			
4.5				9	4.5				
5				10	5	2.5	1		
6				12	6	3			
7				14	7	3.5			
8				16	8	4			
9				18	9	4.5			
10				20	10	5	2	1	
12					12	6			
14					14	7			
15					15		3	1.5	
20					20	10	4	2	1
25							5	2.5	

30			15	6	3	1.5
40			20	8	4	2
50				10	5	2.5
100				20	10	5
150					15	7.5
200					20	10

Fig. I-1 Table for calculation of drug infusion dilution. 1. Select desired drug dosage to be delivered in μg/kg/min (see named bars to right of chart; start at lower end of dose range and adjust according to response) 2. Select infusion rate of syringe pump in ml/hr from table 3. Calculate number of mg of drug to be mixed in 50-ml syringe: wt = patient's weight (kg). If 250-ml bag used, add same mass of drug, but run at 5 × rate quoted in table. For example, a 7-kg infant requires dopamine: from bars on right of chart, range of dosages for dopamine is 2-25 μg/kg/min; start with 2 μg/kg/min. We will opt for rate of fluid infusion of 1 ml/hr. For 1 ml/hr to give 2 μg/kg/min, we need to put 6 × weight (i.e., 42 mg) into 50 ml of solution. (Modified from Shann F: Continuous drug infusion in children: a table for simplifying calculation, *Crit Care Med* 11:462-463, 1983.)

- **Dextrose:** indicated for hypoglycemia (check Chemstrip, blood sugar)
  - D50W 1 ml/kg (0.5 g/kg) IV (use D25W for infants)
- **Atropine:** indicated for bradycardia
  - 0.02 mg/kg IV/ETT (minimum 0.1 mg)
- **Calcium:** indicated in prolonged arrest, hyperkalemia, ventricular arrhythmia, hypocalcemia
  - Calcium chloride 10%, 10 mg/kg (0.1 ml/kg) IV q10-20 min
- **Lidocaine:** indicated for ventricular tachycardia, frequent ventricular premature beats, ventricular fibrillation
  - 1 mg/kg IV/IO/ETT; may repeat once
  - Infusion: 15-50 µg/kg/min (see Fig. I-1)
- **Dopamine:** indicated for hypotension, poor cardiac output
  - Infusion: 5-20 µg/kg/min IV (see Fig. I-1)
- **Bretylium:** indicated for ventricular fibrillation, pulseless ventricular tachycardia unresponsive to epinephrine or lidocaine
  - First dose 5 mg/kg IV; second dose 10 mg/kg IV

Defibrillation
- Indication is ventricular fibrillation (VF), pulseless ventricular tachycardia (VT)
- One paddle on upper right chest below clavicle and other paddle at level of left nipple in anterior axillary line; remember conductive pads or gel
- For VF: nonsynchronized mode
  Dose: 2 J/kg, 4 J/kg, 4 J/kg
  If unsuccessful, give epinephrine +/− lidocaine and repeat with 4 J/kg
  Bretylium may be used in refractory cases (5 mg/kg IV)
- For VT: cardioversion (synchronized mode)
  Dose: 0.5-1.0 J/kg. Double on repeat up to maximum 2 J/kg
- If unsuccessful, correct hypoxemia, acidosis, other metabolic abnormalities, and hypothermia; repeat epinephrine +/− lidocaine and defibrillation (4 J/kg) as necessary

Continuing Support
- If cardiac compressions required, stop intermittently and assess for return of spontaneous rhythm and output
- Maintain ventilation and oxygenation; consider sedation and/or paralysis if necessary
- Monitor and correct abnormalities in blood gases, electrolytes, glucose, and calcium
- Avoid hypothermia (especially in infants and younger children)
- Obtain further history and complete secondary survey of physical exam

SHOCK

DEFINITION

- State of circulatory dysfunction leading to insufficient delivery of oxygen and nutrients to supply needs of tissues
- *Early recognition critical.* Rapid intervention may prevent progression to irreversible shock and/or cardiopulmonary arrest

Clinical Manifestations

- Classical symptoms and signs often absent early on due to compensatory mechanisms
- Early symptoms: poor feeding, fever, lethargy, or irritability; decreased urine output; history of underlying illness
- Early signs:
  1. Resting tachycardia, tachypnea
  2. Normal systolic blood pressure but
     - decreased pulse pressure suggests hypovolemia
     - increased pulse pressure suggests sepsis
  3. Mottling, cool extremities, increased capillary refill time (normal <2 sec)
- Early laboratory: metabolic or mixed acidemia with elevated lactate, hyperglycemia or hypoglycemia
- Some forms of shock have specific clinical features (see Table I-2)
  1. Septic shock (form of distributive shock): early hyperdynamic "warm" phase
  2. Neurogenic shock (form of distributive shock): hypotension without tachycardia or decreased peripheral perfusion
  3. Cardiogenic shock: gallop rhythm with hepatomegaly, cardiomegaly, or dilated neck veins
  4. Obstructive shock: muffled heart sounds or increased resonance with chest percussion

Manifest Shock

- Hypotension: systolic BP <5th percentile for age (<80 mm Hg systolic from 6 wk to 6 yr; see p. 315) or documented decrease of 30% from preshock state

Table I-2   Types of Shock

Type	Primary circulatory derangement	Common causes
Hypovolemic	↓ intravascular blood volume	Hemorrhage, trauma
		Fluid losses, gastroenteritis (see p. 100)
Distributive	Vasodilation → venous pooling → ↓ preload	Sepsis
		Anaphylaxis
	Maldistribution of regional blood flow	CNS or spinal injury
		Drug intoxication
Cardiogenic	↓ Myocardial contractility	Heart surgery
		Congenital heart disease
		Arrhythmias
		Hypoxia, ischemia
Obstructive	Mechanical obstruction to ventricular inflow or outflow	Cardiac tamponade
		Tension pneumothorax
		Coarctation of aorta
Dissociative	O_2 not released from hemoglobin	Carbon monoxide, methemoglobinemia

Adapted from Witte MK, Hill JH, Blumer JL: Shock in the pediatric patient. *Adv Pediatr* 34:139-174, 1987.

- Tachycardia
- Decreased peripheral perfusion: weak peripheral pulses, cool extremities, mottled skin, increased capillary refill time
- Hypothermia
- Decreased urine output (<1 ml/kg/hr)
- Altered mental state: lethargy, confusion, combativeness, coma

Management

Respiratory Support
- O_2 to keep O_2 saturation >90% or PaO_2 >60 mm Hg
- Low threshold for artificial ventilation; reduces work of breathing and cardiac demands, especially in cardiogenic and septic shock

Hemodynamic Support
- Preload (circulating blood volume)
  - Initial: isotonic crystalloid (0.9% saline or Ringer's lactate) 10-20 ml/kg over 15-30 min, then assess for response (heart and respiratory rate, capillary refill, sensorium, urine output); may repeat as necessary
  - If little or no response to fluid or > 40 ml/kg with ongoing requirement, consider
    1. Isotonic colloid (5% albumin) or blood products when specifically indicated
    2. Further boluses of 10 ml/kg as needed
    3. Central venous pressure (CVP) monitoring, especially for distributive or cardiogenic shock (see Table I-2)
    4. Methods to increase contractility and afterload (see the following), avoiding use of large volumes of fluid (especially with distributive and cardiogenic shock)
- Contractility
  - Adequate ventilation and oxygenation
  - Correct pH and other substrate abnormalities
  - $NaHCO_3$ if pH still <7.2 once $PaCO_2$ <40 mm Hg (give weight [kg] × base deficit × 0.15); repeat if necessary
  - Glucose infusion; ensure calcium and electrolytes are normal
  - Dopamine (Fig. I-1) 5-20 μg/kg/min. Note: Dopamine should always be administered through central line when possible because of risk of tissue necrosis, although in emergency setting drug may be administered peripherally (IV or IO) for short period at low doses and preferably through separate line; infusion of inotropes generally requires ICU setting.
  - Epinephrine (Fig. I-1) 0.05-1 μg/kg/min (rarely needed except in severe shock)
- Afterload
  - Will be improved initially with above measures; later, afterload reduction with vasodilators may be necessary

Investigations

- CBC, platelets, coagulation screen, arterial blood gas (ABG), electrolytes, urea, creatinine, calcium
- Blood culture if appropriate
- Cross-match if appropriate

- Chest x-ray
- Sepsis work-up if appropriate

Monitoring

Noninvasive Monitoring

- Vital signs at least every 15 min initially
- Blood pressure
- Pulse oximetry for O_2 saturation monitoring
- Continuous ECG (cardiac monitor)
- Bladder catheterization for urine output
- Arterial blood gases if oximetry not available

Invasive Monitoring

- Central venous line for CVP
- Arterial line for repeated blood sampling, blood pressure monitoring

Further Management

- Specific treatment for underlying illness: antibiotics for sepsis (see p. 257); surgical treatment of hemorrhage, tamponade, or pneumothorax; corticosteroids for suspected adrenal insufficiency
- Nasogastric (NG) tube to empty stomach and decrease risk of aspiration
- Diuretics (furosemide) to promote urine output (when euvolemic)
- Observation for development of multiorgan failure and secondary complications (infection)

COMA AND ALTERED LEVEL OF CONSCIOUSNESS

DEFINITION

- Altered level of consciousness refers to decreased awareness of self and environment; extreme is coma
- Most common pattern of coma in children is diffuse impairment of cerebral hemisphere function; less commonly can be a result of brainstem dysfunction
- Useful mnemonics to remember important causes in children are AEIOU and TIPS (see Table I-3)
- Clinical features: most patients stable at presentation but may have rapidly progressive process and require simultaneous investigations and therapy; occasionally, patients require emergency resuscitation with few initial investigations

Table I-3 Causes of Coma: AEIOU & TIPS

T	Trauma	**A**	Alcohol abuse
I	Insulin/hypoglycemia	**E**	Electrolytes
	Intussusception		Encephalopathy
	Inborn errors of metabolism		Endocrinopathy
P	Psychiatric	**I**	Infection
S	Seizures	**O**	Overdose/ingestion
	Stroke	**U**	Uremia
	Shock		
	Shunt malfunction		

Table I-4 Modified Glasgow Coma Scale*

	Score	<1 yr	>1 yr
Eye opening	4	Spontaneously	Spontaneously
	3	To shout	To verbal command
	2	To pain	To pain
	1	No response	No response
Motor response	6	Obeys	Obeys
	5	Localizes pain	Localizes pain
	4	Flexion withdrawal	Flexion withdrawal
	3	Decorticate	Decorticate
	2	Decerebrate	Decerebrate
	1	No response	No response
	Score	**0-23 mo**	**2-5 yr**	**>5 yr**
Verbal response	5	Smiles, coos, cries	Appropriate words and phrases	Oriented and converses
	4	Cries	Inappropriate words	Disoriented, converses
	3	Inappropriate cry or scream	Cries or screams	Inappropriate words
	2	Grunts	Grunts	Incomprehensible sounds
	1	No response	No response	No response

*Critical Care Unit, Hospital for Sick Children.

Management

Primary Survey

- ABCs (see p. 2) with cervical spine precautions
- Glasgow Coma Scale (Table I-4)
- Measure temperature
- Check for obvious evidence of trauma
- Increased ICP: (see p. 13)
- Hypoglycemia: give glucose 0.5 g/kg (D50W, 1-2 ml/kg IV) empirically if sugar low on Chemstrip
- Narcosis: check pupils; give naloxone (0.1 mg/kg) empirically if small or pinpoint

Secondary Survey

- History: known underlying illness, acute fever, trauma, ingestion
- General and neurologic examination (Tables I-5 and I-6)
  - Look for evidence of infection, intoxication, and metabolic and traumatic causes
  - Oculomotor movements
  - Motor responses (focal signs)
  - Breathing pattern
  - Fundi (retinal hemorrhages), fontanelle, nuchal rigidity, bruits

Investigations

- Depends on knowledge of etiology and clinical condition
- Determine need for urgent computed tomography (CT) scan of head
  1. Diffuse causes (majority): infection, ingestion, metabolic: CT scan not essential immediately
  2. Focal causes (usually trauma): CT scan essential
- Blood: CBC, culture, ABG, glucose, electrolytes, urea, creatinine, calcium, magnesium, liver enzymes, ammonium, clotting screen; blind toxic screen without specific history not generally useful except for acetaminophen ingestion, as most ingestion injuries will present with specific clinical picture (see p. 441)

Table I-5 Distinguishing Diffuse Versus Focal Causes of Coma

	Diffuse	Focal
History	Previous illness	± Previous illness
Consciousness	Gradual ↓	Rapid ↓
General physical exam	Breath, odor, skin color	Trauma
Progression	Affects different levels simultaneously	Rostral-caudal changes
Breathing	↑ then ↓ RR	Ataxic
Pupils	Small, equal, and reactive	Unequal and/or unreactive
Focal signs	Less common	Common
Motor	Myoclonic jerks	Focal oculomotor changes
	Multifocal seizures	Facial asymmetry
	Symmetrically decorticate or decerebrate	Monoparesis or hemiparesis
	Grasping rigidity	↓ Cough or gag

Table I-6 Coma: Level of CNS Involvement and Clinical Correlate

Anatomic site	Pupillary reaction	1. Oculovestibular reflex* (with cold water) 2. Oculocephalic reflex† (Doll's eyes)	Breathing pattern	Posture
Cerebral hemisphere				
Forebrain	Small but reactive	1. Conjugate eye deviation *toward* the lesion 2. Intact (conjugate deviation of eyes *contrary to direction* that head is turned)	Normal or brief periods of apnea followed by voluntary deep breathing	
Deep structures and diencephalon			Cheyne-Stokes (phases of hyperpnea alternating with apnea)	Decortication
Brainstem				
Midbrain	Midpoint and fixed	1. Conjugate eye deviation *away* from the lesion 2. Not intact (conjugate deviation of eyes *in direction* that head is turned)	Central hyperventilation (sustained regular and rapid ventilation)	Decerebration
Pons	Pinpoint		Apneustic (brief respiratory pauses alternating with end respiratory pauses)	Flaccid
Medulla			Apnea	

*In normal, awake person with intact brain stem, normal response is nystagmus with slow component toward ear being irrigated.
† Do not do if suspected C-spine injury.

- Urine: urinalysis, culture, latex agglutination
- Cerebrospinal fluid (CSF): cell count, protein, glucose, Gram's stain, culture, latex agglutination; opening pressures may be useful but difficult to measure accurately in infants and young children; lumbar puncture (LP) contraindicated if profoundly comatose, evidence of raised intracranial pressure (ICP), or hemodynamic instability
- Gastric fluid: toxic screen if specific history
- Radiology: head CT; plain X-rays of chest, cervical spine, abdomen; skeletal survey
- Other: ECG, EEG

Further Management

- Treat underlying problem
- Treat increased ICP (see below)
- Treat seizures
- Maintain homeostasis: O_2, CO_2, fluids, acid-base, electrolytes, nutrition

RAISED INTRACRANIAL PRESSURE (ICP)
Clinical Features

- Early: headache, vomiting, decreased level of consciousness, full fontanelle
- Advanced: decreased HR, increased BP; unequal or unresponsive pupils; papilledema; cranial nerve III, IV, VI palsies; other evidence of herniation

General Management

- Careful handling
- Elevate head of bed to 30° and keep head in midline to decrease pressure on jugular veins
- O_2 (PaO_2 > 100 mm Hg)
- Intubate and hyperventilate ($PaCO_2$, 30-35 mm Hg). Premedication with lidocaine may prevent rise in ICP associated with intubation. Elective intubation in this situation should be carried out by experienced personnel skilled in use of anesthetic agents.
- Maintain cerebral perfusion pressure (mean arterial pressure (MAP) − ICP = CPP)
- Fluid restriction (30%-50% maintenance)
- Normothermia

Pharmacologic Management

- Mannitol 0.2-0.5 g/kg/dose (1-2.5 ml/kg/dose of 20% solution over 10-30 min), q2h prn; monitor urine output
- Dexamethasone 0.1-0.25 mg/kg q6h may be of benefit if edema secondary to space-occupying lesion such as brain tumor

Other

- ICP monitoring (i.e., with intracranial bolt or intraventricular catheter): useful only if risk of rapid increase in ICP
- Surgical decompression for severely increased ICP: only effective if space-occupying lesion or Reye's syndrome

STATUS EPILEPTICUS

DEFINITION

- Single generalized (tonic-clonic, myoclonic, tonic, or absence) or focal (clonic or jacksonian) seizure lasting 30 min or longer; includes any series of seizures without intervening return of consciousness with duration of greater than 30 min

Management

- ABCs (see p. 2)
- NG tube
- Blood for glucose (Chemstrip can be done at bedside), gas, electrolytes, calcium, and magnesium; consider blood culture, CBC, toxic screen, anticonvulsant levels, coagulation parameters, metabolic work-up, and liver function tests as per clinical scenario
- First-line medications (onset of action 1-4 min)
  1. Diazepam 0.1-0.3 mg/kg IV; repeat q5-10 min prn to maximum of three doses
     - Max rate 2 mg/min; push slowly over 5 min
     - May give 0.5 mg/kg pr while obtaining IV access; draw up dose in 1 or 3 ml syringe, dilute with normal saline (NS), administer pr (with or without feeding tube); squeeze buttocks together for 1-2 min)
  2. Lorazepam 0.05 mg/kg IV; repeat q5-10 min prn to maximum of three doses
     - Max rate 2 mg/min; push slowly over 5 min
     - Alternative to diazepam
     - May give rectally at same dose while obtaining IV access
  3. Dextrose 1 ml/kg (0.5 mg/kg) D50W (2 ml/kg D25W) empirically or if hypoglycemic
- Monitor respiratory status; be prepared to manage airway and ventilate if apnea occurs following administration of benzodiazepines
- Second-line medications (maintenance anticonvulsant therapy)
  1. Phenytoin 20 mg/kg IV (maximum 1 g)
     - Max rate 50 mg/min; infuse slowly monitoring for hypotension and bradycardia
     - May give in staged doses of 10 mg/kg up to max of 30 mg/kg
  2. Phenobarbital 20 mg/kg IV (max 800 mg)
     - Consider if seizure activity persists 25-30 min after above-mentioned medications given
     - Max 60 mg/min
     - May give in staged doses of 10 mg/kg up to max of 40 mg/kg
     - Risk of apnea when given concurrently with benzodiazepines
     - In children <2 yr, use as drug of first choice
  3. Paraldehyde 5% solution, 2-3 ml/kg (100-150 mg/kg) IV over 15 min followed by infusion
     - Consider if seizure activity persists after above-mentioned medications given
     - Infusion: 5% solution, 0.4 ml/kg/hr IV (20 mg/kg/hr)

- May give rectally 0.2-0.4 ml/kg/dose of undiluted paraldehyde (200-400 mg/kg/dose) pr; max 10 g/dose
- Dilute in syringe with olive oil; rectal administration as described for diazepam
- May repeat once
4. Sodium chloride 3% solution (0.5 mmol/ml), 3-5 ml/kg IV over 30-60 min
   - Consider if significant hyponatremia found on investigation and believed to be etiology of seizure
- If seizure persists, consider intubation and thiopental infusion in ICU setting with continuous EEG monitoring
- Investigations: depends on history and physical exam but consider:
  - Urgent CT head scan or magnetic resonance imaging (MRI) if history suggestive of focal lesion (i.e., trauma, bleeding, space-occupying lesion) or presence of persistent focal neurologic signs or evidence of increased ICP
  - Lumbar puncture if history consistent with meningitis or encephalitis and no evidence of increased ICP
- See p. 339 for further discussion and long-term management of seizures

---

RESPIRATORY DISTRESS AND/OR FAILURE

DEFINITION

- Respiratory failure: inability of respiratory system to provide sufficient oxygen for metabolic needs or to excrete carbon dioxide produced by body (arterial PaO_2 <50 mm Hg in newborn, 60 mm Hg in infant or older child; arterial CO_2 >60 in newborn, 55 in infant or older child)
- Respiratory distress: increased work of breathing to fulfill body's requirements
- In children, respiratory failure leading to hypoxia and hypercapnia is major cause of apnea/bradycardia and cardiac arrest requiring resuscitation

ETIOLOGY

- Upper airway obstruction (see p. 458): epiglottitis, croup, foreign body, retropharyngeal abscess, subglottic stenosis/web/hemangioma, laryngotracheomalacia, decreased level of consciousness and others
- Lower airway obstruction: asthma, foreign body, cystic fibrosis, bronchopulmonary dysplasia, bronchiectasis, pulmonary edema, and others
- Pulmonary disease: infection (pneumonia, tuberculosis (TB), pertussis), aspiration, cystic fibrosis, vasculitis, interstitial lung disease, toxin aspiration (hydrocarbons), and others
- Pleural disease: pneumothorax, hemothorax, chylothorax
- Chest wall abnormalities: kyphoscoliosis, flail chest
- Other: sepsis, cardiac disease (congestive heart failure [CHF], congenital heart disease), anemia, acidemia (diabetic ketoacidosis [DKA], renal failure, inborn errors of metabolism, liver failure), methemoglobinemia, carbon monoxide poisoning, obstructive sleep apnea, and others

Clinical Manifestations

- Tachycardia, tachypnea
- Cyanosis, retractions, nasal flaring, tracheal tug, grunting, apnea, rib flaring
- Poor perfusion
- Confusion, agitation, restlessness, seizures, coma
- Beware gasping respirations, weakening respiratory effort

Management

- Early identification and management may help prevent progression to respiratory or cardiac arrest
- ABCs (see p. 2) including supplemental O_2
- Blood gas measurement to determine degree of hypoxia and hypercapnia
- Consider elective endotracheal intubation to facilitate oxygenation and ventilation
- Investigations and ongoing management as determined by underlying problem

CHOKING

- If good air exchange (forceful cough, wheezing inspiration, and loud cry), allow child to continue with spontaneous efforts to clear airway; poor air exchange (very weak or nonexistent cough, no cry) or total airway obstruction requires definitive management

CHILD >1 YR

- Six to ten abdominal thrusts (Heimlich maneuver), administered in standing position in older conscious child or by placing heel of one hand on abdomen between umbilicus and rib cage with child in recumbent position; thrusts should be directed inward and upward
- If above maneuvers unsuccessful, use head extension and tongue-jaw lifts (anterior displacement of mandible, using fingers behind mandibular ramus or by gripping mandible anteriorly and lifting forward); if foreign body visualized, finger sweeps may be used to remove it; blind finger sweeps may further impact foreign body and should be discouraged
- When child is unconscious, continue with basic CPR and attempts at ventilation; if ventilation not possible, repeat above maneuvers

INFANT

- In choking infant, abdominal thrusts may be traumatic and should be avoided if other means are effective
- Place infant in 60° head-down position, lying on rescuer's forearm
- Administer four back blows between shoulder blades with heel of rescuer's hand
- If unsuccessful, turn infant over and administer four chest thrusts (as with cardiac compression)
- Attempt to visualize foreign body in mouth; if seen, remove with finger sweeps
- Open airway with tongue-jaw lift technique (see previous discussion)

EMERGENCIES

- Attempt to ventilate
- Repeat above maneuvers until ventilation possible
- If unsuccessful, abdominal thrusts may be attempted

STATUS ASTHMATICUS

DEFINITION

- Asthma: reversible airway obstruction caused by inflammation, bronchospasm, increased mucus production, and airway edema
- Status asthmaticus: prolonged attack of airway obstruction initially minimally responsible to inhaled bronchodilators

Clinical Manifestations

- Dyspnea, tachycardia, pulsus paradoxus
- Cyanosis, intercostal indrawing, tracheal tug, nasal flaring, prolonged expiration, inspiratory and expiratory wheeze, decreased/unequal air entry
- Confusion, agitation, restlessness, drowsiness

Management

- ABCs (see p. 2)
- O_2 by mask
- Medications
  1. Salbutamol (5mg/ml) 0.03 ml/kg (max 1 ml) in 3 ml NS via aerosol; may be given continuously
  2. Ipratropium (250 μg/ml) 0.5-1 ml with salbutamol for first three masks then q4h
  3. Steroids
     Prednisone 2 mg/kg po once or
     Hydrocortisone 4-6 mg/kg IV q4-6h
- Obtain IV access for administration of maintenance fluids and/or medications
- Consider CXR, ABG
- For ongoing and long-term management once stabilized, see p. 462

Complications

- Sudden deterioration: consider pneumothorax (asymmetric air entry, tracheal deviation, hyperresonant chest)
- Normal or elevated $PaCO_2$: consider impending respiratory failure ("tiring out")
- Disappearance of wheezing: consider worsening bronchospasm with decreased air entry

ANAPHYLAXIS

DEFINITION

- Immediate hypersensitivity reaction that can lead to life-threatening cardiorespiratory decompensation brought about by the release of vasoactive amines; hypotensive shock may occur and may be accompanied by laryngeal or bronchial obstruction and cutaneous eruption

Clinical Manifestations

- Anxious
- Hypotension, tachycardia
- Respiratory distress, cyanosis, shortness of breath, stridor, wheeze
- Shock (p. 6)
- Urticaria, edema (periorbital, laryngeal, facial)

Management

- Treat patient at first sign of anaphylaxis; do not wait for evolution of symptoms and signs
- ABCs (p. 2)
- Discontinue any ongoing parenteral medications or blood products
- O_2 by mask
- Medications
  1. Epinephrine
     1:1,000 (1 mg/ml) strength at dose of 0.01 ml/kg (0.01 mg/kg) SC (min 0.1 ml/dose; max 1.0 ml) or
     1:10,000 (0.1 mg/ml) strength at dose of 0.1 ml/kg (0.01 mg/kg) IV/IM (min 1.0 ml/dose; max 10 ml)
     May repeat once in 5 min
  2. Diphenhydramine
     1-2 mg/kg IV/IM (max 50 mg)
  3. Hydrocortisone (if severe reaction)
     1-5 mg/kg IV if severe reaction
- If bronchospasm present, treat as per asthma (see p. 17)
- Observe for recurrence of symptoms over next 24 hr
- For management of anaphylactic reaction once acute episode is over, see p. 43

SMOKE INHALATION

- Consider in *all* fire victims, but especially when history of exposure in confined space, loss of consciousness at scene, or history of deaths at scene; physical markers include facial burns, singed nasal hairs, hoarse voice, carbonaceous sputum
- Multiple mechanisms of injury: hypoxia from decreased atmospheric oxygen, thermal (upper airway edema, obstruction), particulate matter (tracheobronchitis), toxic fumes (alveolitis if distal airways reached); carbon monoxide and cyanide can enter blood and poison cellular respiration

Investigations

- ABG: metabolic acidosis common; PaO_2 does *not* reflect available oxygen in presence of carboxyhemoglobin
- Carboxyhemoglobin level (COHb): elevated levels require treating with 100% O_2; reduces half-life to approximately 60 min
- CXR: essential as baseline but may be normal in first 24 hr in up to 40% of patients

Management

- ABCs (see p. 2)
- *Always give 100% O_2 from time of rescue until proven unnecessary*
- Ensure airway patency (of concern because of delayed development of edema; therefore intubate before edema develops)
- Endotracheal intubation for O_2, humidification, tracheobronchial hygiene, continuous positive airway pressure (CPAP), or intermittent positive pressure ventilation (IPPV) with positive end-expiratory pressure (PEEP)
  - Relatively high ventilation pressures and PEEP may be required because of alveolar capillary leak, reduced compliance, and possible pulmonary edema
  - Bronchial hygiene: humidification, suction, physiotherapy, bronchoscopy (rare) to remove tracheal debris
- Supplemental O_2: high FiO_2 (100% if possible) until COHb levels are <0.05 (5%)
- Hyperbaric O_2 therapy may be considered if available and child is cardiovascularly stable
- Fluids: aim for urine output 1 ml/kg/hr (Note: risk of Adult Respiratory Distress Syndrome (ARDS); careful monitoring essential)

NEAR-DROWNING

- Submersion injury followed by survival
- Major problem is global multiorgan hypoxia
- Most often accidental but may have predisposing problem, including seizures, alcohol or drug ingestion, and accidental or nonaccidental trauma (suicide, child abuse, homicide)
- Associated injuries unlikely unless history of diving, trauma, or abuse
- Hypothermia often present; may improve prognosis but hinders cardiac resuscitation; reliable prognostication not possible until patient rewarmed to >33° C and trend of hemodynamic and neurologic status determined
- Duration of submersion, presence of asystolic cardiac arrest, and extent of resuscitation (i.e., need for resuscitation drugs, cardiac compressions, artificial ventilation) most reliable predictors of outcome

Management

Prehospital Care

- Immediate basic life support (see p. 2), including artificial ventilation +/− compressions
- Remove from water with cervical spine control, since there may be other injuries
- Advanced life support (ABCs), if necessary, once out of the water, including assisted ventilation with 100% O_2 as soon as available, cardiac compressions, and rhythm-appropriate medications

Hospital care
- Reassess ABCs (see p. 2) with cervical spine control
- Indications for immediate intubation (if not yet intubated):
  Apnea
  Tachypnea at rest
  FiO_2 requirement >50% to achieve PaO_2 >90 mm Hg
  $PaCO_2$ >40 mm Hg
  Inability to protect airway
  Significantly altered level of consciousness (determine GCS, p. 10)
- Positive end-expiratory pressure ventilation
- Frequent vital signs, including core temperature; cardiac monitor, O_2 saturation monitor
- IV fluids 50%-80% of maintenance (to minimize fluid overload) unless treating shock (see p. 6)
- NG tube, Foley catheter
- Remove wet clothing, treat hypothermia (see p. 21)
- $NaHCO_3$ (1-2 mmol/kg IV) if prolonged submersion or resuscitation
- Prevention and treatment of increased intracranial pressure (see p. 13)
- Initial investigations: ABG, blood sugar, CXR
- Secondary survey: complete physical exam to rule out other injuries
- Secondary investigations: CBC, electrolytes, urea, creatinine, coagulation, $+/-$ specific drug levels if indicated by history

HYPERTHERMIA AND HEAT ILLNESSES

DEFINITION

- Spectrum of disease that ranges from mild heat edema to potentially fatal heat stroke
- Predisposing factors include young age, dehydration (fluid and electrolyte loss), excess clothing, lack of acclimatization, exercise, abnormalities of skin, fever, and infection; consider thyroid storm, malignant hyperthermia associated with anesthetic, neuroleptic malignant syndrome, cerebrovascular accident, or head trauma

Types and Management

Heat Edema
- Minor edematous swelling of hands and feet in first few days of exposure to hot environment
- Treatment: cooler environment

Heat Cramps
- Muscle cramps occurring in exercised muscles after exertion; usually sweating and replacing losses with hypotonic fluids, therefore salt-depleted
- Treatment: cooler environment, rest, oral electrolyte solution or IV fluids, and salt replacement

Heat syncope
- Syncopal episode in unacclimatized people in early stages of exposure to hot environment
- Treatment: cooler environment, Trendelenburg position, oral electrolyte solution, or IV fluids

Heat exhaustion

- Temperature >39° C; water depletion with lethargy, thirst, headache, vomiting, tachycardia, hypernatremia, increased urine specific gravity; salt depletion may predominate with similar features, as well as weakness, fatigue, muscle cramps, hyponatremia, and increased urine Na
- *Neurologic status remains intact*
- Treatment: cooler environment; monitor vital signs; IV fluids for rehydration (bolus then estimate deficit and ongoing losses, see p. 100); CBC, electrolytes, urea, creatinine, urinalysis; observe in hospital until temperature normal
- *If in doubt, treat as per heatstroke*

Heatstroke

- Life-threatening emergency
- Rectal temperature >41° C
- Neurologic dysfunction (due to cerebral edema), including confusion, delirium, seizures, and coma
- Vomiting, diarrhea
- Hot skin (sweating may stop)
- Tachycardia, tachypnea, hypotension
- Circulatory collapse
- Risk of rhabdomyolysis, acute tubular necrosis, disseminated intravascular coagulopathy (DIC), hepatocellular degeneration
- Sodium normal or increased; CPK increased; Ca increased
- Treatment
  - ABCs (see p. 2)
  - Active cooling (aim for 39° C): remove clothing; air-conditioned room; spray water over body surface; ice packs to head, groin, and axilla; consider immersion in ice bath (difficult with unstable patient)
  - IV fluid replacement with crystalloid to maintain perfusion and urine output (place Foley catheter, consider CVL)
  - CBC, ABGs, electrolytes, urea, creatinine, glucose, calcium, liver function tests, coagulation studies, CPK, blood culture (if sepsis suspected), urinalysis
- Complications
  - Seizures: treat with benzodiazepines (see p. 14)
  - Hypotension: treat with volume +/− inotropes (see p. 6)
  - Myoglobinuria: promote diuresis with furosemide and mannitol
  - Renal failure (see p. 327)
  - Arrythmias: cooling usually reverses
- Note: for malignant hyperthermia, treat with dantrolene and supportive measures in ICU setting

HYPOTHERMIA

DEFINITION

- Core temperature <35° C
- Hypothermic patients with absent vital signs not considered deceased until rewarmed to >33° C with no subsequent response to resuscitation

- Predisposing factors include endocrine or metabolic abnormalities (i.e., hypoglycemia), infection, alcohol or drug ingestion, intracranial pathology (i.e., traumatic), near-drowning

Clinical Manifestations

Cardiac

- Initial increase in BP and HR; decreased HR with prolonged cooling; complete vasomotor paralysis occurs at approx 30° C; ECG shows prolongation of all phases of cardiac cycle, and J wave (elevation of ST segment) may be seen at 33°-32° C
- Sinus bradycardia or atrial fibrillation at 30° C; ventricular fibrillation from 28°-26° C; slow sinus rhythm may be maintained

Respiratory

- Immediate hyperventilation, then normoventilation from 35°-33° C
- Hypoventilation or apnea (especially in premature neonates) at lower temperatures

Neurologic

- Slurred speech, mild incoordination at 35°-32° C
- Progressive decreased level of consciousness; coma occurs at 30°-28° C
- Fixed dilated pupils at <25° C

Muscular

- Early shivering thermogenesis, followed by abolishment of shivering and progressive rigidity at 32°-28° C

Renal

- "Cold diuresis," acute tubular necrosis, hypokalemia, or hyperkalemia

Metabolic

- Lactic acidosis

Management

- ABCs (see p. 2); note that arrhythmias may be resistant to cardioversion until rewarming occurs
- Correct metabolic acidosis (IV fluids and $NaHCO_3$)
- Monitor core temperature, blood pressure, ECG, urine output, and temperature of inspired gases
- CBC, electrolytes, urea, creatinine, glucose (especially in neonates), amylase, blood gases, drug screen, coagulation screen, thyroid function, CXR, ECG

Rewarming

- Mild hypothermia (33°-35° C): passive external rewarming (i.e., remove from exposure, remove wet clothing, cover with warm blankets)
- Moderate hypothermia (30°-33° C): add active external rewarming (i.e., heated water mattress, immersion in warm—37°-40° C—water but not often practical), radiant heater; active core (airway) rewarming: give warm humidified O_2 (40°-45° C by mask or 40° C if intubated) and warm IV fluids
- More severe hypothermia: additional core rewarming (i.e., warm gastric lavage or colonic irrigation with warm normal saline); peritoneal dialysis, hemodialysis, or cardiopulmonary bypass in refractory cases

FROSTBITE

- May accompany hypothermia or may occur independently; usually restricted to head and extremities; frozen part is white and firm
- After core temperature has returned to normal, immerse injured extremity for about 20 min into water kept 37°-40° C (do not start to thaw an extremity if any chance of patient being reexposed to cold)
- Refer patient to plastic surgeon if extensive area of involvement

HYPERTENSIVE EMERGENCIES

DEFINITION

- Severe hypertension: BP >99th percentile for age and sex (see p. 315)
- Accelerated hypertension: BP >95th percentile for age + evidence of end-organ damage

Clinical Manifestations

- Hypertension, +/− tachycardia, +/− tachypnea
- Visual complaints, hypertensive retinopathy
- Left ventricular hypertrophy, cardiac failure
- Seizures, encephalopathy, hemiplegia, facial palsy, cranial bruits

Management

- ABCs (see p. 2)
- Initial aim to reduce BP enough to stabilize patient acutely (i.e., if seizing)
- Subsequent aim to reduce BP *slowly* over 3-4 days after initial stabilization
- Do not acutely drop blood pressure if elevated in response to increased ICP (need increased MAP to sustain CPP, see p. 13)

Medications
- Principles
  - Exclude hypertension due to ↑ ICP
  - *Continuous infusions only*
  - Bolus therapy associated with increased risk of strokes/infarcts
  - Titrate rate to achieve desired BP
  - Base any change in rate of infusion on minimum of two consecutive BP readings
- Labetalol 1-3 mg/kg/hour continuous infusion (see Fig. I-1); do not use in presence of cardiac failure or history of asthma; adverse effects include nausea/vomiting, dizziness, scalp tingling, heart block, burning sensation in throat, liver toxicity
- Nitroprusside 0.5-8 μg/kg/min continuous infusion (see Fig. I-1); avoid if increased ICP, renal failure; adverse effects include nausea/vomiting, diaphoresis, muscle twitching; use for >48 hours may cause cyanide toxicity; medication is photosensitive (needs aluminum-foil covering)

Monitoring
- BP q5-10 min while on infusion
- If BP falls below specified goal then stop infusion and give normal saline in 50-ml boluses until BP recovers; restart infusion at lower rate

Laboratory
- Gas, electrolytes, glucose, urea, creatinine, CBC, blood film
- Urinalysis
- ECG, chest x-ray
- Consider plasma renin (prior to initiation of therapy), urine metanephrine

Further Management

Goals
- Determine etiology of hypertension
- Determine chronicity of hypertension
- Assess for end-organ damage: fundi, brain, heart, kidneys

Etiology
- Renal
  - Reflux nephropathy, obstructive uropathy
  - Renovascular disease, glomerular disease, hemolytic uremic syndrome (HUS)
  - Polycystic renal disease, renal dysplasia
- Cardiac: coarctation of aorta
- Tumors: Wilms' tumor, pheochromocytoma
- Drugs/toxins
  - Sudden withdrawal of antihypertensive agents (e.g., clonidine)
  - Monoamine-oxidase inhibitors, cocaine
- Eclampsia

History
- Symptoms of visual, cerebral, cardiac, and renal dysfunction
- Prior history of hypertension/antihypertensives

Physical Exam
- Vital signs: BP $\times$ 3 with appropriate-sized cuff; four-limb BP
- Glasgow Coma Scale, neurologic exam, fundi
- Cardiovascular exam: apex, brachiofemoral pulse delay
- State of hydration, edema (peripheral and pulmonary)
- Abdominal masses, bruits

HYPERKALEMIA

DEFINITION

- Serum potassium >6.5 mEq/L

Etiology

- Excess input: IV or po
- Cellular breakdown: tumor lysis syndrome, hemolysis, burns, rhabdomyolysis
- Renal failure (see p. 327)
- Systemic acidosis
- Adrenal insufficiency (see p. 97)

Clinical Manifestations

- Life-threatening cardiac toxicity, especially at levels >8.0 mEq/L
- ECG changes:

>6.0 mEq/L	tall, narrow, "tented" T waves
>7.5 mEq/L	long PR interval, widened QRS complexes
>9.0 mEq/L	absent P waves → sinusoidal wave

- Ectopic rhythms and intraventricular block can also occur

Management

- ABCs (see p. 2); if ventricular arrhythmia, may not respond to routine medications or defibrillation until hyperkalemia treated
- Ensure sample not hemolyzed
- ECG; continuous ECG monitoring
- Discontinue any external sources of KCl (i.e., IV additive, po supplements)
- If >8.0 mEq/L or if *any* ECG changes:
  1. Calcium (cardioprotective) with ECG monitoring
     - Calcium chloride 10% (100 mg/ml) 0.2 ml/kg IV over 2-5 min or
     - Calcium gluconate 10% (100 mg/ml) 0.5-1 ml/kg IV over 2-5 min
  2. NaHCO$_3$ 1.5-2 mmol/kg IV (1.5-2 ml/kg of 8.4% solution) over 30 min (shifts K+ into cells, which transiently decreases intravascular K+ concentration)
  3. Glucose 1 g/kg IV (2 ml/kg D50W) +/− insulin 0.1 U/kg IV over 30 min (shifts K+ into cells)
- To *remove* potassium from body:
  1. Dialysis if due to renal failure
  2. Exchange resin (e.g., Kayexalate) 1g/kg pr

ACUTE ADRENAL INSUFFICIENCY

DEFINITION

- Stressed state of steroid (cortisol) +/− mineralocorticoid (aldosterone) deficiency

Clinical Manifestations

- Shock with dehydration (see p. 6)
- Hyponatremia, hyperkalemia, +/− hypoglycemia

Management

- ABCs (see p. 2)
- Treat shock (see p. 6)
  - Fluid resuscitation: use D5NS or NS and give additional dextrose (D25W or D50W) acutely; bolus until hemodynamic stability achieved and acidosis corrected; may be relatively unresponsive to fluids until steroids administered (see below)
  - Dextrose required for hypoglycemia
  - Saline required for Na replacement (if salt-losing state)
  - Do not add KCl to IV solutions
- Treat hyperkalemia if present (see p. 24)

- Steroid replacement: hydrocortisone 100 mg/m^2 stat and then q4h
- Mineralocorticoid replacement: 9-α-fluorohydrocortisone 0.05-0.2 mg/day (required for maintenance in salt-losing states)
- For differential diagnosis and investigations (see p. 97)

CHILD ABUSE

DEFINITION

- Harm resulting from inappropriate or abnormal child-rearing behavior, including physical abuse, sexual abuse, emotional abuse, and neglect
- Physical injury or deprivation of nutrition, care, or affection in circumstances indicating that such injury or deprivation is not accidental
- Age-inappropriate sexual encounter between child and another individual
- Children may be victims of more than one type of abuse

History

- Current allegations made by or on behalf of child; contradictory or no explanation for current injury; explore circumstances and home management of injury; assess appropriateness
- Guardian(s): social risk factors, substance abuse, mental health, present crisis, history of sexual or physical abuse in guardian
- Child: development, past injuries, illness or accidental poisoning, behavior

Physical Examination (Table I-7)

- Must be conducted with patience and sensitivity
- Complete examination essential
- Plot heights and weights on appropriate charts
- Examine fundi of infants; check for retinal hemorrhages
- Examine genitalia and anus; do not do internal examination unless specific indications; *do not* use restraining measures; if child will not cooperate, defer examination or enlist help of subspecialist
- Document all visible trauma—size, shape, color, and location
- Record child's behavior and reactions

Investigation

- Suspected physical abuse
  - Hematology: rule out blood dyscrasia
  - Skeletal survey or bone scan in young children: record location and age of fractures; rule out metabolic bone disease
  - CT scan of head in infants with neurologic symptoms or signs
- Alleged sexual abuse (see p. 28)
  - Forensic specimens; some jurisdictions use sexual assault evidence kit
  - Specimens for sexually transmitted diseases (see p. 28)
  - Pregnancy test
- Color photography: record obvious trauma (important legal documentation)

EMERGENCIES

Table I-7   Child Abuse Indicators*

Physical	Behavioral
1. Injuries not explained by history given	**Child**
2. Poor care and nutrition Inadequate clothing Poor hygiene Failure to thrive Inadequate medical attention	1. Extreme wariness of parents and adults in general 2. Extremes of behavior (e.g., aggressiveness, withdrawal, compliance, fearfulness) 3. Pseudomature behavior
3. Bruises and welts On face, back, buttocks, thighs Multiple, may be at different stages of healing In shape of instrument or hand	4. Self-destructive behavior, including suicide threats or attempts 5. Changes in school performance 6. Running away from home 7. Sexual acting out or age-inappropriate sexual knowledge
4. Burns Cigarette burns Multiple, may be of different ages Immersion burns Burns in shape of instrument Rope burns	8. Functional complaints, particularly abdominal pain **Guardians** 1. Poor self-control, seem under stress 2. Not responsive to child's needs
5. Fractures Skull, ribs, shoulder girdle Multiple, particularly at different stages of healing Spiral and metaphyseal fractures Any fracture in an infant	3. History of physical or sexual abuse as a child 4. Single parent, particularly if young and without support systems 5. Substance abuse 6. Mental illness
6. Retinal hemorrhages	
7. Intracranial hemorrhages, especially subdural	
8. Genitourinary Trauma to the genitals or anus Sexually transmitted diseases Pregnancy	

*Some of these symptoms and behaviors can be caused by events other than child abuse. Also, almost any physical or behavioral symptom can be the result of child abuse. However, those listed above are indicators that, particulary in combination, should raise the suspicion of the examining physician.

Further Management

- Most jurisdictions have laws requiring professionals to report *suspected* child abuse to appropriate authorities *without delay*
- Admit for treatment or protection if indicated
- Treat injuries and other medical problems (e.g., sexually transmitted diseases) as indicated
- Obtain necessary consultations (e.g., social worker, psychiatrist, physician with expertise in child abuse)
- Protection assessment to be carried out by appropriate authorities
- Disposition to be planned with joint medical and social input

SEXUAL ASSAULT

- If assault occurred within 24 hr, then complete examination should be done immediately; otherwise examination can be done at physician's and patient's earliest convenience
- Be patient, reassuring, kind, and calm in manner
- Contact local child protection services and police (if patient < 16 yr)
- Adolescent > 16 yr, contact police if he or she wishes to press charges
- Obtain a brief history from parents or caregivers and full history from patient; use the patient's own words, and keep meticulous records
- Assess and record patient's emotional state
- Obtain written consent before the examination from patient or guardian
- Use sexual assault kit to collect appropriate specimens, and label them carefully; follow enclosed guidelines (e.g., label all slides; put clothing into paper bags), and give evidence directly to police officer; obtain signed receipt for evidence
- Perform complete physical, and record all pertinent data carefully; where possible, illustrate with diagrams, and obtain medical photographs
- Examine following specimens immediately: urine for hemoglobin, RBCs, and sperm; wet mount of vaginal swab for motile sperm
- Take appropriate samples for STDs
    1. Gonococcal swabs: endocervix, vaginal (prepubertal), urethral, rectal, and oral
    2. *Chlamydia:* endocervix, vaginal (prepubertal), oral, rectal
    3. *Trichomonas:* vaginal (postpubertal)
    4. VDRL and follow-up in 8 wk with repeat VDRL
    5. HIV screen and surveillance at 3, 6, and 12 mo
- Gynecology referral if surgical problem is found (e.g., cervical or vaginal tear)
- Pregnancy prevention ("morning after" pill)
    1. Treatment applies to all peri- and postmenarchal women regardless of timing in cycle; given within 72 hr of coitus
    2. Rule out present pregnancy; serum β-hCG is positive at 29 days after last menstrual period
    3. Ovral, 2 tabs PO q12 hr × 2 doses (include antinauseant)
- STD prophylaxis
    1. Ceftriaxone, 250 mg IM × 1
    2. Treat for *Chlamydia* as well (see p. 170)
- Follow-up essential: psychologic/emotional counseling, as well as medical
- Refer to rape crisis center if desired by patient or family; provide rape crisis telephone number
- Offer hepatitis B prophylaxis (see p. 218)

TRIAGE OF THE MULTIPLE-TRAUMA PATIENT

- History of mechanism and force of trauma important in anticipation of possible injuries, which may not be initially apparent
- Common life-threatening problems in immediate period after traumatic

event include acute respiratory failure (e.g., airway obstruction or apnea) and hemorrhagic shock

Immediate Management

- Primary survey and initial resuscitation (ABCs, p. 2): focus on treating immediate threats to life with assessment of airway, oxygenation, ventilation, circulation, and overall neurologic status with appropriate intervention where abnormalities found
- Secondary survey: more thorough physical exam to define presence, type, and severity of injuries
- Additional experienced staff should be alerted
- Consider transfer to a pediatric trauma center after:
  1. Stabilization
  2. Organizing transfer through direct physician-to-physician contact
  3. Appropriate preparation of patient, personnel, and equipment for transfer (see p. 30)

Stablization

- Secure patent airway
  1. Assume that patient has fractured cervical spine
  2. Clear pharynx; chin lift or jaw thrust
  3. Administer O_2 to all patients initially, bag and mask ventilation if necessary
  4. Intubate and assist ventilation if
     Apneic/inefficient ventilation
     Inability to protect airway
     Glasgow Coma Score of 7 or less (see p. 10)
     Severe head injury
     Airway burn or inhalation
     Major maxillofacial injury
- Intravenous access with two wide-bore cannulas (preferably in upper limbs in abdominal trauma)
- Hemostasis and fluid resuscitation
  1. Even in presence of head injury, give initial bolus of 10-20 ml/kg of crystalloid (Ringer's lactate) or colloid (5% albumin) in patient with signs of hypovolemic shock after trauma (see p. 6)
  2. Have sufficient fluid available to continue resuscitation during transport of patient
  3. Transfuse with packed red cells if more than 10% of child's blood volume has been lost (blood volume in child is approximately 80 ml/kg)
  4. Military antishock trousers (MAST) have limited uses and many potential complications (increased vascular resistance, hemorrhage); should not be used in presence of pulmonary edema or myocardial dysfunction and only with caution if there is CNS injury or suspected diaphragmatic rupture; use only if available in pediatric size
- Examine patient thoroughly for significant injury (see assessment below)
- Place NG or orogastric tube (oral mandatory in presence of facial or basal skull fractures)
- Place Foley catheter (unless pelvic injury or blood visible at urethral meatus)

- In hospitals with medium-level trauma care facilities, baseline investigations should be performed before transport to pediatric trauma center: ABG, CBC, cross-match, electrolytes, and CXR
- Chest tube(s) in all ventilated patients with documented pneumothorax or hemothorax
- Measures to avoid hypothermia

Further Assessment

Head
- Laceration, bruising, swelling +/− fracture
- Hemorrhage from nose, mouth, or ears, or clear fluid (CSF) from nose or ears
- Unequal or abnormally reacting pupils, abnormal extraocular movements, penetrating eye injury, visual acuity disturbances

Neck
- Tenderness
- Laryngeal or tracheal injury (abnormal cry, stridor, subcutaneous emphysema)
- Assume there is cervical spine fracture during initial exam

Chest
- Flail segment or penetrating wounds
- Signs of pneumothorax or hemothorax (tracheal deviation, auscultation for reduced air entry, chest expansion)
- Rib fractures, bruising over precordium

Abdomen
- Penetrating wounds
- Bowel sounds
- Guarding
- Peritoneal lavage should not be performed unless discussed with pediatric surgeon

Pelvis
- Instability or pain on compression
- Perineal injury

Extremities
- Fractures, dislocations (*remove clothing*)
- Pulses, perfusion

Back
- Tenderness of spine
- Bruising of flanks

TRANSPORT OF SICK CHILD

- The keys to successful transport include:
  1. Stabilization of patient at base facility
  2. Anticipation of likely complications
  3. Availability of qualified transport personnel (usually nurse, respiratory therapist +/− physician)
  4. Adequate fixation of all lines, drains, and tubes before performing transport
  5. Communication with receiving physician and institution

6. Use of most appropriate transport method
7. Discussion of transport with receiving physician (trauma team leader, general surgeon, ICU, emergency room)
8. Receiving hospital should be requested to retrieve patient if transport facilities available

Modes of Transportation

Land

- Quicker to arrange
- May be stopped en route to perform tasks or diverted to another hospital if patient suddenly deteriorates
- Slower for long journeys; spine fractures a concern (e.g., movement)
- Requires more fluids, drugs, O_2 for trip
- Paramedic assistance may not be available

Helicopter

- Not always available (already in use; bad weather)
- May require land transport to helicopter
- Fast for medium-distance transport
- Usually well equipped
- Paramedic support usually provided

Fixed-wing aircraft

- Slow to arrange
- May not have equipment or personnel provided
- Requires land transport at each end
- Useful for long-distance transport to major facility once patient stabilized
- Transport by helicopter or fixed-wing aircraft may involve transport at altitude; the extra problems include:
  1. Increased gas volume during ascent (e.g., expansion of pneumothorax, air in stomach or intestines, air in inflated cuff of endotracheal tube, air above fluid level in drip chamber of IV line)
  2. Fall in partial pressure of O_2; worse in unpressurized craft
  3. Often increased background noise levels, making auscultation difficult
  4. Vibration of concern in new spine fractures
  5. Confined space, with difficult access to patient, especially if aircraft interior not designed for regular patient transport

Before Transport

- Check equipment
  - Intubation equipment, including bag and mask
  - Adequate O_2 supply
  - Stable IV access; sufficient fluids for maintenance and resuscitation
  - Drugs available, drawn up, and at hand (e.g., anticonvulsants)
  - Suction equipment
  - Humidification (e.g., small condenser humidifier on endotracheal tube)
  - ECG monitor
  - BP cuff or Doppler monitor
  - O_2 saturation monitor if available
  - Precordial or esophageal stethoscope

- Ensure that appropriate personnel accompany child (e.g., MD, transport-trained RN, respiratory therapist, or paramedic)

Respiratory

- Secure airway: endotracheal intubation if necessary; nasal tube preferable to oral tube (more stable); use bite block in orally intubated patients
- Ensure adequate ventilation, oxygenation; check tube placement
- Insert chest tubes if pneumothorax and attach to Heimlich valves to avoid clamping chest drains
- Use condenser humidifier (i.e., Swedish nose)

Cardiovascular

- Stabilize blood pressure and pulse rate before transport
- Two intravenous cannulas advisable; portable syringe drivers preferable to hanging fluid bags because of limited headroom

Other

- NG tube to open drainage
- Aim to maintain normothermia
- Monitor Chemstick for high-risk patients (neonates, fasting, liver failure)
- Keep record of observations during transport

CHAPTER **1**
ADOLESCENT MEDICINE

Susan Campbell and Candice N. Rowe

HISTORY

- Physicians must identify themselves as advocates for teens, ensure privacy and confidentiality for this special population, and provide reassurance and education
1. H = *home,* including relations with parents, family responsibilities, family support and stresses, independence
2. E = *education,* including present performance in school, career goals, relationships, likes and dislikes
3. A = *activities,* including special interests, relationships with friends, job, dating
   A = *antisocial* behavior, including truancy and legal problems
4. D = *drugs,* including smoking and alcohol
5. S = *sexuality,* including pregnancy, birth control, sexually transmitted diseases (STDs)
   S = *suicide*
- Check immunization status, TB test if indicated, Td booster every 10 yr, consider hepatitis vaccine if not already received in school (grade 7 in Canada)

PHYSICAL EXAMINATION

- Growth parameters
- Vision and hearing, using standard screening methods
- Sexual maturity rating (Tanner stage; see pp. 154-156)
- Blood pressure
- Assessment of thyroid
- Assessment of scoliosis (see p. 409)
- Examination of external genitalia in all adolescents
- Pelvic examination in sexually active females or in those with menstrual problems
- Breast examination: explain importance of self-examination in female or gynecomastia, if present, in male
- Testicular examination in males: teach self-examination

LABORATORY INVESTIGATIONS

- CBC, Fe studies as indicated (anemia not uncommon in adolescents)
- Rubella-immune status
- Sexually active females: Pap smear; serologic test for syphilis (VDRL); microscopic examination of discharge; and cultures for gonorrhea, *Chlamydia,* and *Trichomonas* should be done yearly and as clinically warranted
- Sexually active males: VDRL test and cultures when indicated
- Review need for screening for hepatitis and HIV in all teens

CONTRACEPTION

- Oral Contraceptives: see Gynecology (p. 173)
- Remember to discuss abstinence from intercourse as viable option to methods of contraception.
- Morning-after pill: 93%-100% effective; dose: 2 Ovral tablets, repeat in 12 hr; all doses *must be taken within 72 hours* of unprotected intercourse

ANOREXIA NERVOSA

- Criteria that follow adapted from DSM-IV
- Refusal to maintain body weight at or above minimally normal weight for age and height (e.g., weight loss leading to maintenance of body weight less than 85% of that expected or failure to make expected weight gain during period of growth, leading to body weight less than 85% of that expected)
- Intense fear of gaining weight or becoming fat, even though underweight
- Disturbance in way in which one's body weight or shape experienced, undue influence of body weight or shape on self-evaluation, or denial of seriousness of current low body weight
- In postmenarcheal females, amenorrhea (i.e., absence of at least three consecutive menstrual cycles; woman is considered to have amenorrhea if her periods occur only following hormone administration, such as estrogen)

Types

Restricting Type
- During current episode of anorexia nervosa, person has not regularly engaged in binge eating or purging behavior (i.e., self-induced vomiting or misuse of laxatives, diuretics, or enemas)

Binge-Eating/Purging Type
- During current episode of anorexia nervosa, person has regularly engaged in binge eating or purging behavior (i.e., self-induced vomiting or misuse of laxatives, diuretics, or enemas)

Clinical Features

- Psychologic: high achievers with average or above-average intelligence; perfectionistic; low self-esteem; distorted perceptions, particularly of body image
- Behavioral: relentless pursuit of thinness; preoccupations with food, calories, and exercise; decreased sexual interest; denial of weight problem; sleep disturbances
- Physical features: hypothermia and cold intolerance, dry skin, lanugo, easy bruising, yellow skin (carotenemia), hair loss, cold extremities
- Gastrointestinal: slowed gastric emptying; constipation
- Cardiovascular: bradycardia; dysrhythmias; hypotension; ECG shows low voltage, low or inverted T waves, prolonged QTc
- Hematologic: B_{12} deficiency, pancytopenia, ↓ ESR
- Metabolic: features of dehydration, ↓ GFR, ↑ renal stones, ↑ carotene, hypophosphatemia

- Endocrine: amenorrhea, growth retardation (if prolonged starvation during growth spurt), "senile" vaginitis, partial diabetes insipidus, sick euthyroid syndrome (TSH normal, N/↓ T4, ↓ T3, ↑ rT3); GH normal/↑ (somatomedin C ↓), estradiol and testosterone ↓, basal FSH and LH ↓, cortisol normal/↑, osteoporosis

BULIMIA NERVOSA

- Criteria that follow adapted from DSM-IV
- Recurrent episodes of binge eating, characterized by both
  1. Eating, in discrete period of time (e.g., within any two-hour period), amount of food definitely larger than most people would eat during similar period of time and under similar circumstances
  2. Sense of lack of control over eating during episode (e.g., feeling that one cannot stop eating or control what or how much one is eating)
- Recurrent inappropriate compensatory behavior to prevent weight gain, such as self-induced vomiting; misuse of laxatives, diuretics, enemas, or other medications; fasting; or excessive exercise
- Binge eating and inappropriate compensatory behaviors both occur, on average, at least twice a week for three mo
- Self-evaluation unduly influenced by body shape and weight
- Disturbance does not occur exclusively during episodes of anorexia nervosa

Types
Purging Type
- During current episode of bulimia nervosa, person has regularly engaged in self-induced vomiting or misuse of laxatives, diuretics, or enemas
Nonpurging Type
- During current episode of bulimia nervosa, person has used other inappropriate behaviors, such as fasting or excessive exercise, but has not regularly engaged in self-induced vomiting or misuse of laxatives, diuretics, or enemas

Clinical Features
- Psychologic: good peer relations, high energy, talkative, ↑ anxiety and affective disorders, low self-esteem
- Behavioral: self-induced vomiting, laxative and/or diuretic abuse, substance abuse more common, secretive overeating, more likely to be sexually active, distressed by symptoms
- Physical: eroded enamel on posterior aspect of upper incisors and dental caries, parotid enlargement, Russell's sign (calluses on knuckles), edema, conjunctival hemorrhages
- Gastrointestinal: acute gastric dilation, rarely rupture; esophagitis; Mallory-Weiss tears
- Cardiovascular: possible ipecac poisoning (cardiac toxicity; check CPK), ECG shows prolonged QTc
- Metabolic: hypokalemia, hypochloremia, hyponatremia, hyperamylasemia, metabolic alkalosis (may be secondary to vomiting, diuretics, or laxatives)
- Endocrine: menstrual irregularities

Indications for Hospitalization of Patients with Eating Disorders

- Hypothermia $< 36°$ C
- Arrhythmias
- Dehydration
- Significant postural hypotension (drop in systolic blood pressure > 20 mm Hg; increased heart rate > 35 beats/min from baseline)
- Metabolic abnormalities (e.g., hypokalemia)
- Absolute weight $< 75\%$ ideal body weight

Table 1-1 Commonly Abused Substance*

Substance	Characteristics	Effects	Withdrawal	Fetal effects	Treatment principles
Alcohol	Absorption Stomach Small intestine Metabolism 95% liver 5% excreted in kidney	Relaxation, euphoria Blood alcohol levels (BAL): *0.075%-0.15%* *(75-150 mg/dl)* Sedation Hypnotic Impaired judgment Slurred speech Ataxia *0.25%-0.4%* *(250-400 mg/dl)* Apathy Stupor Coma Hypothermia Respiratory distress *0.45%-0.5%* *(450-500 mg/dl)* Death in 50%	Acute alcoholic hallucinoses Wernicke's encephalopathy (thiamine deficiency) Delirium tremens Confusion Hallucinations Sweating Ataxia Seizures	Fetal alcohol syndrome (FAS) Mental retardation Microcephaly Dysmorphic facies Childhood hyperactivity Short stature Cardiac abnormality	Overdose: Airway protection IV fluids, glucose Associated diagnostic possibilities; head injury, hypoglycemia Coexisting illness: GI ulcers, hepatitis, STD Psychologic features: dependency, suicide risk, concomitant drug use
Amphetamines	Absorption Oral Inhalation IV Metabolism Liver	CNS: ↑ Physical and mental alertness, euphoria, gregariousness, hallucinations, intracranial hemorrhages, Gilles de la Tourette's syndrome, seizures	Apathy Depression Lethargy Anxiety Sleep disturbance Myalgias	Unknown	Stabilization of vital signs (VS) Supportive care for agitation, psychosis Seizure control

*See p. 311 for a discussion of neonatal drug withdrawal.

Continued.

Table 1-1 Commonly Abused Substance*—cont'd

Substance	Characteristics	Effects	Withdrawal	Fetal effects	Treatment principles
Amphetamines— cont'd	Excreted in urine	CVS: ↑ BP, ↑ HR, palpitations, arrhythmias GI: Nausea/vomiting Metabolic: Hyperthermia, cardiomyopathy, pulmonary edema, endocarditis GI: Anorexia Pulmonary: Granulomas, fibrosis Musculoskeletal: Rhabdomyolysis Chronic: Anxiety, dysphoria, confusion, depression, nausea, vomiting, headache, sweating, apprehension, confusion, fatigue	Abdominal pain Voracious appetite		

Cocaine	Heroin
Cocaine	**Heroin**
Erythroxylon coca	
"Speedball" (heroin and cocaine)	
"Liquid lady" (alcohol and cocaine)	
"Crack" (free-base cocaine, adulterants removed)	

	Absorption / Metabolism	Effects	Withdrawal	Fetal/Neonatal	Treatment
Cocaine	Absorption Nasal Oral Pulmonary Metabolized in liver and plasma Excreted in urine (↑ with acidic pH), bile	"Fight or flight" response Vasoconstriction Local anesthetic CNS: Euphoria, restlessness, excitement, emotional instability, tremors, seizures Respiratory: ↑ RR → respiratory depression CVS: Tachycardia, VF, hypertension GI: Nausea/vomiting Metabolic: Hyperthermia Eyes: Mydriasis	Agitation, depression Anorexia → hyperphagia Insomnia → hypersomnolence Anhedonia Lack of energy Anxiety	Prematurity IUGR ↓ Interactive behavior Poor response to external stimuli Neonatal cerebral infarction	Stabilization of VS May need activated charcoal, lavage Rx of arrhythmias Temperature control Seizure control Suicide precautions
Heroin	Synthesized from morphine Absorption Inhalation Oral IV SC	CNS: Coma, seizures, ↑ ICP, acute delirium, chronic organic brain damage Musculoskeletal: Rhabdomyolysis, myoglobinuria	Anxiety Yawning Perspiration Lacrimation Insomnia Hypertension Fever Weight loss	IUGR Neonatal withdrawal (Note: secreted in breast milk) ↑ SIDS	Stabilization of VS Gut decontamination Antidote: naloxone Supportive care

Continued.

Table 1-1 Commonly Abused Substance*—cont'd

Substance	Characteristics	Effects	Withdrawal	Fetal effects	Treatment principles
Heroin—cont'd	Converted to MAM (6-monacetylmorphine) in liver, brain, kidneys, blood, lungs Excreted in urine	Pulmonary: Pulmonary edema, respiratory depression, pulmonary arteritis, pulmonary hypertension CVS: Tachy- and bradycardia, paroxysmal atrial tachycardia, VF, QT prolongation Renal: Nephrotic syndrome, amyloidosis Eyes: Miosis	Vomiting and diarrhea		
LSD (Lysergic acid diethylamide)	Absorption Oral (mainly) Nasal	Visual illusions Perceptual distortion and synesthesia	Withdrawal symptoms		Stabilization of VS Supportive care, seizure control

"Acid" "Sunshine" "White lightning"	IV Metabolism Liver		Mydriasis Hyperthermia Depersonalization and derealization Acute anxiety attacks Seizures		Reassurance Reduction of sensory stimuli
Marijuana *(Cannabis sativa)* "Grass" "Pot" Cannabis Hashish (dried resin of plant flower tops) Bhang (dried leaves and stems)	Psychoactive component: tetrahydrocannabinol (THC) Absorption inhalation > oral Metabolized in liver Excreted in feces, urine	Restlessness Sleeplessness ↓ Appetite Nausea Irritability Sweating Dreaming	Acute: Bronchodilation, tachycardia, pupillary constriction, ↓ intraocular pressure, euphoria, relaxation, sleepiness, lethargy, dry mouth, ↑ appetite Chronic: Large AW irritation, gynecomastia, ↓ sperm count Amotivation syndrome: Apathy, passivity, loss of productivity, ↓ energy, tiredness, ↓ frustration tolerance	FAS-like clinical presentation Tremulousness IUGR Facial dysmorphism ↑ Fetal mortality	Stabilization of VS Watch for ARDS, acute renal failure Activated charcoal, gastric lavage Monitor level of consciousness Psychologic features: dependency, suicide risk, concomitant drug use

Continued.

Table 1-1 Commonly Abused Substance*—cont'd

Substance	Characteristics	Effects	Withdrawal	Fetal effects	Treatment principles

Toluene	Present in paints, lacquers, thinners, coatings
	Clear, colorless, flammable liquid
	Absorption
	Inhalation (mainly)
	Oral
	Skin
	Lipid soluble
	Elimination
	80% metabolized in liver
	Small amounts in urine, bile
	18% by lungs
		Exposure to:
		100 ppm: impaired psychomotor and perceptual performance
		500-800 ppm: progressively ↑ headache, drowsiness, nausea, fatigue, weakness, confusion
		> 800 ppm: severe fatigue, convulsions, ataxia, staggered gait
		> 1000 ppm: anesthesia within 1 min
		Renal:
		  Renal tubular acidosis
		CVS:
		  Sudden death, ↓ AV conduction
		Chronic encephalopathy, recurrent headaches, permanent cerebellar ataxia
					Stabilization of VS
					Supportive care

CHAPTER 2

ALLERGY AND IMMUNOLOGY

SUMATHI NADARAJAH

ALLERGY

- Altered reactivity on a second contact with an antigen (type 1 hypersensitivity)

ANAPHYLAXIS

- Acute life-threatening reaction resulting in IgE- or non-IgE–mediated rapid release of mediators from mast cells, basophils, and other inflammatory cells
- See Emergencies (p. 17) for acute management

Clinical Manifestations

- Urticaria, pruritus, angioedema, laryngeal edema, rhinitis, bronchospasm, hypotension, tachycardia, abdominal cramps, nausea, vomiting, diarrhea may occur immediately after parenteral administration of drug or up to several hours after oral administration
- Distinguish from vasovagal reactions: diaphoresis, blanching (rather than flushing), nausea, rapid improvement with recumbency; hypotension may occur in both conditions; bradycardia more likely in vasovagal reactions; tachycardia more likely in anaphylaxis

Etiology

- IgE-mediated: haptens (e.g., penicillin), complete antigens (e.g., foods, latex, insulin)
- Immunologic, non-IgE–mediated (e.g., heterologous immunoglobulin aggregates)
- Nonimmunologic: opiates, dextran, radiographic contrast, aspirin
- Unknown: sulfites

MECHANISM OF ALLERGIC REACTIONS

- Type I: IgE-mediated hypersensitivity (e.g., allergic asthma, hay fever)
- Type II: Cytotoxic reactions (antibody mediated) (e.g., transfusion reaction, hemolytic disease of newborns)
- Type III: Immune complex (e.g., serum sicknesslike or Arthus reactions)
- Type IV: Delayed hypersensitivity (lymphocyte mediated) (e.g., allergic contact dermatitis, tuberculin-type hypersensitivity)

INVESTIGATIONS
Skin Testing

- Skin testing should be carried out with allergens implicated by allergy history; results must be interpreted in context of history

- Preferred method of skin testing is prick method; intradermal tests used less often, but indicated when history highly suggestive and prick test negative
- Positive wheal and erythema reaction occurs within 15 min and enables detection of specific IgE antibodies to applied antigen
- Skin testing is most useful for identification of specific allergens in allergic rhinitis, asthma, insect sting allergy, immediate food reactions, and specific drug allergy; less useful for identification of specific allergens in chronic urticaria, angioedema, and delayed food reactions
- Most antihistamines should be withheld for 72 hr before skin testing; astemizole (Hismanal) should be withheld for 4 weeks; positive histamine control ensures that testing is reliable

In Vitro Testing: Radioallergosorbent Test (RAST)

- Most useful for detection of specific IgE antibodies in patients with life-threatening reactions (anaphylaxis), extensive dermatitis, or severe dermatographism
- No need to discontinue antihistamines before testing
- Expensive and not more reliable than skin testing

Challenge Testing

- Useful for immunologic and nonimmunologic sensitivities to drugs, food, and other biologic products such as vaccines and insulin
- Because of risk of anaphylaxis, tests should be undertaken in controlled setting

Suspicion of Allergic Disorder

- Eosinophilia of $> 5\%$ or $> 0.25 \times 10^9/L$ ($> 250/mm^3$)
- Smear of nasal secretions or bronchial mucus for eosinophils
- Elevated total serum immunoglobulin E level

MANAGEMENT (Box 2-1 and Table 2-1)
Immunotherapy

- Consider in patients poorly controlled on optimal environmental manipulation and pharmacotherapy
- Most important indication: insect venom anaphylaxis
- Not indicated for eczema or food allergy

Other Measures

- Medic Alert bracelet
- Epipen/Anakit and written instruction regarding their use for anaphylaxis
- Identify at-risk children to all school staff

FOOD ALLERGY

- Must distinguish between intolerance, pharmacologic effects, metabolics, and true allergy (uncommon; incidence 5%)
- Most common foods causing food allergy: egg, milk, wheat, peanut, soybean, seafood, and tree nuts; peanuts are most potent allergen (1000 × more potent than other foods) and leading cause of food-induced anaphylaxis

BOX 2-1   Allergen Avoidance

Strategy	Method
I. Identify at-risk infant prenatally or early postnatally	1. Document highly atopic families (biparental, parent and sibling), or
	2. Document elevated cord blood IgE
II. Avoid infant exposure to	
A. Food allergens	
In breast milk	1. Maternal lactation diet without egg, milk, or peanut
	2. Supplement maternal diet daily with 1500 mg elemental calcium
In infant diet	1. Breast-feed for 4-6 mo
	2. Supplement or wean with suitable protein hydrolysate formula
	3. Delay solids until 6 mo, then add least allergenic food first
	4. After 1 yr, add biweekly or monthly, if tolerated: milk, wheat, soy, corn, citrus, egg, peanut, fish; delay egg, peanut, and fish longer in food-atopic infants
B. Inhalant allergens	1. Home dust mite and mold avoidance; dust control in child's bedroom important (regular vacuuming, dusting with damp cloth, removal of feather pillows and comforters, encasing mattresses and pillows in plastic covers, maintaining humidity at 40%, removal of carpeting/using an ascaricide on carpets, frequent cleaning of filters on heating or air-conditioning systems)
	2. Pet avoidance (e.g., cat allergy)
	3. Air conditioners with closed circuit and air purifiers for outdoor allergens will help reduce exposure
III. Avoid nonspecific environmental irritants	1. No smoking prenatally or postnatally
	2. Reduce pollution
	3. Minimize infections (avoid early day care, breast-feed)

From Middleton E, Reed CE, Ellis EF, Adkinson NF, Yuninger JW, editors: *Allergy principles and practice,* ed 3, St Louis, 1988, Mosby.

- Clinical manifestations include gastrointestinal symptoms, urticaria, atopic dermatitis, and angioedema; less commonly other symptoms such as allergic rhinitis, asthma, anaphylaxis
- Symptoms decrease with time, especially to milk and egg; peanut and shellfish allergy is lifelong
- No scientific evidence of immunologic food sensitivity with the following: attention deficit hyperactivity disorder, chronic fatigue syndrome, most headaches
- Symptoms occurring soon after ingestion (within 2 hr) more likely a true allergy
- Physical examination usually noncontributory
- Investigation: double-blind food challenges, skin tests for IgE-mediated reactions

Table 2-1   Pharmacologic Management of Allergic Disorders

Condition	Medication	Comments
Allergic rhinitis	*Antihistamines* Chlorpheniramine Terfenadine Astemizole Loratidine	Newer antihistamines are non-sedating; may be given once daily
	Oral Sympathomimetics Pseudoephedrine	
	Topical Sympathomimetics Oxymetazoline Xylometazoline	Limit use to 3-5 days only; risk of rebound vasodilation
	Topical steroids Beclomethasone Flunisolide Budesonide	Effective in allergic and nonal-lergic rhinitis
	Cromolyn sodium	Prophylactic and therapeutic usage
	Anticholinergics Ipratropium bromide	Especially for rhinorrhea of vasomotor rhinitis
Atopic dermatitis, urticaria	Hydroxyzine Diphenhydramine Ketotifen fumarate Astemizole	
Anaphylaxis	Epinephrine Diphenhydramine Corticosteroids	
Allergic conjunctivitis	Cromolyn sodium Antihistamines	As for allergic rhinitis

Therapy

- Strict elimination of specific food is only proven therapy
- Generalized elimination diets should be restricted

Other Measures

- Food-allergic children should be given classroom designated as allergy free and should not be allowed to trade/share any foods; affected children should eat only home-prepared meals; hand washing before and after eating should be urged; no food should be allowed in crafts and activities; total avoidance in day care
- Medic Alert bracelet
- Epipen/Anakit and written instruction regarding their use for anaphylaxis (must be given at the start of a reaction, repeated in 20 min if anaphylaxis not controlled, and child should be transported to hospital)

ALLERGIC RHINITIS

- Perennial or seasonal sneezing, nasal congestion, nasal discharge, nasal itching, or decreased sense of smell
- Affects approximately 20% of population

- Consider in differential diagnosis of recurrent colds or pharyngitis
- Therapy: avoidance of allergens, pharmacotherapy, and in some cases immunotherapy (see earlier discussion)

ADVERSE DRUG REACTIONS
Nondrug Related

1. Psychogenic (vasovagal, anxiety, fatigue)
2. Coincidental symptoms (viral exanthem)

Drug Related

1. Predictable reactions: usually dose dependent
   a. Known side effects (at usual doses)
   b. Toxic effects (at higher doses)
   c. Drug interactions
2. Unpredictable reactions: usually dose independent, related to individual's immunologic response or genetic susceptibility
   a. Nonimmunologic
      1. Intolerance: lowered threshold to normal pharmacologic action of drugs in susceptible persons
      2. Idiosyncratic reactions: qualitative abnormal response in genetically susceptible persons
      3. Allergic reactions: mediated by definite or presumed allergic reactions
      4. Pseudoallergic reactions: minor allergic reactions but no immunologic mechanism exists (e.g., radiocontrast material, aspirin sensitivity)
   b. Immunologic
      1. Anaphylactic IgE dependent
         - Immediate allergic reactions occur within one hr and consist of pruritus, urticaria, flushing, and other manifestations of anaphylaxis
         - Accelerated reactions occur within 1 to 72 hr of drug administration and consist primarily of pruritus and urticaria, but laryngeal edema may be seen
         - Delayed reactions start three days after initiation of therapy and usually involve the skin with urticarial, exanthematous, or fixed drug eruptions, erythema multiforme or serum sicknesslike reactions; one or more organ systems may be involved

Investigations

- For predictable reactions, good history may be sufficient for diagnosis
- Extremely important to take detailed history as few diagnostic tests are available; history includes time course of reaction, all prescription and nonprescription drugs to which patient was exposed, exact nature of adverse drug reaction, and whether similar reaction had ever occurred in the past
- In vivo/in vitro tests: Skin testing most widely used of in vivo tests (contact sensitivity testing, patch testing, or epicutaneous and intradermal allergy skin testing); delayed hypersensitivity reactions may require in vitro lymphocyte assays

Treatment

- Discontinue suspected medication
- Provide symptomatic relief (epinephrine, antihistamines, corticosteroids)
- When testing is available, test for agents that may have precipitated past anaphylactic episodes
- Educate patient to avoid exposure
- Administer drugs by oral route if feasible
- Require clear indication for drug use
- Observe patient for at least 30 min after injections
- Desensitize patients in controlled clinical setting to any drug known to have caused anaphylaxis if urgently required to treat life-threatening disease and potential efficacy of such desensitization is documented; usually accomplished by administration of gradually increasing amounts of agent to be used, first intradermally, then subcutaneously, and eventually intravenously; for penicillin and aspirin, oral routes of desensitization have proven to be effective and safe; mechanism by which desensitization is effective is unknown; not always effective and it is necessary to repeat process should patient require same agent at later date

SPECIFIC DRUG ALLERGY
Local and General Anesthetics, Steroids, Muscle Relaxants, Select Vaccines, Latex, Insulin, Psyllium, Streptokinase, Chymopapain

- Allergy skin tests available in some form

Penicillin

- Overall incidence 2%-7%
- 80%-95% will skin test negative; no anaphylaxis, but of these, 1.5%-3% will have mild reaction (e.g., urticaria)
- 5%-20% will skin test positive, of which 50%-100% may react severely; desensitize only if penicillin mandatory

Cephalosporins

- 10%-15% cross-reactivity with penicillins; avoid in proven penicillin sensitivity

Sulfonamide

- Up to 5% of patients have side effects, commonly skin rashes
- Urticarial: 1-2 days after onset of treatment; resolves 1-2 days after treatment discontinued
- Idiosyncratic reaction: less common, occurs later (10-12 days) in therapy (e.g., erythema multiforme, Stevens-Johnson syndrome, toxic epidermal necrolysis)

IMMUNOLOGY (Box 2-2 and Table 2-2)

FREQUENCY AND CAUSES OF PRIMARY IMMUNODEFICIENCY DISORDERS (IDDs)

- Selective IgA deficiency occurs in as many as 1/500-1/1000 individuals; other primary immunodeficiencies much less common and occur

---

2

BOX 2-2   Immunodeficiency Disorders (IDDs)

B-Lymphocyte Defects (50%)
  X-linked agammaglobulinemia
  Common variable immunodeficiency
  Selective IgA deficiency
  Transient hypogammaglobulinemia of infancy
T-Lymphocyte Defects (10%)
  Purine nucleoside phosphorylase (PNP) deficiency
  Chronic mucocutaneous candidiasis
  DiGeorge's syndrome: congenital thymic aplasia
Combined B and T-Lymphocyte Defects (20%)
  Severe combined immunodeficiency (SCIDS)
  Wiskott–Aldrich syndrome
  Ataxic telangiectasia
  Adenosine deaminase (ADA) deficiency
Phagocytic Cell Defects (18%)
  Chronic granulomatous disease (CGD)
  Leukocyte adhesion defect (LAD)
  Neutropenia
  Chédiak–Higashi syndrome (defective degranulation)
Complement Deficiencies* (2%)
  C1   deficiency
  C4   deficiency
  C2   deficiency
  C3   deficiency

---

* Early components (C1-C4) associated with collagen vascular disease; late components (C5-C9) associated with recurrent *Neisseria* infection.

with frequency of between 1/10,000–1/100,000; many primary IDDs are genetically determined; some are inherited as autosomal recessive traits, some as X-linked recessive traits, whereas common variable immuno-deficiency and selective IgA deficiency usually occur sporadically

CLINICAL MANIFESTATIONS

- Recurrent pyogenic infections in different sites or more than one severe pyogenic infection (e.g., meningitis, pneumonia, osteomyelitis)
- Prolonged infection with poor response to antibiotics
- Infections with unusual organisms (e.g., *Pneumocystis carinii, Aspergillus*)
- Illness following live viral vaccination (e.g., MMR)
- Failure to thrive
- Hepatosplenomegaly
- Chronic diarrhea, often with malabsorption
- Skin rashes
- Persistent thrush
- Absence of lymph nodes and tonsils
- Frequent URI, sinusitis, otitis media
- Positive family history of early infant deaths, increased susceptibility to infection, autoimmune and rheumatic diseases

DIFFERENTIAL DIAGNOSIS

- Allergy (e.g., asthma, allergic rhinitis)
- Foreign body associated with infection (e.g., foreign body aspiration, central venous line infections)
- Cystic fibrosis (CF)
- Integument defects (e.g., immotile cilia syndrome)
- Infection with resistant organisms
- Continuous reinfection (e.g., contaminated water supply)

MANAGEMENT

- Family studies and genetic counseling; prenatal diagnosis available for some primary IDDs
- Antibiotics: prophylactic (e.g., trimethoprim-sulfamethoxazole) in neutropenia, selective IgA or IgG subclass deficiencies, or after splenectomy
- Avoid exposure to infectious agents
- Immunizations
  1. Avoid live vaccines in T-cell and B-cell disorders and in some secondary IDDs (e.g., generalized malignant disease and immunosuppressive agents, including high-dose corticosteroids); live vaccines can be given when there are neutrophil and complement disorders
  2. Active immunization with pneumococcal vaccine (e.g., before splenectomy or in sickle cell disease)
  3. Passive immunization with gamma globulin especially after exposure to varicella (B-cell, T-cell and some secondary IDDs)
  4. Caution with blood transfusion
- Selective IgA deficiency: washed packed cells to avoid anaphylaxis
- T-cell defects: irradiated blood products to prevent graft-versus-host reaction; use cytomegalovirus-negative blood because of risk of infection
- Specific therapy
  1. Gamma globulin replacement for B-cell defects
  2. Bone marrow transplantation for T-cell and combined defects

---

BOX 2-3   Screening Tests for Primary Immunodeficiency Diseases

---

Panel of Screening Tests
- WBC and differential
  Absolute neutrophil, lymphocyte, and platelet count
- Serum immunoglobulins: IgG, IgA, IgM
- Functional antibody levels
- Delayed-type hypersensitivity skin tests (intradermal skin test with heat-killed *Candida* 1 : 100 dilution)

Disorders Screened for by Panel
- X-linked agammaglobulinemia
- Common variable immunodeficiency
- Selective IgA deficiency
- Severe combined immunodeficiency
- Wiskott–Aldrich syndrome
- Neutropenia

BOX 2-4 Specific Tests for Primary Immunodeficiency Diseases

Tests of B-Lymphocyte Function
Initial
- Quantitative immunoglobulins: IgG, IgA, IgM
- Antibody response to immunizations
    Tetanus, diphtheria, polio, measles, mumps, rubella antibody titers
- Isohemagglutinins (if older than 1 yr) for IgM function
Advanced
- IgG subclasses quantitation
- B-lymphocyte quantitation
- Antibody responses to pneumococcal polysaccharides (IgG subclass 2) and tetanus toxoid protein (IgG subclasses 1 and 3)

Tests of T-Lymphocyte Function
Initial
- Total lymphocyte count
- Delayed hypersensitivity skin tests (intradermal skin test with heat-killed Candida 1:100 dilution)
Advanced
- T-lymphocyte quantitation
    Total T-cells
    T-helper cells (CD4+)
    T-suppressor/cytotoxic cells (CD8+)
- Proliferative responses to soluble antigens, allogeneic cells, and mitogens
- Thymic biopsy
- CXR for thymic shadow
- Include HIV testing in high-risk group

Tests of Phagocytic Cell Function
- Neutrophil count
- Neutrophil morphology
- NBT (nitroblue tetrazolium) to assess metabolic function
- Neutrophil chemotaxis (Rebuck window)

Test of Complement System Function
- CH_{50} (send sample on ice)
- C_3
- C_4

BOX 2-5 Secondary Immunodeficiency

Infections (e.g., HIV, EBV)
Protein-losing states (e.g., nephrotic syndrome, protein-losing enteropathy)
Malignant disease (e.g., leukemia, lymphoma)
Immunosuppressive agents (e.g., antineoplastic drugs, corticosteroids, radiation)
Hematologic disorders (e.g., sickle cell disease)
Metabolic disorders (e.g., diabetes mellitus, severe uremia, galactosemia)
Nutritional deficiencies (e.g., protein-calorie malnutrition)
Splenectomy
Prematurity

Table 2-2 Primary Immunodeficiency Disorders

Syndrome	Specific abnormality	Immune defect	Susceptibility
B-cell Antibody Defects*			
X-linked agammaglobulinemia	Loss of btk tyrosine kinase	No B cells	Encapsulated bacteria (e.g., *pneumococcus*, *H. influenza*, *meningococcus*)
X-linked hyper-IgM syndrome	Defective CD4 ligand	No isotype switching	Encapsulated bacteria
Wiskott–Aldrich syndrome	Unknown: X-linked (thrombocytopenia, otitis media, eczema)	Defective polysaccharide antibody responses	Encapsulated bacteria
Selective IgA deficiency	Unknown: MHC linked	No IgA synthesis	Respiratory infections
Selective Ig deficiencies	Ig constant region gene deletions	Loss of one or more Ig isotypes	Varied
Common variable ID (2nd–4th decade)	Unknown: MHC linked	Defective Ab production	Extracellular bacteria
T-Cell Cellular Defects†			
Severe combined ID	ADA deficiency	No T cells	Gram-neg bacteria, fungi, viruses, protozoa, mycobacteria
	PNP deficiency	No T cells	Gram-neg bacteria, fungi, viruses, protozoa, mycobacteria
	X-linked SCID (IL-2R gamma chain deficiency)	No T cells	Gram-neg bacteria, fungi, viruses, protozoa, mycobacteria
	Autosomal SCID (DNA repair defect)	No T or B cells	Gram-neg bacteria, fungi, viruses, protozoa, mycobacteria
DiGeorge syndrome	Thymic aplasia, hypocalcemia, cardiac defects, unusual facies	No T cells	Gram-neg bacteria, fungi, viruses, protozoa, mycobacteria

Ataxia-telangiectasia	Ataxia; telangiectasia of skin, ears, and conjunctiva; chromosomal breaks
Cartilage-hair hypoplasia	Short-limbed dwarfism; fine, light-colored hair
Phagocytic Disorders‡	
LFA-1 defect	*Staphylococcus*, gram-neg organisms, fungi
	Delayed umbilical cord detachment (> 3 wk) with neutrophilia
Chédiak-Higashi syndrome: partial oculocutaneous albinism	Recurrent staphylococcal infections
	Defective degranulation
Chronic granulomatous disease (CGD)	Recurrent staphylococcal infections
	X-linked, autosomal recessive
Complement Deficiencies§	
C1, C2, C4 deficiency	Lupuslike syndrome
	Encapsulated bacteria
C3 deficiency	Encapsulated bacteria
C5, C6, C7, C8, C9 deficiency	Neisserial infections
	Neisseria

*Common sites and types of infection: sinopulmonary; middle ear infections most common; also skin, gastrointestinal tract involvement; age at presentation 5-6 mo when maternal IgG decreases.
†Common sites and types of infection: candidiasis of skin, mucous membranes, and nails; pneumonitis, enteritis, FTT; age at presentation > 4 months.
‡Common sites and types of infection: skin, lymph nodes, liver (abscess), lung, bone, periodontal, perirectal.
§Common sites and types of infection: meningitis, disseminated gonococcal infection.

CHAPTER 3

CARDIOLOGY

Joel A. Kirsh

COMMON ABBREVIATIONS

AET	atrial ectopic tachycardia
AI/AR	aortic insufficiency/aortic regurgitation
AS	aortic stenosis
ASD	atrial septal defect
AVM	arteriovenous malformation
AVNRT	atrioventricular nodal reentry tachycardia
AVSD	atrioventricular septal defect
BAS	balloon atrial septostomy
BCPA/BCPC	bidirectional cavopulmonary anastomosis/bidirectional cavopulmonary connection
CHF	congestive heart failure
CoA	coarctation of aorta
DORV	double-outlet right ventricle
ECMO	extracorporeal membrane oxygenation
EFE	endocardial fibroelastosis
HLHS	hypoplastic left heart syndrome
HOCM	hypertrophic (obstructive) cardiomyopathy
IAA	interrupted aortic arch
IVC	inferior vena cava
JET	junctional ectopic tachycardia
LBBB	left bundle branch block
LVH	left ventricular hypertrophy
MR	mitral regurgitation
MS	mitral stenosis
MVP	mitral valve prolapse
NSR	normal sinus rhythm
PAB	pulmonary artery band
PAC	premature atrial complex
PAPVR	partial anomalous pulmonary venous return
PDA	patent ductus arteriosus
PFC	persistent fetal circulation
PGE$_1$	prostaglandin E$_1$
PPHN	persistent pulmonary hypertension of newborn
PS	pulmonary stenosis
PVC	premature ventricular complex
RBBB	right bundle branch block
RVH	right ventricular hypertrophy
SBE	subacute bacterial endocarditis
SVC	superior vena cava
SVT	supraventricular tachycardia
TAPVR	total anomalous pulmonary venous return

TCPC	total cavopulmonary connection
TGA	transposition of great arteries
TMI	transient myocardial ischemia
ToF	tetralogy of Fallot
VF	ventricular fibrillation
VSD	ventricular septal defect
VT	ventricular tachycardia
WPW	Wolff-Parkinson-White syndrome

3

HEART MURMURS

- Over 80% of children have an audible murmur at some point in life
- Most murmurs are functional (so-called "innocent murmurs"), without underlying structural abnormalities
- Functional murmurs appear (or become louder) in high-output states (e.g., fever)
- Common functional murmurs:
  1. Still's: vibratory systolic murmur along left sternal border (young children)
  2. Pulmonary flow: soft blowing murmur at upper left sternal border (older children)
  3. Pulmonary flow of newborn: as above, but radiates to back (resolves by 3-6 mo)
  4. Carotid bruit: 2/6 intensity systolic murmur over clavicles and carotids (any age)
  5. Venous hum: continuous murmur over clavicles; disappears when supine (young children)
- Indications that murmur is more likely to be pathologic:
  1. All diastolic murmurs are pathologic
  2. Systolic murmur 3/6 or louder, associated thrill, and/or radiates widely
  3. Abnormal splitting of S2 (see below)
  4. Additional heart sounds (clicks, gallops)
  5. Abnormal pulses (check femorals)
  6. Signs or symptoms of cardiovascular disease
  7. Abnormal heart size or pulmonary vascularity on CXR
  8. Abnormal ECG
- Distinguishing characteristics of heart murmurs:
  1. Intensity (and site of maximal intensity)
  2. Timing: Systolic (early, midsystolic, late, and pansystolic)
     Diastolic (early, middiastolic, and presystolic)
     Continuous
  3. Transmission or radiation (usually systolic murmurs only)
  4. Pitch and quality
  5. Associated click or gallop
  6. Splitting of second heart sound:
     Normally split: single in expiration, split in inspiration (physiologic variation)
     Widely split (varies): RBBB, PS, severe MR, PAPVR
     Widely split (fixed): ASD

Single and loud: pulmonary hypertension
Single: ToF, TGA, truncus arteriosus, tricuspid or pulmonary atresia, HLHS
Paradoxic (reversed) split: LBBB, AS, HOCM

ELECTROCARDIOGRAPHY

- Refer to Fig. 3-1 for proper placement of ECG leads and Table 3-1 for normal ECG values
- Analyze every ECG systematically: rate, rhythm, axis, intervals, chamber enlargement, ST, and/or T-wave changes
- Always consider patient's age and history of heart disease or cardiac surgery
- Rate: At usual speed (25 mm/sec), 1 large square = 0.2 sec, 1 small square = 0.04 sec

$$\frac{60 \text{ sec}}{RR \text{ interval}} = \text{rate (beats/min)}$$

- Rhythm and conduction:
  1. Regular versus irregular and pattern of irregularity
  2. Check for P before each QRS and QRS after each P
  3. Measure PR interval (see AV block in next section)
  4. In AV dissociation, measure both atrial and ventricular rates
- Axis determination (quick check using leads I and aV_F) (Fig. 3-2):

QRS in lead I	QRS in lead aV_F	QRS axis
positive	positive	0° to 90°
negative	positive	90° to 180°
positive	negative	−90° to 0°
negative	negative	−90° to −180°

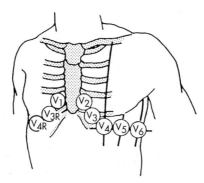

Fig. 3-1 Precordial lead placement. (From Park MK, Guntheroth WG: *How to read pediatric ECGs,* ed 3, Toronto, 1992, Mosby.)

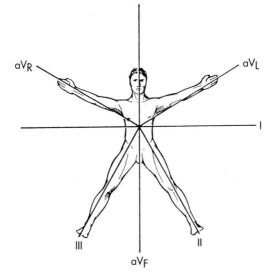

Fig. 3-2 The hexaxial reference system. (Modified from Park MK, Guntheroth WG: *How to read pediatric ECGs,* ed 3, Toronto, 1992, Mosby.)

- Intervals
  1. Measure PR interval, and compare with normal for age (see also AV block)
  2. Measure QRS duration, and look for interventricular conduction disturbance:
     - QRS > upper limit of normal for age:
       0.08 sec if < 2 yr, 0.09 sec if 2-8 yr, 0.10 sec if > 8 yr
     - ECG changes predominantly seen in leads facing affected chamber
     - RBBB: right axis, RSR' in V_{4R}/V_1/ V_2, wide slurred S in lead I/V_5/V_6
     - LBBB: left axis, wide slurred R in lead I/aV_L/V_5/V_6, wide S in V_1/V_2
  3. Measure QT interval and calculate QTc: should not exceed 0.44 sec, although a QTc of up to 0.49 sec may be normal in first 6 mo of life

$$\text{corrected QT (QTc)} = \frac{\text{measured QT}}{\sqrt{\text{preceding RR interval}}}$$

  - Causes of prolonged QT interval: drugs, electrolyte disturbances, myocarditis, CNS injury, and inherited syndromes
- Chamber enlargement
  - Right atrial: peaked P wave of 3 mm (or more) in any lead

Table 3-1 Normal Electrocardiographic Values for Age

Age	Rate 2%-98% (mean) bpm	QRS axis 2%-98% (mean) degrees	PR 98% sec	RV_1 98% mm	SV_1 98% mm	R/S V_1 2%-98% (mean) mm	R+S in V_4 98% mm	RV_6 98% mm	SV_6 98% mm	R/S V_6 2%-98% (mean) mm
< 1 day	93-154 (123)	+59 to −163 (137)	0.16	26	23	0.1-∞ (2.2)	52.5	11	9.5	0.1-∞ (2.0)
1-2 day	91-159 (123)	+64 to −161 (134)	0.14	27	21	0.1-∞ (2.0)	52	12	9.5	0.1-∞ (2.5)
3-6 day	91-166 (129)	+77 to −163 (132)	0.14	24	17	0.2-∞ (2.7)	49	12	10	0.1-∞ (2.2)
1-3 wk	107-182 (148)	+65 to +161 (110)	0.14	21	11	1.0-∞ (2.9)	49	16.5	10	0.1-∞ (3.3)
1-2 mo	121-179 (149)	+31 to +113 (74)	0.13	18	12	0.3-∞ (2.3)	53.5	21.5	6.5	0.2-∞ (4.8)

3-5 mo	106-186 (141)	+7 to +104 (60)	0.15	20	17	0.1-∞ (2.3)	61.5	22.5	10	0.2-∞ (6.2)
6-11 mo	109-188 (134)	+6 to +99 (56)	0.16	20	18	0.1-3.9 (1.6)	53	22.5	7	0.2-∞ (7.6)
1-2 yr	89-151 (119)	+7 to +101 (55)	0.15	17	21	0.05-4.3 (1.4)	49.5	22.5	6.5	0.3-∞ (9.3)
3-4 yr	73-137 (106)	+6 to +104 (55)	0.16	18	21	0.03-2.8 (0.9)	53.5	24.5	5	0.6-∞ (10.8)
5-7 yr	65-133 (100)	+11 to +143 (65)	0.16	14	24	0.02-2.0 (0.7)	54	26.5	4	0.9-∞ (11.5)
8-11 yr	62-130 (91)	+9 to +114 (61)	0.17	12	25	0-1.8 (0.5)	53	25.5	4	1.5-∞ (14.3)
12-15 yr	60-119 (85)	+11 to +130 (59)	0.18	10	21	0-1.7 (0.5)	50	23	4	1.4-∞ (14.7)

Modified from Davignon A, et al: Normal ECG standards for infants and children, *Pediatr Cardiol* 1:123-131, 1979.

Table 3-2 Electrocardiographic Criteria for Ventricular Hypertrophy

	Right ventricular hypertrophy	Left ventricular hypertrophy	Biventricular hypertrophy
Definite:	R in V_1 > 98%ile *or* qR complex in V_1	R in V_6 > 98%ile by 5mm *or* S in V_1 > 98%ile by 5mm	Definite RVH *and* LVH *or* R+S in V_4 > 98%ile
Possible:	R/S ratio in V_1 > 98%ile *or* R/S ratio in V_6 < 2%ile *or* S in V_6 > 98%ile *or* Upright T in V_1 between 1 wk and 8 yr old	R/S ratio in V_1 < 2%ile *or* R in V_6 > 98%ile *or* S in V_1 > 98%ile *or* Inverted T in V_{4-6}	LVH *and* possible* RVH *or* RVH *and* possible* LVH
Supportive:	Right axis deviation	Left axis deviation	

*Using 50%ile voltages.

Modified from Garson A: *The electrocardiogram in infants and children,* Philadelphia, 1983, Lea & Febiger.

- Left atrial: wide ($\geq$ 0.09 sec) bifid P wave in any lead; late negative (1.5 mm) in V_1
- See Table 3-2 for ventricular hypertrophy criteria
- Q wave may normally appear in leads II, III, aV_F, V_5, and V_6
- From birth to 3 days, T wave should be positive in V_1; by 4 days, T wave should be negative in V_1; from this time until age 5-8 yr, positive T wave in V_1 implies RVH
- ST/T-wave changes: seen in hypertrophy/strain, myocarditis, pericarditis
- Compare with previous ECGs, particularly if history of cardiac disease/surgery

IDENTIFICATION OF DYSRHYTHMIAS (Table 3-3)

Note: Always consider morphology of QRS complexes in light of previous cardiac disease or surgery; refer to previous electrocardiograms if available.

Normal Sinus Rhythm (NSR)

- Normal P wave, normal PR interval before each QRS

Premature Atrial Complex (PAC)

- Premature beat with abnormal P wave morphology/axis (ectopic focus)
- Usually normal QRS, but may have wide QRS caused by aberrant conduction
- Causes: normal variation, electrolyte disturbance, hyperthyroidism, cardiac surgery, digoxin toxicity

BOX 3-1 Toxic Effects of Drugs and Electrolytes on the ECG

Drugs

Digoxin	Atrial tachycardias
	AV block
	Junctional tachycardia
	Ventricular dysrhythmias (rare in children)
Type I antiarrhythmics	Sinus bradycardia/arrest/exit block
e.g., quinidine	AV block
procainamide	Long QT
lidocaine	Polymorphic VT
Tricyclic antidepressants	AV block
	Intraventricular conduction delay
	Ventricular tachycardia

Electrolytes

Hyperkalemia	AV block
	Tall, narrow, peaked T waves
	Wide QRS (sine-wave appearance)
	Ventricular fibrillation
Hypokalemia	AV block
	Flat T waves, prominent U wave
	Appearance of long QT (actually QTU)
	Atrial and/or ventricular ectopy
Hypercalcemia	Short QT
Hypocalcemia	Long QT
Hypomagnesemia	Long QT
	Ventricular dysrhythmias (torsades)

Atrial Ectopic Tachycardia (AET)

- Rapid bursts of sustained atrial tachycardia
- P waves usually abnormal and may be multifocal, QRS normal
- May demonstrate "warm-up" and "cool-down" characteristics
- May have periods of AV block

Supraventricular Tachycardia (SVT)

- Rapid rate with normal QRS complex (unless previous cardiac surgery)
- P waves may or may not be visible
- *Wide-complex tachycardia is ventricular tachycardia until proven otherwise*

Atrial Flutter

- Normal QRS with "flutter waves"
- Rapid regular atrial rate, usually with AV block

Atrial Fibrillation

- Normal QRS with irregularly irregular RR interval
- P waves not visible, may see chaotic atrial activity on ECG baseline

Table 3-3   Differentiation of Tachycardia in Children

	Sinus	SVT (reentry)	Atrial flutter	AET	JET	VT
Clinical	Fever Sepsis Shock CHF Catecholamines	Normal heart 50% WPW 25% AVNRT Ebstein's anomaly	90% have dilated atria Mustard/Senning/Fontan Myocarditis Digoxin toxicity	Usually normal heart	Postcardiac surgery	>70% abnormal heart Postcardiac surgery Myocarditis Long QT syndromes Tricyclics Amphetamines Catecholamines Digoxin toxicity (rarely)
Rate	Usually < 200/min	Infants: up to 300/min Children: < 240/min	Atrial rate 250–400/min 2:1, 3:1, or 4:1 AV block	> 200/min	Atrial rate < ventricular Up to 200–300/min	Usually < 250/min
P wave	Normal	May be buried in QRS 60% retrograde P wave	Regular flutter waves	Abnormal but constant	Retrograde P waves	AV dissociation Sometimes retrograde P
QRS	Normal	Normal or aberrant	Normal	Normal	Normal	Wide
Treatment	Treat underlying cause	See text	Digoxin Antiarrhythmics DC cardioversion	33% resolve Antiarrhythmics	Cooling Normalize pH, volume Antiarrhythmics	See text

3

Wolff-Parkinson-White Syndrome

- During sinus rhythm: short PR interval with initial slurring of QRS up-stroke (delta wave) resulting from preexcitation along accessory pathway; QRS slightly prolonged
- During dysrhythmia: usually narrow complex tachycardia with retrograde P wave

First-Degree AV Block

- PR interval > normal for age (see Table 3-1)
- Every P wave followed by QRS (e g., no blocked P waves)
- Causes: normal variation, rheumatic fever, cardiomyopathies, ASD, Ebstein's, AVSD, postcardiac surgery, digoxin toxicity

Second-Degree AV Block

- Mobitz I (Wenckebach): progressive lengthening of PR interval until P wave blocked
- Mobitz II: blocked beats without lengthening of PR interval
- Causes: myocarditis, cardiomyopathy, postcardiac surgery, congenital heart disease, digoxin toxicity

Third-Degree Heart Block (AV Dissociation)

- No consistent relationship between atrial and ventricular activity
- Atrial rate faster; presence of slower junctional or ventricular escape rhythm
- Causes: Congenital: idiopathic, maternal SLE, congenitally corrected TGA
  Acquired: cardiac surgery, myocarditis, postinfarction

Premature Ventricular Complex (PVC)

- Usually wide QRS complex (always different from QRS in NSR)
- T wave deflection opposite to QRS

Ventricular Tachycardia (VT)

- Greater than 3 PVCs at a rate > 120 beats/min
- Usually wide QRS complex
- Do not assume SVT with aberrancy; 95% of wide-complex tachycardias are VT

TREATMENT OF COMMON ACUTE DYSRHYTHMIAS (Table 3-3)

- See previous section for diagnostic features of dysrhythmias
- Assess ABCs (see p. 2) and intervene if unstable
- In stable patient, serial 12-lead ECGs (both during dysrhythmia and then following conversion) are crucial for diagnosis
- Continuous cardiac monitoring with printed rhythm strip during all diagnostic and therapeutic maneuvers

ATRIOVENTRICULAR BLOCK

- ABCs (see p. 2)
- Management influenced by ventricular rate and evidence of symptoms
- Therapy aimed at increasing rate, improving AV conduction, and supporting BP
- Atropine 0.02 mg/kg/dose, maximum two doses
- Isoproterenol infusion 0.05-1 µg/kg/min
- May require inotropes for BP support (see p. 8)
- Consult cardiology for transthoracic or transvenous pacing

SUPRAVENTRICULAR TACHYCARDIA (REENTRANT MECHANISMS)

- Note: *wide complex tachycardia should be treated as VT* (see the following)
- ABCs (see p. 2)
- For unstable patients: synchronized cardioversion 0.25-1 J/kg
- Vagal maneuvers: Valsalva, unilateral carotid sinus massage, gagging
- Ocular pressure should *not* be used in children
- Ice bag to face should only be used in infants
- Adenosine 0.05 mg/kg IV rapid bolus, may increase dose by 0.05 mg/kg every two min to maximum of 0.25 mg/kg (side effects: flushing, severe chest pain)
- Adenosine induces brief (< 10 sec) AV block and terminates reentrant dysrhythmias; in nonreentrant dysrhythmias, adenosine assists in diagnosis by unmasking underlying atrial rhythm
- Neostigmine 0.01-0.04 mg/kg IV; use atropine (0.01 mg/kg) if cholinergic side effects
- Phenylephrine 0.01-0.10 mg/kg IV slowly (rarely used)
- Verapamil 0.1-0.3 mg/kg IV (have $CaCl_2$ on hand in case of toxicity)
- Verapamil is contraindicated in infants
- Overdrive pacing (esophageal or wire), if available
- Elective synchronized cardioversion
- Recurrent/incessant SVT: procainamide 10-15 mg/kg IV over 1 hour, followed by infusion

VENTRICULAR TACHYCARDIA

- Note: Some patients may require a combination of electrical and drug therapy
- ABCs (see p. 2)
- For unstable patients: synchronized cardioversion 0.5-2.0 J/kg
- Lidocaine 1 mg/kg then 0.5 mg/kg IV (maximum 2.0 mg/kg), followed by infusion (see the inside front cover)
- Procainamide 10-15 mg/kg IV over one hr, followed by infusion
- Elective synchronized cardioversion
- Treat underlying cause (e.g., electrolyte disturbances)

CONGENITAL HEART DISEASE (Tables 3-4 to 3-6)

CLINICAL FEATURES, INVESTIGATIONS, AND MANAGEMENT

- Approach to diagnosis based on presentation, physical findings, CXR, and ECG
- Physical findings can range from none to nonspecific to pathognomonic
- CXR: Look at pulmonary vascularity and cardiomegaly
- ECG: Look for abnormal QRS axis or evidence of ventricular enlargement
- Three major modes of presentation of heart disease in neonatal period:
  1. Heart murmur (see Table 3-7)
  2. Congestive heart failure (Table 3-8)
  3. Cyanosis (central) (Table 3-9)

Table 3-4 Chromosomal Abnormalities Associated with Congenital Heart Disease

Chromosomal abnormality	% Risk of heart disease	Associated lesion(s)
Trisomy 13	90	VSD, ASD, PDA
Trisomy 18	95	VSD, DORV, PDA
Trisomy 21	40	AVSD, VSD, ASD, ToF
Tetrasomy 22 (cat-eye)	40	TAPVR, ToF, VSD
Deletion 4p	50	ASD, VSD, PDA
Deletion 5p (cri-du-chat)	30	VSD, ASD, PDA
Deletion 22q (various)	85	Conotruncal anomalies
45 XO (Turner)	15	CoA
47 XXY (Klinefelter)	50	VSD, PDA, MVP, ToF
Fragile X	50-75	MVP (in older patients)

Modified from Freedom RM, Benson LN, Smallhorn JF, eds: *Neonatal heart disease*, New York, 1992, Springer-Verlag.

Table 3-5 Maternal Factors Associated with Congenital Heart Disease

	% Risk of heart disease	Associated lesion(s)
Maternal Diseases		
Rubella infection	35	PDA, peripheral PS
Diabetes (poor control)		HOCM, TGA, CoA, VSD
Phenylketonuria	25-50	ToF
Lupus erythematosus	20-40	Complete heart block
Maternal Drugs		
Alcohol	25-30	ASD, VSD
Phenytoin	2-3	VSD, ASD, PS, AS, CoA
Valproate		CoA, HLHS, AS, VSD
Trimethadione	15-30	TGA, ToF, HLHS
Retinoic acid (vitamin A)	3.6	Conotruncal anomalies

Modified from Freedom RM, Benson LN, Smallhorn JF, eds: *Neonatal heart disease*, New York, 1992, Springer-Verlag.

Table 3-6   Syndromes Associated with Congenital Heart Disease

Syndrome	% Risk of heart disease	Associated lesion(s)
Alagille		Peripheral PS
Apert's	10	VSD, ToF
Asplenia/polysplenia	almost 100	AVSD, TGA, TAPVR
CHARGE	60-70	ToF, AVSD, DORV, VSD
Crouzon's		PDA, CoA
Cutis laxa		PS, pulmonary hypertension
DiGeorge's (deletion 22q)	90	Conotruncal anomalies
Ehlers-Danlos (some types)	50	MVP, dilated aortic root
Ellis-van Creveld	50-60	Common atrium, ASD
Goldenhar's	15	ToF, VSD
Holt-Oram	100	ASD, VSD, AV block
Hurler/Hunter/other MPS		Valvular insufficiency
Kartagener's	100	Dextrocardia or normal
LEOPARD	50	PS
Marfan's	60-80	MVP, AI, dilated aortic root
Noonan's	50	PS
Osteogenesis imperfecta	5-10	Aortic incompetence
Rubenstein-Taybi		VSD
Smith-Lemli-Opitz		VSD, PDA
TAR	20	ToF, ASD
Tuberous sclerosis	30	Cardiac rhabdomyoma
VATER/VACTERL		VSD, ToF, ASD, PDA
Williams (deletion 7q)	90-100	AS, PS, renal stenosis

Modified from Freedom RM, Benson LN, Smallhorn JF, eds: *Neonatal heart disease*, New York, 1992, Springer-Verlag.

Table 3-7   Congenital Heart Lesions Presenting as a Heart Murmur

| ECG | Chest x-ray | |
	Increased pulmonary vascularity	Normal pulmonary vascularity
Normal	PDA	Small VSD
or	VSD	Small PDA
mild RVH	ASD	PS
or	AVSD	AS
mild LVH		Acyanotic ToF
		AVM
		AV valve regurgitation
		Peripheral pulmonary branch stenosis
		Functional murmur

Modified from Freedom RM, Benson LN, Smallhorn JF, eds: *Neonatal heart disease*, New York, 1992 Springer-Verlag.

- Noncardiac causes of neonatal cyanosis:
  - Sepsis, cold, hypoglycemia: usually peripheral, poor perfusion
  - Polycythemia, methemoglobinemia: normal arterial pO_2
  - Lung disease/hypoventilation: abnormal CXR, elevated pCO_2
- Hyperoxic test to exclude cyanotic congenital heart disease:
  1. Infant in 100% FiO_2, breathing or ventilated to normal pCO_2

Table 3-8 Congenital Heart Lesions Presenting as Congestive Heart Failure

| | Chest x-ray | | | |
ECG	Increased pulmonary vascularity	Pulmonary venous congestion*	Normal pulmonary vascularity	Decreased pulmonary vascularity
RVH	HLHS	Obstructed TAPVR	CoA (early)	PS
	CoA	Mitral stenosis	AVM	Ebstein's anomaly
	IAA	Cor triatriatum		
	AS			
	Truncus arteriosus			
	TAPVR			
	AVSD			
	DORV			
	ASD			
	AVM			
LVH	PDA	AS	AS (early)	Pulmonary atresia
	Truncus arteriosus			
	AS			
	Single ventricle			
CVH	VSD		AS	
	PDA			
	AVSD			
	Truncus arteriosus			
	DORV			
	AVM			
	Single ventricle			

*Pulmonary venous congestion may be seen in *any* lesion with severe congestive heart failure.
Modified from Freedom RM, Benson LN, Smallhorn JF, eds: *Neonatal heart disease,* New York, 1992, Springer-Verlag.

Table 3-9 Congenital Heart Lesions Presenting as Cyanosis

| | Chest x-ray | |
ECG	Decreased pulmonary vascularity	Normal or increased pulmonary vascularity
RVH	ToF	TGA
	TGA with VSD and PS	TAPVR
	Severe PS with intact septum	HLHS
	DORV with PS	DORV without PS
	Pulmonary atresia	Single ventricle
	Ebstein's anomaly	
	Tricuspid regurgitation	
	Single ventricle with PS or atresia	
LVH	Pulmonary atresia	Tricuspid atresia
	Tricuspid atresia	Double-inlet LV
	Hypoplastic right ventricle	
	Single ventricle with PS or atresia	
CVH	Single ventricle with PS or atresia	Truncus arteriosus
	Truncus with pulmonary hypoplasia	DORV without PS
		Single ventricle (LV type)
		TGA (rarely)

Modified from Freedom RM, Benson LN, Smallhorn JF, eds: *Neonatal heart disease,* New York, 1992, Springer-Verlag.

2. Measurement of preductal and postductal pO_2 by ABG or transcutaneous probe
3. $pO_2 \geq 250$ mm Hg excludes cyanotic congenital heart disease
4. $pO_2 \geq 160$ mm Hg strongly against cyanotic congenital heart disease
5. Preductal and postductal pO_2 useful in assessing right-to-left ductal shunting

- Prostaglandin E_1 to maintain patency of ductus arteriosus:
  - Indicated in any duct-dependent lesion, both cyanotic and noncyanotic (e.g., TGA, tricuspid/pulmonary atresia, Ebstein's anomaly, ToF, CoA, HLHS)
  - Starting dose 0.1 μg/kg/min (500 μg PGE_1 in 80 ml at 1 ml/kg/hr), then wean as able to minimize side effects: apnea (12%), fever (10%), hypotension (4%), seizures (4%)
  - Consider elective intubation and ventilation before transporting infants on PGE_1

CYANOTIC SPELLS IN TETRALOGY OF FALLOT

CLINICAL FEATURES

- Paroxysmal dyspnea with cyanosis; rapid, deep (Kussmaul's) breathing
- Diminished or absent pulmonary ejection murmur due to increased right-to-left shunting
- Hypotonia, although may initially be agitated
- Progression (rarely) to loss of consciousness, seizures, death

INVESTIGATIONS

- Not usually done during acute spell; increased patient agitation may aggravate episode
- ABG: acidosis with hypoxia
- CXR: decreased pulmonary blood flow
- ECG: increased P wave

TREATMENT

- Quiet, calm environment; spell may resolve by settling in parent's arms
- Knee-chest position (increases afterload and thus decreases right-to-left shunt)
- Oxygen (blown to face or by mask/hood)
- Morphine 0.1 mg/kg IV or SC (may depress respiration)
- Propranolol 0.05-0.1 mg/kg slow IV push (3 to 5 min)
- $NaHCO_3$ 1-2 mEq/kg IV, for correction of metabolic acidosis
- Phenylephrine 0.01-0.10 mg/kg/dose IV (increases afterload, decreases shunt)
- May need general anesthesia if severe and/or prolonged spell
- Interim prophylactic treatment with propranolol while awaiting surgery

CONGESTIVE HEART FAILURE

CLINICAL FEATURES AND INVESTIGATIONS

- Four key features: tachycardia, tachypnea, cardiomegaly, and hepatomegaly

- Other features: diaphoresis, poor feeding, failure to thrive, gallop rhythm, weak pulses
- Pulmonary venous congestion is marked by exertional dyspnea (e.g., during feeding), orthopnea, wheezing, and crackles; history of "asthma" or recurrent chest infections
- CXR typically shows cardiomegaly $\pm$ venous congestion
- ECG may be normal, but does *not* rule out CHF
- May see electrical alternans in severe CHF

MANAGEMENT
General Measures

- Sitting up to relieve respiratory distress, NPO if severe
- Humidified oxygen if hypoxic or distressed and monitor O_2 saturation
- Treat associated causes/complications (dysrhythmias)
- Address confounding factors (anemia, fever, infection)

Diuretics

- Acute: furosemide 1 mg/kg/dose PO or IV
- Chronic: hydrochlorothiazide-spironolactone $\pm$ furosemide
- Monitor electrolytes and renal function

Vasodilators

- ACE inhibitors
- Watch for hypotension as a "first-dose" effect (give small test dose under supervision)

Digoxin

1. Digoxin not universally indicated in CHF and use should be individualized, in consultation with cardiologist; initial IV administration in severe CHF; less distressed infants may be treated orally; all patients should be switched to oral therapy as soon as feasible; check digoxin dosing carefully in age-appropriate formulary. Note: IV dosage is only 70%-80% of amount used orally
2. In cardiomyopathies, renal failure, or in presence of drugs that increase digoxin levels (e.g., quinidine, amiodarone, propafenone, erythromycin):
   - Digitalization dose reduced to 50%, maintenance dose reduced to 33%-50%
   - Monitor with serial ECGs plus serum digoxin levels
3. Digoxin is *contraindicated* in HOCM, cardiac tamponade, and AV block
4. Digoxin has low therapeutic safety index; noncardiac symptoms of toxicity include anorexia, nausea, vomiting or diarrhea, restlessness, fatigue, and visual disturbance (older children)
5. ECG changes in digoxin toxicity include AV block, sinus bradycardia or sinoatrial block, and supraventricular dysrhythmias (particularly in presence of AV block); ventricular dysrhythmias rare in children; assume that any rhythm or conduction disturbance occurring in patient on digoxin is most likely due to digoxin
6. Treatment of toxicity: hold digoxin, ECG monitor, normalize serum K, consider Fab fragments (Digibind) in presence of severe rhythm disturbance

Intensive Care Management

- Consider in any case of severe/refractory CHF
- Mechanical ventilation
- Inotropic support (dopamine, dobutamine, amrinone)
- Afterload reduction (nitroprusside, nitroglycerine)

MYOCARDIAL FAILURE IN STRUCTURALLY NORMAL HEART

CLINICAL FEATURES AND INVESTIGATIONS

- Generally presents as signs of CHF, prominent cardiomegaly, and abnormal ECG
- Specific findings dependent on underlying etiology (see below)

DIFFERENTIAL DIAGNOSIS

- Primary cardiomyopathies:
  - Endocardial fibroelastosis
  - Idiopathic dilated cardiomyopathy
  - Hypertrophic cardiomyopathy (with or without obstruction)
- Secondary cardiomyopathies:
  - Metabolic disorders: Pompe's disease, carnitine and mitochondrial disorders
  - Toxins: chemotherapy (Adriamycin), radiotherapy
  - Malnutrition: protein-calorie malnutrition, anorexia nervosa
  - Neurologic disorders: muscular dystrophy, Friedreich's ataxia, myotonic dystrophy
  - Hematologic disorders: sickle cell anemia, thalassemia major, hemochromatosis
  - Endocrine disorders: hypothyroidism, pheochromocytoma
- Myocarditis (see next section)
- Coronary artery disease:
  - Anomalous origin of left coronary artery from pulmonary artery
  - Kawasaki syndrome
  - Other vasculitis syndromes
- Miscellaneous conditions:
  - Transient myocardial ischemia (asphyxiated neonate)
  - Chronic dysrhythmias
  - Cardiac tumors (extremely rare)

ACUTE MYOCARDITIS

ETIOLOGY

- Usually viral infection: enterovirus most common (up to 50% coxsackie B), adenovirus, CMV, influenza (A and B), measles, rubella, mumps, hepatitis (A and B), varicella zoster
- Other causes: Kawasaki syndrome, rheumatic fever, collagen vascular diseases, toxins

CLINICAL FEATURES AND INVESTIGATIONS

- Symptoms: fatigue, malaise, exercise intolerance, exertional dyspnea, palpitations, chest/abdominal pain, anorexia, vomiting
- Signs of CHF: tachycardia, tachypnea, gallop rhythm, hepatomegaly
- ECG: low-voltage QRS, ST changes, T wave inversion, prolonged QT, dysrhythmias
- CXR: cardiomegaly, pulmonary venous congestion
- Echocardiography: ventricular dysfunction and dilatation, AV valve regurgitation

MANAGEMENT

- Close observation and continuous monitoring, as may deteriorate suddenly
- Treatment of dysrhythmias
- Treatment of CHF (may require intensive care, inotropes, ECMO)
- Transfer to pediatric center for cardiologic consultation
- Role of endomyocardial biopsy and immunotherapy remains controversial

PERICARDITIS AND PERICARDIAL EFFUSION

ETIOLOGY

- Most commonly viral (see myocarditis above)
- Bacterial, fungal, or mycobacterial infection
- Collagen vascular disease, particularly SLE and JRA
- Oncologic disease and/or complications of chemotherapy or radiation
- Postpericardiotomy syndrome following cardiac surgery
- Uremia (chronic renal failure)

CLINICAL FEATURES AND INVESTIGATIONS

- Fever
- Precordial pain (may vary with posture)
- Pericardial friction rub (may vanish with effusion)
- Distant heart sounds (with effusion)
- Signs of cardiac tamponade (large effusion): tachycardia, pulsus paradoxus, hepatomegaly, venous distension
- ECG: normal or low-voltage QRS, ST elevation, or T wave changes if myocarditis present
- CXR: cardiomegaly and effusion, increased pulmonary venous markings
- Echocardiography: diagnostic for pericardial effusion or developing constriction
- Cardiac tamponade is clinical diagnosis and requires urgent intervention

MANAGEMENT

- Resuscitation: ABCs (see p. 2); optimize preload by giving intravascular volume; *do not diurese*
- Pericardiocentesis mandatory for cardiac tamponade; send sample for culture

- Consider surgical pericardiectomy or window in bacterial infection or loculation
- Treat underlying medical condition and/or infectious etiologies
- ASA and steroids may have role in noninfectious pericarditis
- Digoxin is *contraindicated* as it blocks compensatory tachycardia
- Follow for late development of constrictive pericarditis

INFECTIVE ENDOCARDITIS

ETIOLOGY

- *Streptococci* (usually *viridans* group), followed by *staphylococci,* then *enterococci* account for up to 80% of childhood infective endocarditis
- *Staphylococci* (both *aureus* and *epidermidis*) most common postcardiac surgery
- Gram-negative and fungal infections uncommon unless associated with immunosuppression or catheter-related sepsis
- Up to 10% of infectious endocarditis is culture negative

CLINICAL FEATURES

- Fever (mean of 90% among published studies)
- Underlying heart defect (90%)
- Splenomegaly (55%)
- Cutaneous manifestations (secondary to microemboli); most commonly petechiae (33%); Osler's nodes, Janeway's lesions, and classic splinter hemorrhages are rare (5%) in children
- Embolic phenomena (30%):
  - Pulmonary emboli
  - CNS emboli and/or abcesses
  - Hematuria, glomerulonephritis, renal failure
- Heart failure (30%)
- New or changing murmur (25%)

INVESTIGATIONS

- Blood cultures (three separate cultures before therapy yields 95% sensitivity)
- CBC, ESR, urea, creatinine
- Urinalysis (hematuria in 30%)
- Transthoracic echocardiography only detects vegetations $\geq$ 2 mm and is not effective screening test; negative echocardiogram does not rule out endocarditis
- If endocarditis truly suspected clinically, transesophageal study must be considered
- Culture-negative endocarditis (10% of cases) usually caused by previous antibiotics, unusual organisms, anaerobes, or right-sided endocarditis

MANAGEMENT

- Empiric antibiotics depending on clinical scenario:
  1. Postoperative cardiac surgery (up to 60 days): vancomycin + gentamicin

2. Community-acquired or > 60 days postoperative: cloxacillin + gentamicin
- Antibiotic regimen refined by identification, sensitivities, and clinical response
- Use of vancomycin should be limited to organisms resistant to other antibiotics
- Early surgical treatment indicated for persistently positive cultures, serious septic embolic events while on therapy, myocardial abscess, progressive intractable cardiac failure unresponsive to medical management, or fungal endocarditis (rare)

PREVENTION

- See Formulary section for endocarditis prophylaxis regimens (p. 632)

RHEUMATIC FEVER (Table 3-10)

MANAGEMENT

- Antibiotic therapy:

Initial treatment course:	Benzathine penicillin G 0.6-1.2 million U IM
	or penicillin VK 125-250 mg PO tid-qid × 10 days
	or erythromycin 20-40 mg/kg/day (÷ bid or tid) × 10 days
Continued prophylaxis:	Benzathine penicillin G 0.6-1.2 million U IM monthly
	or penicillin VK 125-250 mg PO bid
	or erythromycin 250 mg bid-tid
	or sulfadiazine 0.5-1 g PO daily

(Low dose for patients < 30 kg, high dose for patients > 30 kg)

Table 3-10   Revised Jones Criteria for Diagnosis of Rheumatic Fever*

Major manifestations	Minor manifestations
Carditis	*Clinical*
Polyarthritis	Fever
Chorea	Arthralgia
Erythema marginatum	Previous rheumatic fever
Subcutaneous nodules	*Laboratory*
	Increased ESR/CRP/WBC
	Anemia
	Prolonged PR or QT intervals

*Two major criteria or one major and two minor criteria, in the presence of supportive evidence of preceding streptococcal infection (positive throat culture, recent scarlet fever, or increased antistreptococcal antibodies) indicate high probability of rheumatic fever; *failure to meet Jones criteria does not exclude rheumatic fever.*

Modified from Behrman RE, Vaughan VC, eds: *Nelson textbook of pediatrics,* ed 13, Toronto, 1987, W.B. Saunders.

- Bed rest then gradual ambulation as inflammation subsides (follow ESR)
- ASA 100 mg/kg/day × 2 wk, then 40 mg/kg/day and wean as inflammation subsides
- Prednisone 1-2 mg/kg/day only for moderate to severe carditis (e.g., with cardiomegaly)

CARDIAC SURGICAL PROCEDURES

- Bidirectional cavopulmonary anastomosis: SVC to pulmonary artery connection
- Blalock-Hanlon: surgical atrial septectomy
- Blalock-Taussig shunt: subclavian artery to pulmonary artery
- Fontan: connection of right atrium to pulmonary artery
- Glenn shunt: SVC to right pulmonary artery (with disconnection from MPA)
- Jatene: arterial switch for correction of TGA
- Mustard: intraatrial baffle or patch (pericardium) for palliation of simple TGA
- Norwood: First of three-stage palliation for HLHS and other forms of complex CHD with systemic outflow obstruction
- Potts shunt: descending aorta to left pulmonary artery
- Rashkind: transcatheter balloon atrial septostomy
- Rastelli operation (for TGA with VSD and PS):
  1. Placement of valved conduit-graft between right ventricle and pulmonary artery
  2. Left ventricular blood directed to aorta via VSD and intraventricular tunnel
- Ross: Aortic valve replacement with pulmonary autograft, then pulmonary homograft
- Senning: modified Mustard-type repair of simple TGA by intraatrial baffle
- Total cavopulmonary connection (TCPC): redirection of SVC and IVC flow to pulmonary arteries
- Waterston shunt: ascending aorta to right pulmonary artery

CHAPTER 4

DENTISTRY

SEAN GODFREY

- Parent education and prevention most important: discourage bedtime bottle to prevent "nursing caries" or "baby bottle" syndrome
- Encourage parents to clean child's teeth (initially with gauze swab and later with soft toothbrush) as soon as they appear
- First teeth eruption: central mandibular incisors at approximately 6 mo; varies with sex and race
- Recommend regular dental visits, beginning not later than 24 mo
- See Table 4-1 for chronology of human dentition

DENTAL TRAUMA

- Displacement of deciduous teeth interferes with development and eruption of adjacent permanent teeth
- Never replant primary teeth
- Interference with blood supply secondary to trauma may result in pulpal necrosis (indicated by blue-black discoloration of crown) and infection
- Space preservation unnecessary in anterior segment but imperative in posterior segments of deciduous dental arch until age 9-10 years
- All cases require referral to dentist

Management

- Clean site of blood, debris for maximum visualization
- Determine time of accident; age of patient; whether tooth is deciduous or permanent; whether tooth is loose, out, intruded, or fractured; and whether dental pulp (pinkish coloration or direct visualization of blood) visible
- Therapy depends on type of injury and tooth affected
  1. Loosened or displaced anterior teeth
     - Deciduous: removal of injured tooth
     - Permanent
       a. Consult dentist immediately (affected tooth may be immobilized with wire splint)
       b. Every 6 wk observe the tooth for signs of pulpal necrosis due to interference with neurovascular supply (less likely in younger children and where dental trauma has been treated promptly)
  2. Fractured permanent anterior teeth
     - Early referral (especially if temperature sensitive)
     - Even small enamel fractures in teeth may have associated root fractures, which may require rigid stabilization for minimum of 6 wk
     - Pulp (pink area) exposure requires urgent treatment

Table 4-1 Chronology of Human Dentition

	Calcification		Eruption		Shedding	
	Begins at	Complete at	Maxillary	Mandibular	Maxillary	Mandibular
Primary or Deciduous Teeth						
Central incisors	5th fetal mo	18-24 mo	6-8 mo	5-7 mo	7-8 yr	6-7 yr
Lateral incisors	5th fetal mo	18-24 mo	8-11 mo	7-10 mo	8-9 yr	7-8 yr
Cuspids (canines)	6th fetal mo	30-36 mo	16-20 mo	16-20 mo	11-12 yr	9-11 yr
First molars	5th fetal mo	24-30 mo	10-16 mo	10-16 mo	10-11 yr	10-12 yr
Second molars	6th fetal mo	36 mo	20-30 mo	20-30 mo	10-12 yr	11-13 yr
Secondary or Permanent Teeth						
Central incisors	3-4 mo	9-10 yr	7-8 yr	6-7 yr		
Lateral incisors	Max., 10-12 mo Mand., 3-4 mo	10-11 yr	8-9 yr	7-8 yr		
Cuspids (canines)	4-5 mo	12-15 yr	11-12 yr	9-11 yr		
First premolars (biscupids)	18-21 mo	12-13 yr	10-11 yr	10-12 yr		
Second premolars (biscuspids)	24-30 mo	12-14 yr	10-12 yr	11-13 yr		
First molars	Birth	9-10 yr	6-7 yr	6-7 yr		
Second molars	30-36 mo	14-16 yr	12-13 yr	12-13 yr		
Third molars	Max., 7-9 yr Mand., 8-10 yr	18-25 yr	17-22 yr	17-22 yr		

From Behrman RE, Vaughan VC, eds: *Nelson textbook of pediatrics*, ed 15, Philadelphia, 1996, WB Saunders.

3. Avulsed teeth
   - Deciduous
     a. No treatment required except radiographic search for remnants in jaw, lips, or lungs, if indicated
     b. Never replant avulsed primary tooth
   - Permanent
     a. Ask patient to bring tooth along ASAP!
     b. *Keep tooth moist in cold milk or ice water*
     c. Early referral for replanting and immobilization
     d. Prognosis dependent on length of time out of mouth (extraalveolar period < 30 min has > 90% chance of long-term retention), contamination of tooth (should avoid handling root surface), and age of patient

DENTAL PAIN

- Most dental pain requires referral to dentist
- Simple pulpal hyperemia resulting from trauma or large restorations
- Pulpitis caused by dental caries
  - Serous pulpitis: tooth sensitive to cold, pain relieved by heat
  - Suppurative pulpitis: tooth sensitive to heat, cold may relieve pain
- Pulpal necrosis with abscess
  - May occur without facial swelling or systemic signs
  - Management: analgesics, antipyretics, antibiotics (penicillin), possible removal of offending tooth
- Periodontal abscess
  - Usually pain (localized or referred) with associated facial swelling and fever
  - Uncommon in children, more common with orthodontic braces
  - Management: analgesics, antipyretics, surgical drainage, antibiotics

DENTAL POSTOPERATIVE HEMORRHAGE

- Definition: bleeding longer than 4 hr or delayed recurrent bleeding

Management

- Apply pressure: have patient bite firmly on folded, moistened 2 × 2 gauze pack positioned over surgical site
- Recheck in approximately 10 min for hemostasis
- If above unsuccessful:
  1. Local infiltration of 2% lidocaine with epinephrine 1:200,000 and curette socket
  2. Topical hemostatic agents (e.g., Gelfoam, bovine thrombin)
  3. Further therapy (suturing)

ACUTE HERPETIC GINGIVOSTOMATITIS

- Self-limiting disease lasting 10-14 days

Management

- Mainly supportive
  1. Topical analgesic mouthwash (e.g., benzydamine, Tantum)
  2. Topical antiseptics (antiseptic mouthwash) (e.g., dequalinium, Dequadin)
  3. Topical anesthetics (e.g., benzocaine) not usually required; apply carefully with cotton swabs to affected areas; may be used as oral rinse (risk of methemoglobinemia if swallowed)
  4. Acetaminophen for pain and fever
  5. Systemic antibiotic only for secondary bacterial infection
  6. Soft bland diet with extra fluids encouraged

Sᴀɴᴅʀᴀ Aʀɴᴏʟᴅ

ACNE

- Acne vulgaris
- Two types of lesions:
  1. Noninflammatory: comedones (open, closed)
  2. Inflammatory: papules, pustules, cysts, nodules

GENERAL MEASURES

- Diet is noncontributory
- Do not use moisturizers, steaming, or saunas
- Use oil-free makeup

TOPICAL MEDICATION
Benzoyl Peroxide (2.5% to 20%)

- Oxidizer; inhibits *Propionibacterium acnes*
- Mild comedolytic
- Apply qhs; start with 5%-10%; then increase % prn
- May cause localized drying and peeling; start with brief applications

Vitamin A Acid (0.01%, 0.025%, 0.05%) Cream and Gel

- Reverses follicular retention and hyperkeratosis, thereby decreasing comedone formation
- May worsen initially; may be associated with photosensitivity (wear sunblock); may also cause redness and peeling
- Apply qhs; start at 0.025% cream for 1 hr; increase slowly by weeks
- Minimum of 6 wk required before effect seen

Antibiotics

- For inflammatory lesions; 2% clindamycin solution in Duonalc solution, erythromycin (Staticin) bid

ORAL MEDICATION (FOR INFLAMMATORY ACNE)
Antibiotics

- Bacteriostatic for *P. acnes;* inhibits lipases, which produce free fatty acids
- Tetracycline (do not use if under 8 yr or pregnant), 250 mg tid for 3 wks and then 500 mg daily (may be divided bid); or minocycline, 100 mg bid for 1 wk and then 100 mg/day; or erythromycin, 250 mg tid for 3 wks; can be maintained long-term on 250 mg bid until acne resolves
- With prolonged use of antibiotic (1.5-2 yr) and decreasing effect, may switch to another antibiotic or discontinue; patient may have quiescent disease at this point.

Isotretinoin (Accutane)

- Oral synthetic vitamin A
- Antiinflammatory; decreases sebaceous gland secretion; normalizes keratinization of follicular epithelium
- Best used only by dermatologist or physician familiar with drug
- For nodulocystic, scarring acne resistant to oral antibiotics
- Use oral erythromycin or topical antibiotics while patient is receiving Accutane to reduce scarring, since acne will likely worsen before it improves
- Five-mo course and laboratory tests at 3 and 10 wks (liver function tests, urinalysis, CBC, cholesterol, and triglycerides)
- Must avoid pregnancy during and for 1 mo after treatment finished (mandatory pregnancy test, where appropriate, before starting Accutane)
- Use oral contraceptives during course of treatment, where appropriate
- Side effects: cheilitis (100%), xerostomia, xerosis ophthalmia, conjunctivitis, myalgia, facial dermatitis, headache (all reversible when drug discontinued); teratogenic
- Rise in AST, cholesterol, and triglycerides
- If necessary, dermatology referral for intralesional steroid injections of cysts and scars

ALOPECIA

- Five most common causes of patchy nonscarring alopecia in children are alopecia areata, trichotillomania, tinea capitis, telogen effluvium, and hair shaft abnormalities
- Examine entire skin, mucosal surfaces, nails, and teeth
- Depending on etiology, fungal, or other microbiologic studies, Wood's light examination of scalp, light microscopic examination of hair, or scalp biopsy may be indicated

ALOPECIA AREATA

- Smooth, sharply demarcated bald areas; exclamation mark hairs at edges
- Rarely may be associated with autoimmune disease
- For prolonged disease, potent topical steroids (e.g., fluocinonide 0.05%—Lidex or Topsyn Gel—tid) or intralesional steroids if patient can tolerate injections and areas are small

TINEA CAPITIS

- Most frequent organisms: *Trichophyton tonsurans* and *Microsporum canis*
- Nonscarring alopecia with associated scale
- "Black dot alopecia" (hairs very short because they break at scalp level)
- Kerion (boggy granulomatous reaction) may cause scarring
- Very contagious: spreads through family and school
- Wood's light fluorescence of hair (green) if *M. canis* (dandruff appears white); *T. tonsurans* does not fluoresce
- Fungal culture
- Treatment: Griseofulvin orally for 8 wk to 3 mo; topical treatment alone is inadequate

DERMATITIS

ATOPIC DERMATITIS

- Acute: pruritus, erythema, vesicles, exudation, and crusts
- Chronic: pruritus, xerosis (dry skin), scaling, lichenification
- Distribution:
  - Infant: cheeks, forehead, scalp, extensor surfaces
  - Child: antecubital and popliteal fossa, wrists, and ankles

General Measures

- Carefully explain to parents that atopic dermatitis is a relapsing and remitting disease that tends to improve with age; treatment does not cure but provides good control
- Prevent overheating: wear cotton clothes, ensure adequate control of ambient temperature (air-conditioning if necessary)
- Humidification: humidifier in bedroom
- Daily bath: od to bid; add oilated Aveeno, Alpha Keri, or baby oil to bath; use emollient while skin still damp
- Chemical: use mild or no soap (e.g., Dove or baby soap); wash clothes in Ivory, and rinse well; no bleach or fabric softener

Topical Agents

- Steroids (see Table 5-1): hydrocortisone 1% ointment on face, Betnovate 0.05% ointment to body (*not* to face or groin) tid; apply first before emollient
- Emollients: Vaseline in winter, Nivea or other moisturizing cream (e.g., Complex 15, Lachydrin, or Nutraplus) in summer
- Antihistamines: hydroxyzine or diphenhydramine may help (especially if child cannot sleep because of itchiness)
- Antibiotics: erythromycin or cloxacillin po for clinical infection (do not treat surface swab growth of *Staphylococcus* unless clinical infection)
- Avoid systemic steroids

DIAPER DERMATITIS

- Irritant dermatitis: due to urine, feces, and maceration; creases are spared; if severe, may be erosive; more common with cloth diapers washed at home
- Seborrheic dermatitis: greasy, yellow scales and erythema commonly affecting diaper area; if seborrheic dermatitis fails to respond to treatment, consider possibility of histiocytosis X
- *Candida:* pink papules with superficial scale or erythematous patch with peripheral scale; may have associated oral thrush; creases involved; may complicate irritant dermatitis

Management

- Use disposable diapers or diaper service; change diaper frequently and expose buttocks to air
- 1% hydrocortisone ointment tid for contact dermatitis, seborrheic dermatitis
- If *Candida,* 1% hydrocortisone in Canesten cream tid is best choice
- Apply barrier ointment (zinc oxide) over top of topical medication

SEBORRHEIC DERMATITIS

- Greasy yellow scales with erythema typically on scalp (cradle cap), behind ears, diaper area, axillae, and flexural creases
- Scalp: daily tar shampoo; 1% hydrocortisone lotion or cream tid
- Body: 1% hydrocortisone ointment tid; oatmeal baths

POISON IVY CONTACT DERMATITIS

- Potent steroid cream (e.g., Betnovate 0.1% cream tid)
- Use prednisone if extensive (start at 1 mg/kg/day po with maximum 40-60 mg daily; taper over 2-3 wk period)

PAPULOSQUAMOUS DISORDERS

PSORIASIS

- Erythematous plaques with silver scale on extensor surfaces, scalp, and groin; nails often have pits; guttate lesions associated with antecedent streptococcal infections
- May have associated seronegative arthropathy (rare)

Management

1. Topical steroids
2. Tar (crude cool tar: used in hospital only) with UV light; may use 5%-10% LCD topically mixed with steroid or glaxal base
3. Scalp: 5%-10% salicylic acid qhs to lift thick scale followed by steroid lotion tid

PITYRIASIS ROSEA

- "Herald patch" followed in 5-10 days by multiple, erythematous, scaling patches; unknown etiology
- Lasts 6-8 wks and resolves spontaneously
- If pruritic, use oilated baths and topical steroids

TINEA CORPORIS

- Dermatophyte infection of any part of skin
- Predominant species: *Trichophyton tonsurans, Trichophyton rubrum, Trichophyton mentagrophytes,* and *Microsporum canis*
- Erythematous papules expand to form plaques with scaling; annular in shape; may have central clearing; pruritic; skin does not fluoresce so Wood's light not helpful
- Fungal culture
- Topical antifungal first
- Systemic antifungal if topical therapy fails (e.g., griseofulvin, Lamisil)

BACTERIAL INFECTIONS

CELLULITIS

- See p. 242

IMPETIGO

- Contagious infection by *S. aureus* and Group A beta-hemolytic *Streptococcus*
- Child not systemically ill

Staphylococcal Impetigo

- Bullous; often begins in folds (neck, groin); eroded areas in flexures
- *Staphylococcus* reservoir: upper respiratory tract

Streptococcal Impetigo

- Honey-colored crusts ("classic impetigo")
- Poststreptococcal glomerulonephritis can occur after impetigo; rheumatic fever does not

Management

- Cool compresses to dry lesions
- Cloxacillin or erythromycin po for 10 days for *S. aureus*
- If streptococcal impetigo, use penicillin or erythromycin po; may use cephalexin to cover both
- If localized, topical therapy with Fucidin or Bactroban

STAPHYLOCOCCAL SCALDED SKIN SYNDROME (SSSS)

- Superficial epidermal blistering caused by epidermolytic toxin produced by *S. aureus*
- Cloxacillin for 7-10 days
- Emollients when dry
- Heals without scarring

VIRAL INFECTIONS

MOLLUSCUM CONTAGIOSUM

- Dome-shaped, umbilicated papules
- Occurs anywhere on children; mostly axillae and genital area
- Usually asymptomatic; some develop a surrounding pruritic dermatitis
- Lesions last from a few weeks to 2 yr; will resolve spontaneously if left untreated

Management

- Children: topical cantharidin (0.7%) applied by physician to lesions (avoid surrounding skin); warn patients to expect blistering
- Older children: can use cantharidin (0.7%) or curettage
- Repeat treatment as new crops of lesions arise

VERRUCAE
Verruca Vulgaris

- Caused by human papillomavirus (HPV) 1,2,4,7
- Apply 75% salicylic acid in petrolatum, cover with adhesive bandage,

and leave on for 1 wk, then debride in office; may use daily topical salicylic acid preparation (Soluver) available over the counter
- Repeat until all warty tissue removed
- Liquid nitrogen every third week until tissue scabs and heals; usually not tolerated in children (very painful)
- Plantar warts (*verruca planteris*) managed in same way

Condyloma Accuminatum

- Caused by HPV 6,11,16,18,31
- Apply (in office only) 25% podophyllin and leave on 4-6 hr (avoid contact with normal surrounding skin)
- Patient washes it off at home with soap and water
- Repeat weekly
- In children, have index of suspicion for sexual abuse (although rare)

INFESTATIONS

LICE

- *Pediculosis capitis* (head louse): adult louse is 3-4 mm long, eggs (nits) are 1 mm, usually white, and firmly adherent to hair shafts; postauricular and occipital regions are most common sites
- *Pediculosis pubis* (crab louse): smaller than head and body louse; found on eyelashes and pubic hair; transmitted by sexual contact or rarely by shared clothing and bed linen
- For head lice, permethrin (Nix) can be used: wash, rinse, and towel dry hair; apply Nix as cream rinse for 10 min, then rinse; Nix is ovicidal, therefore nits do not have to be combed out; contraindicated in individuals with allergy to chrysanthemums; Nix is very expensive
- Gamma benzene hexachloride 1% (Kwellada) shampoo to affected hair-bearing site; lather for 10 min and rinse; repeat 1 day later and in 7 days
- Eyelash involvement with *Pediculosis pubis:* apply petrolatum to eyelashes bid or tid for 10 days
- Nits can be removed with vinegar soaks (vinegar mixed with water 1:1) and fine-toothed comb
- Soak combs, brushes, barrettes in Kwellada shampoo for 10 min
- Clothing and bed linen should be washed in hot water or dry-cleaned

SCABIES

- Caused by *Sarcoptes scabiei humanis*
- Incubation period: 3-6 wk; primary lesion is burrow 2-10 mm in length, with female mite at end
- Sites of predilection: finger webs, axillae, genitalia, periumbilical area; palms, soles, nape of neck, and axillae in infants; face usually not involved except in infants and Norwegian (extensive) scabies
- Nodular lesions common in axillae and groin

Management

1. Under 2 yr or in pregnancy: 5% permethrin cream applied from neck down and rinsed off after 8-14 hrs; repeat in 5-7 days

2. Over 2 yr: Kwellada (gamma benzene hexachloride) cream applied from neck down, washed off after 8 hr (overnight ideal); repeated in 5-7 days
3. Wash all bed and personal clothing used recently
4. Advise that pruritus and rash may persist for several weeks after mite eradicated
5. Nodular lesions may persist for months after active infection controlled (topical steroids may be beneficial)
6. Treat all household contacts simultaneously as above, whether itchy or not

MISCELLANEOUS

ERYTHEMA MULTIFORME

- 1-2 cm erythematous papules, target lesions, may have one or two mucous membranes involved

Etiology

- Infection (currently believed to be most likely etiology) (e.g., herpes simplex, mycoplasma)

Management

- No specific treatment for eruption
- In recurrent *erythema multiforme minor* with herpes, can often abort episode by use of acyclovir or prednisone for 2 wk

STEVENS-JOHNSON SYNDROME

- Bullous lesions; severe (oral, nasal, conjunctival, and genital) mucous membrane involvement
- Drugs: sulfa, phenytoin, penicillin, and phenobarbital are most commonly implicated
- Supportive treatment with IV fluids, pain control, ophthalmology consult; prednisone use controversial
- Stop medication implicated in etiology

HEMANGIOMAS AND VASCULAR MALFORMATIONS
Capillary (Strawberry) Hemangioma

- Often mixed capillary and cavernous
- Immature capillaries may not be present at birth (50% usually appear within first 2 wk); increase in size for several months out of proportion to body growth; usually start to involute by end of second year; 90% regress by 9 yr

Cavernous Hemangioma

- Deeper and larger vessels than capillary type; may be present at birth
- Regress by age 9 yr: may leave redundant skin

Vascular Malformations

- May consist of capillaries, arteries, veins, or lymphatics
- Port-wine stain: vascular malformation of mature capillary vessels; present at birth; grows in proportion with patient

Salmon Patch (Stork Bite, Angel's Kiss)

- Dilated embryonal dermal capillaries; pink macular lesion found on nape of neck, glabella, forehead and eyelids; present at birth; disappears with time except patches on back of neck

Complications and Associated Syndromes

- Ulceration and secondary infection
- May enlarge very quickly (bleeding into hemangioma)
- May develop Kasabach-Merritt syndrome (platelet sequestration by large hemangioma and coagulopathy)
- May affect important organs, especially eyes (amblyopia, glaucoma, strabismus) or airway
- Klippel-Trenaunay-Weber syndrome: vascular malformation with underlying soft tissue and bony hypertrophy of limb
- Neonatal hemangiomatosis: multiple cutaneous and visceral hemangiomas, which may lead to high-output cardiac failure and GI hemorrhage
- Sturge-Weber syndrome: port-wine stain in distribution of cranial nerve V_1; underlying meningeal vascular malformation; seizures; mental retardation

Management of Capillary and Cavernous Hemangiomas

- Generally, no treatment necessary
- Prednisone, 1-3 mg/kg/day (may require several months of treatment with careful follow-up) if:
  1. Enlarges very quickly
  2. Affects vital structures, respiratory tract, eye
  3. Kasabach-Merritt syndrome
- Cosmetic treatment: pulsed dye laser; makeup
- Embolization

URTICARIA

- Typical wheal; may coalesce, may clear centrally
- Angioedema may be associated with pharyngolaryngeal edema and anaphylaxis (see p. 17)
- History and physical examination to eliminate obvious causes (e.g., medications). Often no offending agent found; routine lab tests not necessary
- Symptomatic treatment: oral antihistamines (diphenhydramine, hydroxyzine) continuously for 10 days or risk of relapse
- If chronic, consider CBC, differential, ESR, urinalysis, stool for ova and parasites

Table 5-1 Examples of Topical Steroids

Potency	Brand name	Generic name
Nonfluorinated, lowest potency		Hydrocortisone (1%)
Nonfluorinated low potency	Tridesilon	Desonide (0.05%)
	Westcort	Hydrocortisone valerate (0.2%)
Intermediate potency	Betnovate (0.05%, 0.1%)	Betamethasone valerate (0.05%; 0.1%)
	Valisone scalp lotion	Betamethasone valerate (0.1%)
		Fluocinolone acetonide (0.025%)

TOPICAL STEROIDS (Table 5-1)

- Use cream, lotion or gel on scalp (e.g., Betnovate 0.1%)
- Ointments are used more in winter (to prevent drying) and on dry lesions
- Creams are used more in summer and on moist lesions
- Avoid using fluorinated steroids on face and in flexural areas
- Rule of thumb: 30 g (1 oz) of medication will cover entire adult body once
- Side effects of prolonged topical steroid are minimal if used appropriately

CHAPTER 6

ENDOCRINOLOGY

JILL HAMILTON

DIABETES MELLITUS

NEWLY DIAGNOSED DIABETES

- Diagnosis: random blood glucose > 11 mmol/L, glycosuria ± ketonuria
- Symptoms: polyuria, polydipsia, polyphagia, weight loss, approximately 25% of children present in diabetic ketoacidosis (see below)

Management of New Stable Diabetic (No DKA)

- Admission to hospital indicated only to correct ketoacidosis or if other factors (distance, language, psychosocial) make ambulatory care difficult; stabilization and initiation of diabetes education for child and family can be achieved on outpatient basis

Insulin

- On day of diagnosis: Regular insulin (0.1-0.25 U/kg) is given q4-6 hr for symptomatic relief; usually NPH/Lente insulin is added before evening meal
- Next day, start mixture of NPH/Lente and Regular insulins before breakfast and supper (children under 5 yr), or NPH and Regular insulin prebreakfast, Regular insulin presupper, and NPH at bedtime (children over 5 yr); all insulins are biosynthetic human insulin
- NPH starting dose is approximately 1 U/yr prebreakfast and ¼-½ of this dose at supper/bedtime; Regular insulin dose is approximately ¼-⅓ of NPH dose at each time
- Monitor blood glucose level before meals, before bed, and at specific additional times as indicated during periods of adjustment
- In younger age group and during initial diabetes education period, blood glucose levels should be kept between 6-12 mmol/L; once patient and family familiar with monitoring and treatment, optimal glucose target range can be decreased to 4-8 or 4-10 mmol/L, depending on individual child
- Anticipate decrease in insulin requirements in first few weeks postdischarge with increased activity and honeymoon period
- Comprehensive outpatient educational program and ongoing communication with diabetes team essential in long-term management of children with IDDM

Diet

- Exchange-type diabetes diet:
  - To start, 1000 kcal + 100 kcal/yr of age; individualize according to age, appetite, activity

- Children under 4-5 yr are started on low-concentrated carbohydrate diet appropriate for age with no total caloric intake restrictions
- Timing of meals and snacks should be consistent
- Composition:
  1. 50%-55% carbohydrate (3/4 complex carbohydrate)
  2. 30%-35% fat (polyunsaturated to saturated ratio: 1.2 : 1)
  3. 15%-20% protein

DIABETIC KETOACIDOSIS (DKA)
Classification

Mild: pH 7.2-7.3
Moderate: pH 7.0-7.2
Severe: pH < 7.0

- Causes: new onset DM, insulin omission, intercurrent illness

Diagnosis

- Vomiting, abdominal pain, dehydration, rapid or Kussmaul respiration, altered level of consciousness
- Measure blood glucose, pH, pCO_2, HCO_3, electrolytes, urea, urine ketones
- Calculate:
  1. Anion gap = $[Na - (Cl + HCO_3)]$
  2. Serum osmolality = $(2 \times Na) + glucose$
  3. Corrected serum Na (mmol/L) = (measured Na [mmol/L]) + 1.5 × (glucose [mmol/L] ÷ 5.5)

Management

- Monitoring:
  1. NPO until recovered
  2. Careful hourly documentation of vital signs, level of consciousness, accurate intake and output
  3. Blood glucose q1-2 hr, biochemistry as above q4 hr; ensure that "corrected" Na does not decrease over first 12 hr, then no faster than 1 mmol/L/hr
- Fluids: Initially: 0.9% saline at 10 ml/kg/hr × 1 hr, then 5 ml/kg/hr until acidosis corrected
- Potassium: Add KCl to IV (20-40 mmol/L or 3-5 mmol/kg/day) after patient voids (or immediately if serum K^+ < 4 mmol/L)
- Glucose: Add to IV fluids when blood glucose < 15-17 mmol/L by changing IV solution to 5% dextrose in normal saline (D5/0.9NS)
- Insulin:
  1. Start insulin infusion immediately; dose: 0.1 U/kg/hr; dilute 25 U regular insulin in 250 ml saline as second IV line or in Y tubing and run at weight in ml/hr (e.g., 30 kg = 30 cc/hr = 0.1 U/kg/hr)
  2. Maintain insulin infusion at 0.1 U/kg/hr and increase glucose concentration in IV fluid as blood glucose levels fall below 15-17 mmol/L; continue until acidosis resolved; if blood glucose level falling too rapidly, insulin infusion may also be decreased to 0.02-0.05 U/kg/hr
- Bicarbonate: Generally given as $NaHCO_3$ when plasma HCO_3 < 12

mmol/L and pH < 7.2; dose $= (12 - [HCO_3]_{plasma} \times$ weight (kg) $\times$ 0.6; give half IV over 10-20 min and infuse remainder over 2 hr

Complications of DKA and its Treatment

- Hypoglycemia
- Hypokalemia: potassium < 3.0 mmol/L
- Persistent acidosis: if not correcting, check to make sure child is getting insulin appropriately (e.g., long IV line in small child)
- Cerebral edema: warning symptoms: headache, irritability; examine pupillary response and fundi; monitor GCS closely if any concerns; follow serum sodium and infusion rates closely

MANAGEMENT OF INTERCURRENT ILLNESS
(Table 6-1)

- Measure blood glucose and urine ketones immediately and q4 hr around the clock until recovered
- If child unable to eat, offer sugar-containing fluids such as soda pop or juice
- Antipyretic as indicated: treat underlying illness
- Should vomiting develop twice in 4-6 hr period, child should be assessed in emergency department; if child has been vomiting clear fluids and is nauseated, keep NPO, and establish IV to provide maintenance fluids and glucose
- *Do not stop insulin!* May have to decrease dose if glucose levels low, or increase dose if levels high or ketones are present

HYPOGLYCEMIA IN DIABETES MELLITUS

- Can occur secondary to excess insulin administration; missed, delayed, or decreased meals; and increased physical activity without adequate caloric compensation
- Early warning symptoms: tremors, sweating, palpitations, hunger, pallor, dizziness, blurred vision
- Neuroglycopenia: irritability, confusion, coma, seizures
- All patients should have clear instructions regarding management of hypoglycemia, including use of glucagon

Treatment

1. Mild:
   - Concentrated carbohydrate (60-120 ml juice, 2-4 glucose tablets): 10-15 g; if not resolving in 10-15 min, repeat carbohydrate intake
   - If recurrent, may need diet or insulin adjustment
2. Severe:
   - Treat initially at home with glucagon 1 mg SC for age > 5 yr, 0.5 mg SC for age < 5 yr
   - Needs medical assessment if has seizures, hemiparesis, altered level of consciousness (may require hospitalization)
   - At hospital: if altered level of consciousness or history of seizure, give glucose 0.5 g/kg (1 ml/kg D50W, 2 ml/kg D25W) IV push
   - Continue dextrose solution (5% or 10%) for several hours until clinical improvement noted
   - Adjust diet and insulin; counsel regarding prevention methods

6

Table 6-1 Guidelines for Insulin Adjustment During Intercurrent Illness

Sickness profile	A	B	C	D	E
Blood glucose in mmol/L	≥ 4-6* and ≤ 13	≥ 13 and < 17	≥ 17	≥ 13	< 4-6
Urine ketones	Neg. or pos.	Neg.	Neg.	Pos.	Neg. or pos.
Action	Wait; continue to monitor carefully	Wait; if condition persists, increase insulin next day by 10%-20%/day until aims achieved	Give extra regular insulin q4h, equal to 10%-20% of total daily dose until urine ketones clear and/or blood sugar < 11 mmol/L; then proceed as for regimen in columns A and B		Decrease daily insulin by 20%/day until blood glucose is between 4-11 mmol/L

*Depending on target range.

Management During Surgery

- For minor procedures, patient can be admitted on day of surgery for IV insertion and preoperative monitoring; if major procedure planned, admit patient on day before to ensure adequate preoperative control

Minor Procedures (< 1 hr)

- Patients will be able to take fluids shortly after procedure
- IV 3.33% dextrose and 0.3% saline (⅔-⅓) or 5% dextrose in 0.45% saline (D5/0.45) plus KCl at maintenance rates (start at 7:30 AM)
- Insulin ⅔ daily dose given as intermediate-acting insulin only (NPH/Lente) SC; no fast-acting insulin given
- Blood glucose preoperatively and immediately postoperatively; monitor as necessary
- Regular insulin given postoperatively as necessary to maintain blood glucose at 5-15 mmol/L
- Usual dose of insulin resumed when child able to take normal diet

Major Procedures (> 1 hr)

- Patient unlikely to drink shortly after procedure
- No SC insulin on day of surgery
- NPO postoperatively
- IV as above
- Insulin infusion, 0.02 U regular insulin/kg/hr
- Adjust insulin infusion to maintain blood glucose at 5-15 mmol/L
- Monitor blood glucose hourly intraoperatively, q4 hr postoperatively, urine ketones bid
- When tolerating fluids PO (usually next day):
  1. Discontinue insulin infusion
  2. Start SC insulin (⅔ usual dose and increase as indicated)
- For emergency procedures, surgery should be delayed, if possible, until acidosis and dehydration are corrected

HYPOGLYCEMIA (Table 6-2)

- Hyperinsulinemic hypoglycemia is the common cause of hypoglycemia in children below 1 yr; ketotic hypoglycemia is the common cause in children over 1 yr old
- Critical blood sample for diagnosis: glucose, blood gas, electrolytes, insulin, growth hormone, lactate, cortisol, beta-hydroxybutyrate, free fatty acids, and urine for ketones
- Treat with glucose 0.5 g/kg (1 ml/kg of D50W or 2 ml/kg of D25W) IV bolus, plus continuous glucose infusion to maintain glucose level in normal range
- More detailed investigation may require admission for monitored starvation challenge
- Neonates: see p. 296

Table 6-2 Major Differential Diagnoses of Hypoglycemia

	Hyperinsulinism	Substrate deficiency (e.g., glycogen storage disease)	Ketotic hypoglycemia (including GH and cortisol deficiency)
Glucose	Low	Low	Low
Insulin	High	Low	Low
Lactic acid	Normal to low	High	Normal
β-hydroxybutyric acid	Low	High	Very high

From Aynsley-Green A: *Hypoglycemia* in infants and children, *Clin Endocrinol Metab* 11:170, 1982.

BOX 6-1 Differential Diagnosis of Hypocalcemia

I. **Decreased PTH Secretion**
   A. *Neonatal Hypocalcemia*
      1. Transient hypocalcemia
         a) Early onset
         b) Late onset (> 3 days)
      2. Transient hypoparathyroidism secondary to maternal hyperparathyroidism
      3. Deletion 22q11 (DiGeorge's/Velocardiofacial syndrome)
      4. Primary hypomagnesemia
   B. *Congenital Hypoparathyroidism*
      1. Aplasia/hypoplasia of parathyroid gland
      2. Hypoparathyroidism (X-linked, autosomal recessive)
   C. *Acquired Hypoparathyroidism*
      1. Idiopathic
      2. Polyglandular autoimmune disease
      3. Postsurgical
      4. Secondary to iron loading (e.g., thalassemia major)
II. **Inadequate Target Tissue Response to PTH**
   A. *Vit D deficiency (decreased intake, malabsorption, or block in metabolism leading to decreased 1,25-(OH)$_2$ Vitamin D)*
   B. *Pseudohypoparathyroidism Types I and II*
   C. *Magnesium deficiency*
III. **Increased Protein Bound Calcium (e.g., alkalotic states)**

Modified from Harrison HE, Harrison HC: *Disorders in calcium and phosphate metabolism in childhood and adolescence,* Philadelphia, 1979, Saunders.

HYPOCALCEMIA (Box 6-1)

NORMAL CALCIUM RANGE

- Premature infants:
   0-3 days → 1.8-2.5 mmol/L
   3 days-2 months → 2.0-2.75 mmol/L
- Term infants 0-2 months → 2.0-2.75 mmol/L
- Child → 2.25-2.62 mmol/L
- Adult → 2.12-2.62 mmol/L

- If hypoalbuminemia present, measured Ca may be falsely low:
  Adjusted Ca (mmol/L) = [Ca (mmol/L) − albumin(g/L)/40] + 1
- Measure ionized Ca if serum protein or pH is abnormal
- History: neck surgery/trauma, family history, diet, sunlight exposure, GI, hepatobiliary or pancreatic disease, renal disease
- Symptoms/signs : muscle cramps, carpopedal spasm (Trousseau's sign), facial twitch (Chvostek's sign), paresthesias, tetany, seizures, laryngeal stridor, ECG abnormalities
- Investigations: phosphate, magnesium, ALP, PTH, 25-(OH)-Vitamin D; 1,25-(OH)$_2$ vitamin D, ± renal, and liver function tests, serum pH, total protein/albumin

Management

- Most mild hypocalcemia can be managed without IV calcium infusion
- If IV calcium infusion is required (Ca gluconate, Ca chloride), administer as diluted solution (e.g., 10% Ca gluconate diluted to 2% solution)
- 10 ml of 10% Ca gluconate contains 90 mg of elemental Ca (2.25 mmol); add 10 ml of 10% Ca gluconate to 40 ml of saline to obtain 2% solution; this dilution contains Ca 0.04 mmol/ml
- For serious hypocalcemia (convulsions and arrythmias), give Ca 0.1 mmol/kg/hr
- For less severe cases (muscle cramps, paresthesia) give Ca 0.05 mmol/kg/hr
- Never give IV bolus calcium to correct hypocalcemia
- Adjust infusion rate q4h based on plasma Ca level; aim for > 2 mmol/L; reduce infusion rate slowly once desired level reached
- All patients receiving IV calcium should be on cardiac monitor
- Monitor IV site: high risk of extravasation burns and venous thrombosis
- Do not administer calcium and NaHCO$_3$ in same IV tubing
- Never give Ca IM or SC
- Maintain oral intake of 100 mg elemental Ca/kg/day; use supplement if needed (e.g., calcium lactate/gluconate/carbonate)
- Start vitamin D metabolites: 1,25-(OH)$_2$ vitamin D$_3$ or 1α(OH) vitamin D$_3$ if more than 3-4 days of IV calcium are anticipated

HYPERCALCEMIA

- Definition: Ca > 2.75 mmol/L
- Symptoms/signs: generally nonspecific weakness, anorexia, polyuria, polydipsia, mental status changes

Differential Diagnosis

- Caused by either increased intestinal calcium absorption or increased resorption of bone
  1. Hyperparathyroidism
  2. Familial benign hypercalcemia (hypocalciuric hypercalcemia)
  3. Medication related: excess vitamin D, vitamin A, thiazide diuretics, lithium
  4. Neoplasia related

5. Immobilization
6. With other endocrinopathies (Addison's, hyperthyroidism, pheochromocytoma)
7. With granulomatous disease (subcutaneous fat necrosis in newborn, sarcoid)

Management

- Low Ca, high-fluid diet for all patients
- For emergency treatment give IV fluids to increase extracellular fluid volume (0.9% saline at 2.5 × maintenance) ± furosemide ± steroids
- May require calcitonin or bisphosphonate in refractory cases
- Oral phosphate may be used if serum phosphate concentration low

AMBIGUOUS GENITALIA (Fig. 6-1, Box 6-2)

- Psychosocial emergency: timely sex determination important
- Sex assignment generally based on phallic size and not genetic makeup
- History: pregnancy (hormones, medications), family history
- P/E: palpation for gonads, rectal exam
- Investigations
  1. Biochemistry:
     - Electrolytes (salt-wasting congenital adrenal hyperplasia [CAH]), renin level
     - 17-α-hydroxyprogesterone (may not be reliable until day 3)
     - Androgens
     - Follicle stimulating hormone (FSH), lutenizine hormone (LH)
  2. Karyotype
  3. Anatomic:
     - Pelvic/abdominal ultrasound (US) (look for uterus)
     - Cystogram/cystoscopy

BOX 6-2   Differential Diagnoses of Ambiguous Genitalia

Female Pseudohermaphrodite (XX)
Virilizing CAH (21-hydroxylase deficiency commonest cause)
Maternal androgen ingestion/virilizing condition
Fetal/Placental aromatase deficiency
Nonandrogen-induced structural malformation
Male Pseudohermaphrodite (XY)
Impaired Leydig cell activity (inborn errors of testosterone biosynthesis, Leydig cell hypoplasia)
Impaired peripheral androgen metabolism (5α-reductase deficiency, androgen receptor insensitivity)
LH/hCG unresponsiveness
Nonandrogen-induced structural malformations
Mixed Pattern
True hermaphrodite
Mixed gonadal dysgenesis

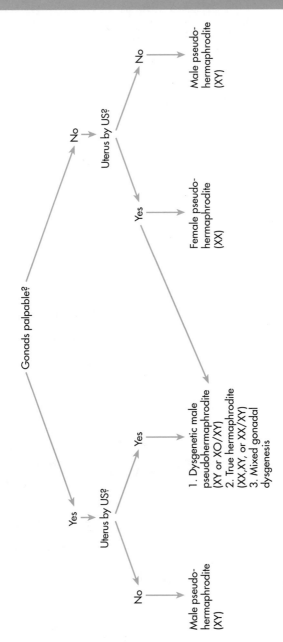

Fig. 6-1 Ambiguous Genitalia (See also Box 6-2.) (From Rudolph AM, Kamei RK: *Rudolph's fundamentals of pediatrics*, New York, 1994, Appleton & Lange.

ADRENAL INSUFFICIENCY

- For management of acute adrenal insufficiency (see p. 25)
- Major cause in neonatal period is congenital adrenal hyperplasia
- Addison's disease rare; iatrogenic adrenal suppression may occur in children taking pharmacologic doses of adrenal steroids
- Children with diseases of the hypothalamic-pituitary axis (e.g., craniopharyngioma) are also at risk for adrenal insufficiency during intercurrent illness

Clinical

- Acute: shock with dehydration, decreased Na, increased K, ± decreased glucose
- Chronic: fatigue, weight loss, abdominal pain, salt craving, hypoglycemia, increased pigmentation

Investigations

- Measure plasma cortisol, renin, aldosterone, electrolytes before treatment
- If newborn (especially with ambiguous genitalia), 17α-hydroxyprogesterone most important investigation (done after 48 hrs of age)
- May need abdominal US, head CT, ACTH studies, adrenal antibody titers

ANTIDIURETIC HORMONE

DEFICIENCY (DIABETES INSIPIDUS)

- Clinical: polyuria, polydipsia, usually no weight loss, family history, CNS symptoms (if central DI)
- Presence of urine SG $\leq$ 1.005, hypernatremia, increased serum osmolality
- Do water deprivation test to differentiate central diabetes insipidus from nephrogenic diabetes insipidus and psychogenic polydipsia
- Treat underlying cause; give DDAVP, 0.025-0.1 ml (2.5-10 μg) intranasally q12-24 hr for symptomatic control (monitor by urine output, specific gravity, thirst); allow free access to water

EXCESS (SYNDROME OF INAPPROPRIATE ANTIDIURETIC HORMONE [SIADH])

- Generally caused by CNS disorder (infection, trauma, tumor), but also caused by drugs (vincristine, vancomycin) and respiratory and paralytic diseases
- Hallmark is hyponatremia, with decreased serum osmolality in face of elevated urine SG; urine Na > 20 mmol/L; urine osmolality > plasma osmolality (e.g., urine Na and osmolality higher than expected for serum levels)
- Treatment: fluid restriction (e.g., 50%-60% maintenance or insensible water losses—400 ml/m^2/day—+ ½ urine output); rarely requires 3% NaCl + diuresis (furosemide) for symptomatic hyponatremia (see p. 104)

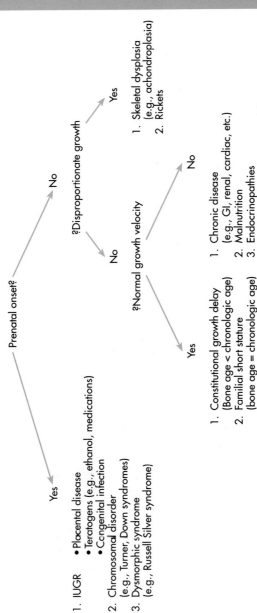

Fig. 6-2 Differential Diagnosis of Short Stature

SHORT STATURE (Fig. 6-2)

- Growth velocity less than 4-5 cm/yr between ages 3-10 yr is abnormal; during the first three yr of life, rapid shifts in growth rate occur; at puberty, may see decline in growth rate just before adolescent growth spurt
- Accurate measurements over time intervals at least 6 mo apart most important part of assessment
- Investigate if abnormal growth rate, height significantly less than genetic potential, or height less than 3rd percentile
- Disproportionate failure in weight gain should direct investigations to conditions associated with undernutrition (e.g., "occult" anorexia nervosa) or to possibility of parental deprivation
- More retarded the bone age, greater the likelihood of organic disease, particularly long-standing hypothyroidism, and greater the potential for "catch-up"
- Bone age also useful to distinguish constitutional (bone age < chronologic age) from genetic/familial (BA = CA) growth delay
- Chromosomal analysis should be performed in any girl measuring less than 3rd percentile in height to exclude Turner's syndrome
- Hormonal causes of short stature (GH or thyroid hormone deficiencies, hypercortisolism) relatively uncommon (< 15% of cases)
- Cortisol administration in excess of hydrocortisone 25 mg/m^2/day (prednisone, 5 mg/m^2/day) will retard normal somatic growth
- Rough estimate of final height of normal child can be made by calculating midparental height (MPH):

$$\text{for boys} = \frac{\text{father's Ht (cm)} + 13 \text{ cm} + \text{mother's Ht (cm)}}{2}$$

$$\text{for girls} = \frac{\text{father's Ht (cm)} - 13 \text{ cm} + \text{mother's Ht (cm)}}{2}$$

- Note: 13 cm is inherent mean difference in final height between men and women
- One standard deviation is 2.5 cm
- Measure upper to lower segment ratio (lower = symphysis pubis to ground, upper = height − lower segment) and arm span (should be within 5 cm of height) to determine if growth delay is proportionate

Initial Investigations

- Complete blood count and sedimentation rate
- Thyroid function tests: serum-free T$_4$, TSH
- Urea, creatinine
- Karyotype in girls or in any child with dysmorphic physical features
- Urinalysis (pH, protein, blood, glucose, WBC, RBC)
- Radiologic investigations: bone age, skull radiographs (CT or MRI) if CNS disorder suspected

CHAPTER 7

FLUIDS AND ELECTROLYTES

WENDY H. EDWARDS

CONVERSIONS

- millimole (mmol) to mg = number of mmol × molecular weight (e.g., 1 mmol NaCl = 1 × [23 + 35.5] = 58.5 mg; 2 mmol Ca = 2 × 40 mg = 80 mg (Box 7-1)
- mmol to milliequivalent (mEq) = number of mmol × valence (e.g., 1 mmol Na^+ = 1 mEq; 1 mmol Ca^{2+} = 2 mEq)
- milliosmoles (mOsm) = mmol × number of particles produced by dissociation (e.g., 1 mmol $CaCl_2$ = 3 mOsm)
- To calculate estimated serum osmolality: 2 × Na (mmol/L) + glucose (mmol/L) + urea (mmol/L)
- Normal plasma osmolality 280-295 mosm/kg

MAINTENANCE FLUID AND ELECTROLYTE REQUIREMENTS/24 HR (Table 7-1)

- Based on body weight in kg and usual insensible, urinary, and fecal losses; does not account for replacement of ongoing losses or previous deficits (see next section)
- Water
  - 1st 10 kg (0-10) = 100 ml/kg
  - 2nd 10 kg (11-20) = 50 ml/kg
  - Any additional kg = 20 ml/kg
  - or, 1500 ml/m², for children > 10 kg (see p. 314 for BSA calculation)
- Example: 25 kg child needs (100 × 10) + (50 × 10) + (20 × 5) = 1600 ml/24 hr
- Electrolytes
  - Sodium: 2-3 mmol/kg
  - Potassium: 2-3 mmol/kg
- Suggested maintenance solutions: 5% dextrose and 0.2% saline with 20 mmol/L of KCl, or 3.33% dextrose and 0.33% saline (2/3:1/3) with 20 mmol/L KCl
- For neonatal requirements, see p. 293
- Fever: add 12% to total maintenance requirements per 1° C rise above 37.5° C rectally

DEHYDRATION (Table 7-2)

- Infants and children at high risk of hypovolemic shock from increased losses and decreased intake of any cause; for assessments and management of shock, see p. 6

BOX 7-1 Molecular Weights

Calcium (Ca) 40.1	Nitrogen (N) 14.0
Carbon (C) 12.0	Oxygen (O) 16.0
Chlorine (Cl) 35.5	Phosphorus (P) 31.0
Hydrogen (H) 1.0	Potassium (K) 39.1
Magnesium (Mg) 24.3	Sodium (Na) 23.0

Table 7-1 Average Normal Values for Various Body Compartments (L/kg)

	Newborn	Child	Adult Male	Adult Female
TBW*	0.75	0.65	0.60	0.55
ICF	0.40	0.40	0.40	0.40
ECF	0.35	0.25	0.20	0.15
Blood volume (ml/kg)	(70-90)	(70-90)	(70-80)	(70-80)

*TBW, Total body water; ICF, intracellular fluid; ECF, extracellular fluid.

History

- Type and frequency of losses (i.e., diarrhea, vomiting, gastroenteritis most common cause of childhood dehydration)
- Type of replacement fluids given (H_2O, juices, boiled formula with increased Na)
- Frequency and concentration of urine
- Changes in weight
- Known cardiac or renal disease

Investigations

- Serum electrolytes, venous gas, glucose (high in hypernatremia), calcium (low in hypernatremia, alkalemia, and hyperphosphatemia), urea, creatinine, CBC
- Determine type of dehydration, based on serum Na level and calculated osmolality (see above):
  1. Isotonic: [Na] = 130-150 mmol/L
  2. Hypertonic: [Na] > 150 mmol/L
  3. Hypotonic: [Na] < 130 mmol/L

Treatment

- ABCs (see p.2)
- Restore circulating volume
  1. Normal saline or Ringer's lactate 20-40 ml/kg IV over 20-40 min (Note: Ringer's lactate contains 4 mmol/L of KCl and metabolism is limited in hypovolemic shock; do not use with renal failure)

Table 7-2 Clinical Features of Dehydration*

Severity	Age < 1 yr		Age > 1 yr		Clinical signs
	% Water deficit	Water deficit†	% Water deficit	Water deficit	
Minimal	<5		<3		Thirst, mild oliguria
Mild	5	50 ml/kg	3	30 ml/kg	Dry mucous membranes, axilla, groin, concentrated urine
Moderate	10	100 ml/kg	6	60 ml/kg	Loss of skin turgor, severe thirst, sunken eyeballs and fontanelle, oliguria
Severe	15	150 ml/kg	9	90 ml/kg	Low BP, poor circulation, CNS changes, fever

*In hypernatremic dehydration, water deficit may be difficult to assess; neurologic features predominate early, whereas ECF volume is preserved; skin feels doughy.
†Refers to deficit requiring replacement.

2. Plasma and/or blood (if anemic) or 5% albumin 10-20 ml/kg over one hr
- If circulating volume is still inadequate after 40 ml/kg, consider CVP monitoring and other causes of ineffective circulating volume (see p. 6)
- Calculate fluid and electrolyte requirements: maintenance, deficit (Table 7-3), and ongoing losses (Table 7-4)
- Subtract resuscitation fluid volume and electrolytes from calculated

Table 7-3   Practical Approach to Correction of Fluid and Electrolyte Deficits

		Deficit	
Type	Component	5%	10%
Isotonic	Water	50 ml/kg	100 ml/kg
	Na	4-5 mmol/kg	8-10 mmol/kg
	K	2-3 mmol/kg	4-5 mmol/kg
	Suggested solution*: 3.33% dextrose and 0.33% saline with 20 mmol/L KCl		
Hypotonic	Water	50 ml/kg	100 ml/kg
	Na	5-6 mmol/kg	10-12 mmol/kg
	K	3 mmol/kg	5 mmol/kg
	Suggested solution*: 5% dextrose and 0.45% saline with 20 mmol/L KCl		
Hypertonic	Water	50 ml/kg	100 ml/kg
	Na	2-4 mmol/kg	2-4 mmol/kg
	K	2-4 mmol/kg	2-4 mmol/kg
	Suggested solution*: 5% dextrose and 0.2% saline with 40 mmol KCl/L, or 5% dextrose and 0.45% saline with 40 mmol/L KCl (once urine output established) and adjust based on serum sodium		

*Suggested solutions most closely approximate ideal solution to correct both fluid and electrolyte deficits; can also be calculated, see examples.

Table 7-4   Approximate Electrolyte Composition of Gastrointestinal Fluids

	mmol (mEq)/L				
Fluid	H^+	Na^+	K^+	Cl	HCO_3
Gastric	80	40 (20-80)	20 (5-20)	150 (100-150)	0
Small intestinal	0	130 (100-140)	20 (5-25)	120 (100-130)	30
Pancreatic	0	135 (120-140)	15 (5-15)	100 (90-120)	50
Diarrheal	0	40 (10-90)	40 (10-80)	40 (10-110)	40

- For NG or vomiting losses use 0.45% saline with 20 mEq/L KCl as replacement fluid.
- For diarrhea losses alone use D5W with 40 mEq/L KCl and 40 mEq/L $NaHCO_3$ as replacement fluid.
- Adjust replacement fluids according to reassessed blood electrolye values.

Table 7-5   Composition of Some Common Parenteral Solutions
            (mmol or mEq/L)

Solution	Na$^+$	K$^+$	Cl$^-$	HCO$_3$*	Comments
Isotonic (0.9%) NaCl (normal saline)	154		154		
Hypertonic (3%) NaCl	513		513		
3.33% Dextrose and 0.33% NaCl (⅔:⅓)	51		51		Contains 33.3g/L dextrose; useful maintenance and replacement fluid for Na$^+$
5% Dextrose + 0.2% NaCl (D5: 0.2)	34		34		Contains 50 g/L dextrose; useful Na$^+$ maintenance fluid
8.4% NaHCO$_3$ (1 mmol [mEq/ml]	1000			1000	1 mmol of Na$^+$ and bicarbonate/ml
Lactated Ringer's	130	4	109	28	Calcium 1.5 mmol/L
½ normal saline (0.45%)	77		77		
5% Dextrose (D$_5$W)					50 g/L dextrose

*Bicarbonate or potential bicarbonate.

24-hr fluid requirement, or reassess degree of dehydration and electrolyte disturbances after initial resuscitation
- Correct metabolic acidosis with NaHCO$_3$ if pH ≤ 7.2 or HCO$_3$ < 12 mEq/L; rehydration alone may correct acidosis if pH > 7.2 (see p. 109)
- First 8 hr (repletion phase: replacement of extracellular deficits): give maintenance fluids plus 50% of calculated deficit plus replace ongoing losses (see following section)
- Next 16 hr (recovery phase: replacement of intracellular deficits): continue maintenance fluids and replacement of ongoing losses, and replace remaining 50% of calculated deficit (see following section)
- Hold potassium replacement until patient voids and/or if renal disease present; replace potassium over 2 days
- Monitor fluid, electrolyte, and acid-base status frequently, especially in hypernatremia
- See Table 7-5 for composition of common parenteral solutions

SPECIFIC APPROACH TO CORRECTION OF FLUID AND ELECTROLYTE DEFICITS (see Table 7-3)

Isotonic Dehydration
- See Example 7-1

Hypotonic Dehydration (Fig. 7-1, Example 7-2)
- In addition to correction of volume deficit, correct hyponatremia to isotonic state using Table 7-3 (estimate), or calculate exact deficit:

[Na$^+$]$_{deficit}$ = ([Na$^+$]$_{desired}$ − [Na$^+$]$_{actual}$) × body wt (kg) × total body water (L/kg)

EXAMPLE 7-1 Isotonic Dehydration

12-kg child, 10% dehydrated, Na=135
Given 240 ml normal saline bolus
Ongoing diarrheal losses

Requirements	H_2O	Na	K
Maintenance	1100 ml	24-36 mmol	24-36 mmol
Deficit	1200 ml	96-120 mmol	48-60 (give half)
Ongoing losses	replace losses 1:1 with D5W with added KCl 40 mEq/L and $NaHCO_3$ 40 mEq/L		
	2300	≈ 138 (120-156)	48-66
	−240	−37	
	2060	101	≈ 57

The IV solution should contain 101 mmol Na^+ and 57 mmol of K^+ in 2060 ml (or 49 mmol Na^+/L and 28 mmol of K^+/L); ⅔:⅓ or D5:0.45 saline with 20 mEq/L KCl closely matches these needs; run at 129 ml/hr for 8 hr, then 64 ml/hr for 16 hr.

EXAMPLE 7-2 Hypotonic Dehydration

12 kg child, 10% dehydrated, Na = 110
Given 240 ml normal saline bolus

Requirements	H_2O	Na	K
Maintenance	1100 ml	24-36 mmol	24-36 mmol
Deficit	1200 ml	20 × 12 × 0.65 = 156 mmol	60 mmol (give half)
Ongoing losses	nil		
	2300	≈ 186 (180-192)	54-66
	−240	−37	
	2060	149	≈ 60

The IV solution should contain 149 mmol Na^+ and 60 mmol K^+ in 2060 ml (or 72 mmol Na^+/L and 29 mmol K^+/L); D5:0.45 saline with 20 mEq/L KCl closely matches these needs; run at 129 ml/hr for 8 hr then 64 ml/hr for 16 hrs.

if [Na] ≥ 105 mmol/L: correct to 125-130 mmol/L as desired Na^+
if [Na] < 105 mmol/L: correct by 20 mmol/L maximum
- When deficit known, correct by ~ 50% over first 8 hr and remainder over next 16 hr; knowing Na^+ deficit and fluid deficit, select appropriate Na^+-containing fluid (generally, 5% dextrose and 0.45% saline with 20 mmol/L KCl)
- Rate of rise of Na should not exceed 2-4 mmol/L q4h or 20 mmol/L/24 hr
- For symptomatic hyponatremia (seizures), correct serum sodium to 125 mmol/L over 0.5-4 hr, that is, (125 − measured [Na^+] × body wt × total body water) to calculate deficit; use hypertonic saline 3%-5% (3% = 0.5 mmol/ml, 5% = 0.855 mmol/ml)

Hypertonic Dehydration (Fig. 7-2, Example 7-3)

- Clinical evaluation of dehydration can be difficult; look for doughy or velvety skin and CNS disturbances, especially irritability; minimal signs of intravascular volume depletion

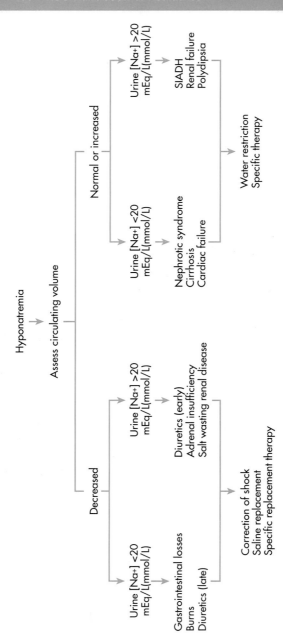

Fig. 7-1 Differential diagnosis of hyponatremia and approach to therapy. Hyponatremia can also be factitious, as in hyperlipidemia (caused by measurement techniques in some labs) or hyperglycemia (for every elevation of glucose 5.5 mmol/L above baseline of 5 mmol/L, Na^+ will decrease by 1.6 mmol/L.) (From Perkin RM, Lewin DL: *Pediatr Clin North Am* 27:573, 1980.)

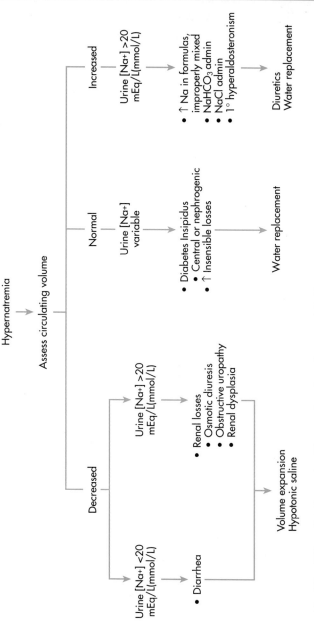

Fig. 7-2 Differential diagnosis of hypernatremia and approach to therapy.

EXAMPLE 7-3   Hypertonic Dehydration

12-kg child, Na = 150
Given 240 ml normal saline bolus

Requirements	H_2O	Na^+	K
Maintenance 75%	825 ml	24-36 mmol	24-36 mmol
Deficit	40* × 12 = 480ml	24-48 mmol	24-48 mmol (give half)
Ongoing losses	nil	nil	nil
	1305	≈ 66 (48-84)	36-60
	−240	−37	
	1065	29	≈ 48

The IV solution should contain 29 mmol Na^+ and 48 mmol of K^+ in 1065 ml (or 24 mmol Na/L and 45 mmol of K^+/L); D5:0.2 saline with 40 mEq/L KCl closely matches these needs; run at 44 ml/hr.

*Using rule of thumb (see text).

- Occurs with increased Na (boiled milk feeds) or, more commonly, decreased free water (diabetes insipidus, high fever, or in infants or handicapped children who have no access to free water)
- Avoid rapid rehydration because of risk of cerebral edema and seizures (correct fluid deficit over 48-72 hr, depending on degree of hypernatremia)
- Restore circulating volume and urinary output as priority
- Lower serum sodium by 10-15 mmol/L/day maximum
- Calculate water deficit to be replaced so as to lower serum sodium by predictable amount:

$$H_2O = [(Na^+ \text{ actual} - Na^+ \text{ desired})/Na^+ \text{ desired}]$$
$$\times \text{ total body water (L/kg)}$$

- Or use rule of thumb: 4 ml/kg of free water lowers serum sodium by 1 mmol/L (i.e., 40 ml/kg H_2O lowers Na^+ 1O mmol/L)
- Fluids for 24 hr = 75% maintenance (due to risk of SIADH) + water deficit + ongoing losses; subtract Na^+ of resuscitation fluid in calculations
- Avoid use of insulin for hyperglycemia as this rapidly lowers extracellular osmolality and may cause cerebral edema
- For jitteriness: monitor rate of fall of $[Na^+]$, check $[Ca^{2+}]$ and glucose; monitor CNS status (e.g., subdural hematoma with hypertonic state)
- If Na^+ drops too quickly, treat water intoxication with 3% NaCl 4-6 ml/kg over 30 min-1 hr

Salt Poisoning

- Serum $[Na^+] > 200$ mmol/L may occur, with increase in total body load of sodium
- If [Na] > 180 or renal function poor, dialysis may be necessary
- Furosemide 1 mg/kg, while replacing urine output with 5%-10% dextrose, can be used when renal function good and electrolytes properly monitored

Hypokalemia

- Serum $[K^+] < 3$ mmol/L
- Causes include poor intake (e.g., TPN) or excess losses (vomiting, diarrhea, NG suction, diuretics, renal tubular acidosis, Fanconi syndrome, increased renin, increased mineralocorticoid)
- Clinical features include weakness, hyporeflexia, paresthesia, ileus, polyuria, polydipsia, dysrhythmias, low amplitude T waves, ST depression, and U waves (see p. 61)
- Investigations should include ECG, electrolytes, urinalysis, urine electrolytes, osmolality, and creatinine
- Cardiac monitor if $[K^+] < 3$ or patient receiving digoxin (see p. 69)
- Ensure intake of maintenance potassium; replace ongoing losses (e.g., prophylactic supplementation for patients receiving diuretic therapy)
- Replace potassium deficits (difficult to estimate as potassium is intracellular)
- Maximum potassium concentration in peripheral IV = 40 mmol/L; for concentrations of 60-80 mmol/L or greater, use CVL and ECG monitoring; maximum rate = 0.5 mmol/kg/hr

Hyperkalemia

- Serum $[K^+] > 6.5$ mmol/L in infant or > 5.5 mmol/L in child
- Causes include increased extracellular potassium (cell breakdown, metabolic acidosis) or decreased excretion of potassium (renal failure, hypoaldosteronism)
- See p. 24 regarding recognition and treatment
- See p. 314 regarding transtubular potassium gradient (TTKG), a measurement of aldosterone activity

ACID-BASE DISORDERS

- Normal pH = 7.38-7.42
- Vital organ dysfunction occurs at pH < 7.1 or > 7.6
- Measure serum pH, pCO_2, HCO_3, and electrolytes
- For acidosis, calculate unmeasured anion gap: $Na^+ - (Cl^- + HCO_3)$
  Normal value = 12 ± 4.

Metabolic Acidosis (Fig. 7-3)

- Treat if pH < 7.2 or $[HCO_3] < 12$ mmol/L
- Calculate bicarbonate deficit (mmol)

$$\text{bicarbonate deficit} = (\text{desired } HCO_3 - \text{actual } HCO_3)$$
$$\times \text{ body weight (kg)} \times 0.6$$

(for desired HCO_3 use 18-24 mmol/L depending on age)
or
< 5 kg: (base excess $\times$ wt $\times$ 0.05) mmol
> 5 kg: (base excess $\times$ wt $\times$ 0.03) mmol

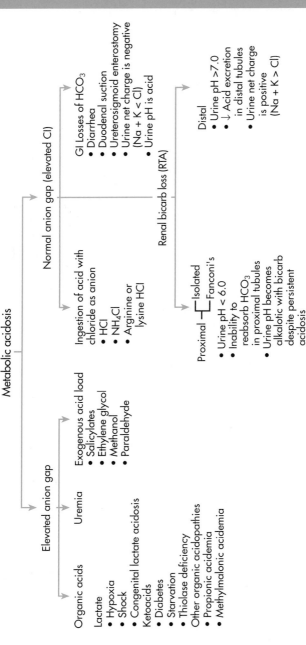

Fig. 7-3   Differential diagnosis of metabolic acidosis.

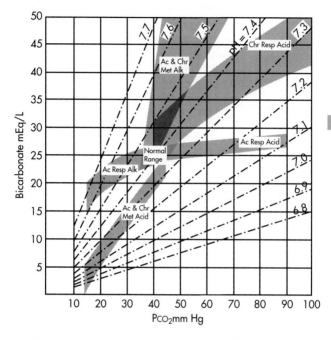

Fig. 7-4 **An in vivo acid-base nomogram for clinical use.** Usually acid-base values falling within a shaded band indicate a single disturbance. Occasionally they may indicate a mixed disturbance. Acid-base values falling outside shaded bands indicate there are at least two acid-base disturbances. (From Arbus GS: *Can Med Assoc J* 109:291, 1973.)

Table 7-6 Common Patterns of Blood Gas Abnormality

	HCO$_3$	pCO$_2$
Metabolic acidosis	↓ 1 mmol/L	↓ 1 mm Hg
Metabolic alkalosis	↑ 1 mmol/L	↑ 0.7 mm Hg

	pCO$_2$	HCO$_3$
Respiratory acidosis		
• Acute	↑ 1 mm Hg	↑ 0.1 mmol/L
• Chronic	↑ 1 mm Hg	↑ 0.4 mmol/L
Respiratory alkalosis		
• Acute	↓ 1 mm Hg	↓ 0.2 mmol/L
• Chronic	↓ 1 mm Hg	↓ 0.5 mmol/L

- Give half calculated bicarbonate deficit over 2-4 hr, then reassess (bolus with 1 mmol/kg bicarbonate IV over 15-30 min, then remainder over 1.5-3.5 hr)

Blood Gas Interpretation (Fig. 7-4, Table 7-6)

- Check pH: acidic or alkalotic
- Check pCO_2: elevated (resp. acidosis), normal or low (resp. alkalosis)
- Check HCO_3 (and base excess): elevated (met. alkalosis), normal, or low (met. acidosis)
- Even with chronic compensations, pH will never return completely to normal

CHAPTER 8

GASTROENTEROLOGY

MARIA SANDE-LEMOS AZCUE

DIARRHEA (Fig. 8-1).

ACUTE DIARRHEA

- Most commonly due to enteric infection

Investigations

- History and physical examination, assess degree of dehydration (see p. 100)
- Rectal examination for stool consistency, fecal leukocytes (microscopy)
- Stool for bacterial cultures, virology (electron microscopy and cultures), ova and parasites. *Clostridium difficile* toxin identification must be specifically requested
- Blood tests (if severe): CBC, differential, electrolytes, blood gases, urea, creatinine, ± blood culture, urine culture, *Yersinia* titer

Management

- Prevention and treatment of dehydration most important: replacement of fluid deficit + maintenance + ongoing losses (see p. 100)
- Antibiotic therapy for specific organisms and systemic infection when present
- Oral rehydration therapy (small frequent volumes if vomiting); Pedialyte approximates fecal losses in most common infections. Note: vomiting is not contraindication to oral rehydration therapy; usually transient and overcome by giving small volumes frequently (e.g., 15 to 30 ml q30min)
- IV required for moderate to severe dehydration (see p. 100)
- Early refeeding advisable
  1. Continue breast-feeding when possible
  2. Allow child to eat solids as soon as tolerated and appetite has returned; most solids are acceptable; sugar-containing foods and drinks should be avoided initially
  3. Transient lactose intolerance may occur secondary to villous damage; avoidance of lactose-containing formulas and foods *may* be required for 48-72 hr
- Antidiarrheal medications not indicated
- Specific therapy:
  C. difficile
    Metronidazole, vancomycin
  Campylobacter
    Erythromycin
  Shigella
    Amoxicillin, trimethoprim-sulfamethoxazole (sensitivities may vary)

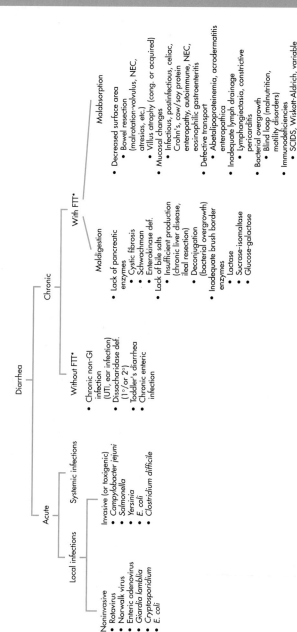

Fig 8-1   Differential diagnosis of acute and chronic diarrhea.
*Failure to thrive.

Diarrhea

Acute

Local infections

Noninvasive
• Rotavirus
• Norwalk virus
• Enteric adenovirus
• Giardia lamblia
• Cryptosporidium
• E. coli

Systemic infections

Invasive (or toxigenic)
• Campylobacter jejuni
• Salmonella
• Yersinia
• E. coli
• Clostridium difficile

Chronic

Without FTT*
• Chronic non-GI infection (UTI, ear infection)
• Dissacharidase def. (1° or 2°)
• Toddler's diarrhea
• Chronic enteric infection

With FTT*

Maldigestion
• Lack of pancreatic enzymes
  • Cystic fibrosis
  • Schwachman
  • Enterokinase def.
• Lack of bile salts
  • Insufficient production (chronic liver disease, ileal resection)
  • Deconjugation (bacterial overgrowth)
• Inadequate brush border enzymes
  • Lactase
  • Sucrase-isomaltase
  • Glucose-galactose

Malabsorption
• Decreased surface area
  • Bowel resection (malrotation-volvulus, NEC, atresias, etc.)
  • Villus atrophy (cong. or acquired)
• Mucosal changes
  • Infectious, postinfectious, celiac, Crohn's, cow/soy protein enteropathy, autoimmune, NEC, eosinophilic gastroenteritis
• Defective transport
  • Abetalipoproteinemia, acrodermatitis enteropathica
• Inadequate lymph drainage
  • Lymphangiectasia, constrictive pericarditis
• Bacterial overgrowth
  • Blind loop (malnutrition, motility disorders)
• Immunodeficiencies
  • SCIDS, Wiskott-Aldrich, variable hypogamm, DiGeorge, AIDS
• Neoplasms (pheo, neuroblastoma)
• Other (laxatives, heavy metal poisoning)

Giardia lamblia
   Metronidazole, furazolidone
Yersinia
   Trimethoprim-sulfamethoxazole, chloramphenicol, tetracycline (age >
   9 yr)

CHRONIC DIARRHEA

- Diarrhea lasting more than 14 days

Investigations

- Serial heights and weights, growth percentiles; note that with nonspecific diarrhea of infancy, child is growing well and thriving
- Nature of stool also helpful: watery versus bulky versus bloody
- *Without failure to thrive,* consider giardia, disaccharidase deficiency, "Toddler's diarrhea"
- *With failure to thrive,* consider malabsorption conditions (see the following discussion)

Management

- Most otherwise healthy children require minimal diagnostic work-ups
- Nonspecific diarrhea of infancy (Toddler's diarrhea) is most common diagnosis in children from 6 mo to 3 yr; often begins after acute gastroenteritis; requires no specific therapy (avoiding high sorbitol-containing fruit juices (e.g., apple juice) helps; avoid elimination diets; stools will form by 3 yr or when toilet trained
- Children with pathologic chronic diarrhea may require electrolyte and water replacement; critical to consider protein, calorie, and other nutrient requirements (e.g., postinfectious diarrhea is most common cause of this group of disorders and although requires no specific therapy, adequate protein and calorie replacement factors most in recovery)
- Specific therapy may be required for other etiologies

MALABSORPTION

- Implies generalized malabsorption of fat, protein, ± carbohydrates
- Suspect if poor weight gain or falling-off growth curves, ± chronic diarrhea
- Assess caloric intake
- Think of causative disease entities in terms of intestinal, pancreatic, and biliary

Investigations

- Rectal examination for stool consistency, pH, reducing substances; microscopy for fecal leukocytes, fat crystals or globules, blood (visible or occult)
- Urinalysis
- Stool collection (multiple samples): ova and parasites, cultures, *C. difficile* toxin, 3-day fecal fat, α-1-antitrypsin clearance, electrolytes; alkalinization: pink color indicates phenolphthalein (present in some laxatives)
- CBC, differential, ESR, smear, electrolytes, total protein, albumin, immunoglobulins

- Biochemical assessment of absorptive and nutritional status: albumin, Ca^{2+}, PO_4, Mg, Zn, iron, ferritin, folate, fat-soluble vitamins, PT, PTT; if warranted, consider liver function tests, cholesterol, triglycerides, trypsinogen
- If indicated, thyroid function tests, urine VMA and HVA, HIV testing, lead levels
- Radiologic examinations: upper GI series $\pm$ follow-through to evaluate for inflammatory lesions of bowel
- Specialized tests:
  1. Small bowel biopsy $\pm$ aspiration
  2. Upper and lower GI tract endoscopy and biopsy
  3. Quantitative exocrine pancreatic testing

PROTEIN-LOSING ENTEROPATHY

- General term that describes hypoproteinemia secondary to gastrointestinal protein leakage; suspect in child with edema, hypoproteinemia, but no proteinuria
- Confirmation by fecal α-1-antitrypsin clearance
- Common causes: milk-soy protein intolerance, celiac disease, inflammatory bowel disease; less common: malrotation, Hirschsprung's disease, Ménétrier's disease, Henoch Schönlein Purpura (HSP), lymphangiectasia, Congestive heart failure (CHF), restrictive pericarditis, eosinophilic gastroenteritis
- Cow's milk protein intolerance most common; classic presentation: infant 10-18 mo with edema, hypoalbuminemia, and iron deficiency anemia; responds promptly to removal of antigenic protein; site of intestinal lesion not always identifiable; 50% also react to soy protein; most children tolerate cow's milk by 2 yr; may have peripheral eosinophilia; IgE and RAST usually normal; younger infants (2-4 mo) more often present with proctocolitis (even if breast-fed with mother on dairy/soy products)
- Investigations include urinalysis, α-1-antitrypsin clearance, CBC, smear, WBC and differential, ESR, albumin, globulins, Fe studies
- Cow's milk protein intolerance should not be confused with lactose intolerance, which is result of mucosal lactase deficiency

INFLAMMATORY BOWEL DISEASE (IBD)

- Chronic inflammation in GI tract in absence of detectable pathogenic agent
- Initial assessment aimed at distinguishing Crohn's disease from ulcerative colitis (UC) and assessing extent of disease

Pathological Distinction

Crohn's disease	UC
• Any part of GI tract	• Colon only
• Segmental disease with skip lesions	• Continuous disease, worse distally
• Transmural inflammation	• Mucosal inflammation
• Granulomas present	• Crypt abscess common

Differential Diagnosis

- Infections
  - Usually self-limited but must be considered in the first 4-6 wk after onset of symptoms:
    C. jejuni, Yersinia, Entamoeba histolytica, Salmonella, Shigella, C. difficile
- Henoch-Schönlein purpura (HSP)
- Hemolytic uremic syndrome (HUS)
- Eosinophilic gastroenteritis
- Allergic colitis, necrotizing enterocolitis, Hirschsprung's disease
- Behçet's disease

CROHN'S DISEASE

- Rarely manifests before age 5 yr; mean age of onset with pediatric population 12 years, 18%-30% present before age 20 yr
- Genetic predisposition: around 25% positive family history
- Major presenting features: recurrent abdominal pain (most common single presenting symptom), anorexia, diarrhea, weight loss, anemia, recurrent fever, growth retardation, pubertal delay, and perianal disease; extraintestinal manifestations include arthritis and arthralgias, mouth ulcers, erythema nodosum, uveitis, clubbing

Management (Table 8-1)

- Surgery: reserved for complications of Crohn's disease (obstruction, abscess); *not* curative but often necessary

ULCERATIVE COLITIS

- 5% of UC patients present before age 20 yr; does occur in very young children
- More uniform clinical presentation: bloody diarrhea (most common sign) ± urgency, tenesmus, abdominal pain, weight loss; extraintestinal manifestations similar to Crohn's disease
- 60% β-ANCA positive

Management (see Table 8-1)

- Mild disease may require 5-ASA PO ± distal treatment
- Moderate disease requires prednisone
- Severe disease requires hospitalization; NPO and IV steroids
- In severe pancolitis, 50% will not respond to medical treatment; monitor for toxic megacolon (physical exam, electrolytes, plain abdominal x-rays); if toxic megacolon suspected, barium enema studies and morphine-derivative analgesics are contraindicated
- Colectomy if not settled within 7-10 days (curative procedure)

PROGNOSIS FOR IBD

- Both diseases have relapsing course with exacerbations and remissions
- In more severe forms, disease activity is continuous and chronic; colectomy is curative for UC, whereas resection for Crohn's disease, while necessary, is never curative
- Cancer risk increases in both diseases after 8-yr duration of disease; an-

Table 8-1 Pharmacologic Treatment of Inflammatory Bowel Disease

	Treatment of active disease	Maintenance of remission
Ulcerative colitis (enemas intended for distal disease or as adjuncts in more extensive disease)	Sulfasalazine (50-75 mg/kg/day up to 3-4 g daily) Oral 5-ASA* (50-60 mg/kg/day up to 4 g daily) Corticosteroids (Prednisone 1 mg/kg/day up to 40-60 mg daily) (IV hydrocortisone 4 mg/kg/day for acute severe disease) 5-ASA enemas (4 g nightly or bid) Hydrocortisone/budesonide enemas	Sulfasalazine (50 mg/kg/day up to 3 g daily) Oral 5-ASA (50 mg/kg/day up to 3 g daily) 5-ASA enemas (2g/4g) nightly or every other night
Crohn's disease Small bowel only	Corticosteroids (1mg/kg/day up to 40-60 mg/day prednisone) Oral 5-ASA (Pentasa or Salofalk most suitable) (60 mg/kg/day up to 4 g/day) 6MP† (1.5 mg/kg/day)‡ Azathioprine (2 mg/kg/day)‡	Oral 5-ASA 6MP/azathioprine (same dose as active disease)
Colon only	Sulfasalazine Oral 5-ASA Metronidazole (10-20 mg/kg/day up to 1 g daily) Corticosteroids ?5-ASA enemas§ 6MP/azathioprine‡	?Sulfasalazine Oral 5-ASA 6MP/azathioprine
Ileocolonic	Same as for small bowel and colon	Same as for small bowel and colon
Perianal	Metronidazole (10-20 mg/kg/day) 6MP/azathioprine‡	Metronidazole (10-20 mg/kg/day)

*5-ASA = 5-aminosalicylic acid.
†6MP = 6-mercaptopurine.
‡Delayed onset of action.
§Not subjected to controlled clinical trial.
(From Griffiths, A: Inflammatory bowel disease, *Adolesc Med* 6(3):359, 1995.)

nual surveillance colonoscopy with biopsy for dysplasia recommended for patients with UC; recommendation for Crohn's disease less clear

RECURRENT ABDOMINAL PAIN (RAP)

DEFINITION

- Three or more attacks of abdominal pain severe enough to affect normal activities over at least a 3-mo period
- Common in children 5-15 yr
- More than 90% no organic cause found, labeled RAP or psychophysiologic pain
- Features suggesting organic causes (red flags):
  Age < 5 yr
  Location other than periumbilical
  Night pain, night awakening
  Vomiting, diarrhea, weight loss
- Features suggesting RAP:
  Vague, variable, periumbilical pain
  Often other somatic complaints (headache, limb pain)
  General appearance of good health
  School absenteeism

Management

- All patients deserve full history, thorough physical exam
- CBC, differential, ESR, urinalysis, stool for occult blood, further tests only as specifically indicated
- Should proceed to explanation, reassurance; avoid overinvestigation
- Conditions that may masquerade as RAP: IBD, intestinal obstruction (malrotation with intermittent volvulus), recurrent pancreatitis, Peptic ulcer disease, lactose intolerance, constipation

VOMITING (Fig. 8-2)

- Causes often nongastrointestinal
- Look for evidence of bile or blood (visible, occult) in vomitus

Investigations

- Urinalysis, microscopy, ± culture
- CBC, differential, ESR, electrolytes, blood gases, urea, creatinine
- Radiologic investigations, other GI procedures if indicated

Management

- Prevention and treatment of dehydration and electrolyte imbalance (see p. 100)
- Antiemetic medications should be used with caution: rule out surgical causes of vomiting
- Bowel rest (depends on cause)
- Always consider mechanical obstruction (intermittent, persistent)

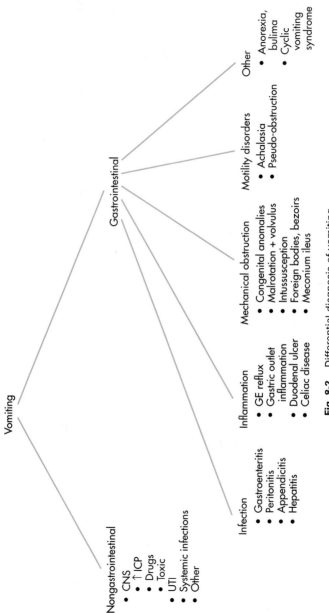

Fig. 8-2 Differential diagnosis of vomiting.

GASTROESOPHAGEAL REFLUX (GER)

- Benign GER extremely common in infancy; requires no investigation on thriving baby
- Following is indicative of pathologic reflux, requiring investigation/intervention:
  1. Failure to thrive
  2. Recurrent pneumonia, bronchospasm
  3. GI blood loss

Investigations

- Upper endoscopy and esophageal biopsies for suspected esophagitis
- 24 hr pH probe when presence of GER not obvious clinically or to assess efficacy of antireflux therapy
- UGI to rule out anatomic causes; not reliable to document reflux

Management

- Conservative therapy: small, frequent feeds; thickened feeds; positioning prone at 45 degrees during sleep and postfeeding
- Medical therapy: short-term enteral feedings to enhance weight gain; proton-pump inhibitor (omeprazole) or H_2 blockers indicated when esophagitis present; prokinetics (domperidone, cisapride) may also be indicated
- Surgical therapy: indicated for failure of medical therapy

GASTROINTESTINAL BLEEDING (Fig. 8-3)

UPPER GI BLEEDING
Investigations

- Physical exam: hemodynamic status, evidence of oropharyngeal bleeding or chronic liver disease (splenomegaly, spider nevi, ascites, jaundice)
- Nasogastric aspirate: test for blood (Note: gastric acid may interfere with Hemoccult testing), pH, Apt test in newborn (distinguishes maternal from fetal red blood cells [RBC])
- CBC, hematocrit, smear, platelets, PT, PTT, urea, creatinine, urinalysis; liver function tests if indicated. Follow CBC, reticulocytes

Management

- Acute stabilization
  1. ABCs (see p. 2)
  2. Reclining at 45° angle
  3. Vitamin K, 5-10 mg IV (if suspected liver disease)
  4. Volume and blood replacement (urgent cross-matching for adequate volumes)
  5. NG saline lavage (omit if source known to be esophageal varices)
  6. H_2 blocker (ranitidine IV), proton-pump inhibitor (omeprazole IV)

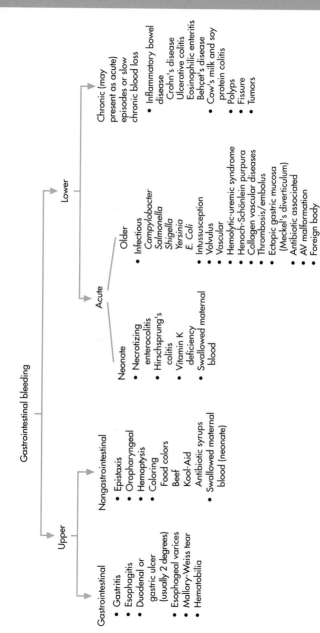

Fig. 8-3   Causes of GI bleeding.

- Once stabilized: diagnostic endoscopy; radiologic examinations of little benefit
- If continues unstable
  1. Vasopressin 0.2-0.3 U/kg/dose IV over 20 min; repeat in 1-2 hr if bleeding continues
  2. Intervention endoscopy, balloon tamponade, angiography with embolization, surgery

LOWER GI BLEEDING
Investigations

- Differential diagnosis of black stools: iron, bismuth, spinach
- Physical exam: hemodynamic status, evidence of growth failure, fevers
- Anal and rectal examination: tags, fissures, anal fistulas, polyps, trauma, foreign bodies, blood (visible, occult), stool appearance (gross blood, streaking), and microscopy for leukocytes
- Nasogastric aspirate: upper GI bleed may present as melena or hematochezia
- Stool cultures, *C. difficile* toxin, urinalysis, and microscopy
- CBC, smear, differential, platelets, ESR, electrolytes, urea, creatinine, PT, PTT, Apt test (newborn), albumin, iron studies, amoeba titers
- Radiologic investigations: plain abdominal x-rays to rule out obstruction
- Specialized tests according to suspected diagnosis
  1. Ultrasound (US)
  2. Air enema
  3. Diagnostic endoscopy ± biopsy
  4. Meckel's scan
  5. Angiography
  6. ^{99}Tc RBC scan

Management

- Acute stabilization
  1. ABCc (see p. 2)
  2. Volume and blood replacement
  3. Bowel rest: npo, nasogastric tube to suction
- If continued instability:
  1. Angiography with embolization
  2. Surgery

PEPTIC ULCER DISEASE (PUD)

- May be present in children and teenagers, common when secondary to systemic illness (shock, sepsis, burns) or drugs (aspirin, NSAIDs)
- Primary duodenal ulcer: almost always *H. pylori* positive; consider ampicillin, bismuth, Flagyl, omeprazole × 14 days; if *H. pylori* negative: ranitidine 6-8 wk
- *H. pylori* not associated with secondary PUD

CONSTIPATION

- Infrequent passage of hard stools with difficulty
- Usually functional ($> 95\%$)
- Most children have voluntary retention-type constipation and require minimal investigation; consider further investigation in patients with onset at < 3 mo of age and nonresponders to conventional treatment; check urine to exclude UTI, which can complicate chronic constipation
- Consider hypothyroidism, neurogenic bowel (spinal dysraphism, tethered cord), abnormal motility (Hirschsprung's disease, pseudoobstruction), polyuric states with chronic dehydration

Management

- Education: toilet training, regular attempts just after meals, proper position (hips flexed, feet flat; may need support for feet)
- Diet: increased fiber and fluids
- Initial evacuation in chronic encopretic children: enemas (saline or hypertonic phosphate, 10 ml/kg) or GI lavage: Peglyte electrolyte solution
- Maintenance: mineral oil, 15 ml/15 kg, increase by 1 tsp every 3 days until oil is leaking from anus; continue 4-6 mo before weaning; avoid use in infants < 1yr and neurologically impaired because of risk of aspiration; lactulose is alternative
- No role for irritative suppositories or prokinetic agents for voluntary retention

ACUTE PANCREATITIS (Box 8-1)

- Presents as abdominal pain lasting hours, usually with vomiting; pain characteristics not as precise as in adults; serum amylase usually but not always elevated
- US usually diagnostic

Management

- Acute: NPO; analgesia, NG suction, IV calcium supplements as required
- Increased amylase found in pancreatitis, pancreatic pseudocyst, parotitis, biliary tract disease, duodenal ulcer, burns, and stress

EXOCRINE PANCREATIC INSUFFICIENCY

- Causes: CF, Schwachman syndrome, Johanson-Blizzard, protein-calorie malnutrition, chronic pancreatitis

Management

- Treat underlying cause as appropriate
- High-energy, high-fat diet
- Pancreatic enzyme supplement in quantity sufficient to normalize stools;

BOX 8-1   Etiology of Acute Pancreatitis

Trauma
Infection
- Virus: mumps, coxsackie B, EBV, hepatitis A, influenza A
- Bacteria: mycoplasma
- Parasites: malaria

Drugs: multiple (Lasix, steroids, Imuran)
Obstruction
- Gallstones
- Choledocal cyst
- Pancreas divisum
- Sclerosing cholangitis

Systemic diseases
- Cystic fibrosis (pancreatic sufficient)
- IBD
- Vasculitis (HSP, SLE)
- Hyperparathyroidism, hypercalcemia
- Hyperlipoproteinemia I, IV

Idiopathic

8

too much supplement may result in tenesmus and colonic strictures in CF
- Fat-soluble vitamin supplements

GI TESTS

BIOCHEMICAL (transport, surface area)
Fat

- Gold standard: 3-day fecal fat, with careful records of dietary fat intake; newborn period nonabsorbed fat is 10%-15%. Adult normal up to 7%
- Stool microscopy: fat globules with black or red Sudan; useful screening test for pancreatic exocrine insufficiency (positive only if being fed)
- Serum carotene: from enteral ingestion of carotene (not in formula); low in fat malabsorption but poor sensitivity and specificity

Carbohydrates

- Stool for reducing substances (Clinitest): detects most dietary sugars, except sucrose, if malabsorbed
- Stool pH: usually pH < 6 if carbohydrate intolerant (organic acids produced by bacterial breakdown of nonabsorbed sugar)
- Breath hydrogen test: hydrogen concentration in expired air after enteral dose of sugar (2g/kg, max 50 g); rise in breath hydrogen > 20 ppm in 2 hr is abnormal; patients on antibiotics and small percentage of population do not have hydrogen-producing flora
- D-xylose test: monosaccharide (pentose) absorption in duodenum and jejunum, minimal metabolism, excreted in urine (concentration in urine depends on absorption): some false positives and negatives

Protein

- α-1-antitrypsin clearance: enteric protein loss in 24 hr
- > 25 ml/day is abnormal

Vitamins

- Vitamin A, D, E, K absorption dependent on intake and fat absorption
- B_{12} absorption: Schilling test
- Folate in serum

PANCREATIC FUNCTION TESTS

- Double lumen tube in duodenum, IV infusion of secretin and CCK: measurement of HCO_3, water content, enzyme activity (trypsin, lipase, colipase)
- Serum trypsinogen increased in newborn with CF; with pancreatic damage, levels decrease to below normal
- Bentiromide: synthetic tripeptide; oral bentiromide is cleaved by chymotrypsin, releasing PABA, which is then absorbed; measurement of serum PABA at 90 min
- Breath tests: carbon-labeled triolein taken orally; digested by pancreatic lipase with release of labeled CO_2.

CHAPTER 9

GENETICS

SHEILA UNGER

APPROACH TO CHILD WITH MULTIPLE CONGENITAL ABNORMALITIES OR MENTAL RETARDATION AND DYSMORPHISM

PHYSICAL EXAM

- Diagnosis of syndromes is based on pattern of dysmorphic features and organ involvement; following is outline of dysmorphologic exam
- Growth parameters (e.g., microcephaly in fetal alcohol syndrome, overgrowth in Beckwith-Wiedemann syndrome)
- Skull (contour and symmetry) (e.g., tall, narrow skull caused by craniosynostosis in Apert's syndrome)
- Hair
  1. Texture (e.g., woolly hair of Noonan's syndrome)
  2. Pattern (> 1 whorl may reflect brain dysgenesis)
- Neck: redundant nuchal skin/webbed neck are thought to be result of fetal edema
- Facial gestalt (e.g., myopathic facies)
- Ears
  1. Structure (including pits and tags) (e.g., cup-shaped ears of CHARGE association)
  2. Size (e.g., large ears of fragile X syndrome)
  3. Placement and rotation (normally during fetal development, ears migrate upward and anteriorly; thus failure of this process will result in low-set posteriorly rotated ears)
- Eyes and adnexa
  1. Distance apart (e.g., hypotelorism of holoprosencephaly sequence)
  2. Orientation (e.g., upslanting palpebral fissures of trisomy 21)
  3. Eyebrows and eyelashes (e.g., synophrys and lush eyelashes of de Lange's syndrome; absence/hypoplasia in ectodermal dysplasias)
  4. Any folds or creases (e.g., epicanthal folds of trisomy 21)
  5. Coloboma (e.g., inferior coloboma of iris in cat-eye syndrome)
  6. Fundus (e.g., cherry red spot of Tay-Sachs disease)
- Nose
  1. Nasal bridge (e.g., low nasal bridge of achondroplasia)
  2. Nostrils (e.g., anteverted nostrils of Miller-Dieker syndrome)
- Philtrum (length and shape) (e.g., smooth philtrum of fetal alcohol syndrome)
- Mouth
  1. Lips
  2. Palate (e.g., submucous cleft palate of microdeletion 22)
  3. Teeth (e.g., missing in ectodermal dysplasia)
- Chin (e.g., retrognathia in Pierre Robin syndrome)

- Thorax
  1. Shape (e.g., pectus excavatum with inferior pectus carinatum of Noonan's syndrome)
  2. Size (e.g., small size/bell shape in lethal skeletal dysplasias)
  3. Nipple spacing
- Hands and feet
  1. Creases (e.g., single palmar crease of trisomy 21)
  2. Structure (including position, number of digits, syndactyly) (e.g., arachnodactyly of Marfan's syndrome)
  3. Nails (e.g., hyperconvex and/or deep-set nails of Turner's syndrome)
- Limbs
  1. Proportions (e.g., rhizomelic shortening in achondroplasia)
  2. Reduction defects (e.g., hypoplastic or aplastic radius in Fanconi anemia)
  3. Amputations (e.g., amniotic band sequence)
- Spine (e.g., scoliosis in Marfan's syndrome and other connective tissue diseases)
- Genitalia (e.g., ambiguous genitalia of Smith-Lemli-Opitz syndrome, congenital adrenal hyperplasia)
- Skin (e.g., café au lait spots in neurofibromatosis type 1)
- General physical examination (e.g., visceromegaly in Beckwith-Wiedemann syndrome, mucopolysaccharidoses, and other lysosomal storage disorders)

DIAGNOSTIC CATEGORIES

- Once anomalies are known, thorough differential diagnosis can be generated by considering various possible etiologies

Classic Mendelian Inheritance (traditional single-gene disorders)

- Autosomal dominant (e.g., tuberous sclerosis)
- Autosomal recessive (e.g., cystic fibrosis, β-thalassemia)
- X-linked recessive (e.g., Duchenne's muscular dystrophy)
- X-linked dominant (e.g., X-linked hypophosphatemic rickets)

Non-Mendelian Inheritance

1. Trinucleotide repeat expansions: group of disorders caused by unstable expansions of trinucleotide sequence (e.g., fragile X syndrome, Huntington's disease, myotonic dystrophy)
2. Mitochondrial diseases: Mitochondria have circular chromosome that contains several genes, most of which are involved in energy metabolism and mitochondrial structure; this genetic material is passed to offspring only from mother (maternal inheritance); consider mitochondrial disorders in cases of unusual neuromuscular diseases with encephalopathy and unexplained lactic acidosis (e.g., MELAS [mitochondrial encephalomyopathy, lactic acidoses, and strokelike episodes])
3. Genomic imprinting and uniparental disomy: Genomic imprinting refers to differential expression of genetic material depending on whether inherited from male or female parent; it explains why certain mutations at same gene locus may cause different effects (e.g., most Prader-Willi syndrome cases result from deletion of 15q11-q13 on paternally

inherited chromosome, but apparently identical deletions on maternally inherited chromosome 15 cause Angelman's syndrome); approximately 25% of Prader-Willi syndrome cases caused by inheritance of both chromosomes 15 from mother (i.e., uniparental disomy of chromosome 15)

Chromosomal Abnormalities

1. Aneuploidy (abnormal number of chromosomes): All trisomies, (e.g., 21, 13, 18); Klinefelter's syndrome 47, XXY; monosomy X (e.g., Turner's syndrome 45, X)
2. Unbalanced structural rearrangement (loss or gain of chromosomal material)
   a. Visible deletion (e.g., $5p^-$): Cri du chat syndrome (usually visible microscopically)
   b. Submicroscopic deletion (microdeletion) (e.g., del(22)(q11.2q11.2) has several phenotypic effects due to deletion of multiple genes on this chromosome) (e.g., conotruncal heart defect, cleft palate, and learning disability)
3. Apparently balanced structural rearrangements; this type of chromosomal change may or may not have phenotypic consequences; major types are Robertsonian translocations, reciprocal translocations, and inversions; carriers should get genetic counseling because they may be at risk of having unbalanced offspring
4. Other chromosomal: Chromosomal breakage syndromes (e.g., Fanconi anemia, which is actually single-gene disorder that has chromosomal effects)

MULTIFACTORIAL INHERITANCE

- Combination of genetic and nongenetic influences
- This category probably accounts for most common birth defects as well as majority of normal human traits; genetic predisposition probably related to multiple gene loci (multigenic); examples include neural tube defect, club foot, VSD

TERATOGENS

- Congenital infections (e.g., TORCH, varicella, parvovirus)
- Drugs (e.g., thalidomide, anticonvulsants [phenytoin], retinoic acid, warfarin, alcohol)
- Metabolic diseases (e.g., maternal diabetes, which has been associated with several birth defects, including congenital heart disease and caudal dysgenesis)

CHROMOSOME ANALYSIS

- Indicated for confirmation of clinical diagnosis or when chromosomal abnormality suspected (e.g., when two or more major congenital anomalies or one anomaly and developmental delay present); chromosome analysis can be done within a week on heparinized peripheral blood leukocytes; urgent cases should be discussed with geneticist; for additional information, or where mosaicism suspected, fibroblasts (cultured from skin biopsy tissue) or other tissue can be used; prenatal diagnosis by chromosomal analysis of amniocytes (amniocentesis) or chorionic villi (chorionic villus sample) is available

- Small deletions may be difficult to detect; if high index of suspicion exists for specific deletion syndromes, fluorescent in situ hybridization (FISH) technology should be considered; a small fluorescently labeled DNA probe, which will bind to its complementary sequence, is used to detect specific deletion (e.g., for microdeletion 22); only one fluorescent tag will be visible because probe can hybridize only with nondeleted chromosome 22; FISH must be ordered specifically from cytogenetics laboratory (e.g., 7q11 for Williams syndrome, 15q12 for Prader-Willi syndrome, 17p13 for Miller-Dieker syndrome, 22q11.2 for microdeletion 22); FISH is likely to have other clinical applications in near future

MOLECULAR DIAGNOSTICS

- More commonly ordered tests from molecular laboratory include mutation analysis for Duchenne's muscular dystrophy and cystic fibrosis; lab can also test for myotonic dystrophy and fragile X (both trinucleotide expansion disorders); if necessary, twin zygosity can be determined; for more information, a geneticist should be contacted

APPROACH TO DYING CHILD OR STILLBIRTH WITH SUSPECTED GENETIC SYNDROME OR INBORN ERROR OF METABOLISM (IEM)

- Every attempt should be made to make accurate diagnosis to enable accurate counseling; remember IEM even in cases of so-called sudden infant death syndrome (SIDS)
- Autopsy: Whenever possible, obtain consent after death for full postmortem examination or at least limited examination or biopsy of organs of interest as soon as possible
- Photographs essential to document abnormalities
- Radiologic investigations: full skeletal survey for any suspected or obvious skeletal dysplasia; may be useful for metabolic diseases (e.g., storage), as well; US of heart and kidneys, especially if full autopsy not performed
- Collect following samples:
  1. Sterile skin biopsy for fibroblast culture for metabolic work-up, chromosome analysis, and possible future DNA analysis; about 0.5 cm^2 of full-depth skin is required and should be stored in fresh tissue culture medium at 4° C until processed; biopsy is preferable before death to avoid bacterial contamination
  2. Sterile blood: peripheral or by cardiac puncture; 5-10 ml clotted blood for serum and 5-10 ml heparinized blood for plasma should be centrifuged, separated, and stored at −20° C for enzyme and biochemical work-up as indicated; 5 ml heparinized blood for lymphoblast line and karyotype analysis: may keep at room temperature but should be processed as soon as possible; if ACD tube (yellow stopper) available, it is preferable for lymphoblast lines
  3. Urine: as large volume as possible (± 30 ml) and store at −20° C for metabolic screen, organic acids, mucopolysaccharide and oligosaccharide screening, and other tests as indicated by clinical findings
- Contact genetics or metabolics consultant as soon as possible

CHAPTER 10

GROWTH AND DEVELOPMENT

Vᴉᴄᴋʏ Lᴇᴇ

- See Tables 10-1 to 10-3 and Figures 10-1 to 10-17 for normal patterns of growth and development

PERVASIVE DEVELOPMENTAL DISORDERS (PDD)

- Characterized by severe and pervasive impairments in several developmental areas: reciprocal social interaction skills; communication skills; or the presence of stereotyped behaviors, interests, and activities (DSM-IV)
- Includes autistic disorder, Rett's syndrome, childhood disintegrative disorder, Asperger's disorder, and pervasive developmental disorder not otherwise specified (PDD NOS)
- Incidence: 12.5 per 10,000 children

AUTISM (Table 10-4)

- First described by Kanner in 1943
- Incidence: 2-5 per 10,000 children
- Differential diagnosis: other PDD, sensory deficits, tic disorder, elimination disorder, eating disorder, communication disorder, obsessive-compulsive disorder, Rett's syndrome, general medical conditions (e.g., encephalitis, fragile X)
- See Table 10-5 for information on stimulant medications used for treatment

LEARNING DIFFICULTIES

- Learning disability: average or greater-than-average intelligence, but selective learning weaknesses (i.e., reading, spelling, mathematics, memory, visual-spatial, language)
- General learning problem: lower overall level of intellectual functioning, with consequent limited potential to acquire school learning skills
- Potential causes of learning problems are multiple and complex:
  1. Biomedical: mental retardation, autism, chronic illness, genetic-familial considerations, attention and memory disorders, neuromigrational disorders, ADHD (Box 10-1)
  2. Biosocial: poverty, social dislocation, deprivation of proper care, poor or lack of learning or language model, family dysfunction, interpersonal/intrapsychic factors
  3. Associated organic conditions: head injury/CNS infection, asthma, allergies with decongestant use, seizure disorder with anticonvulsant

Text continued on pg 144.

Table 10-1 Emerging Patterns of Behaviour from Birth to Five Years

	Gross motor	Fine motor	Social	Language	Self-help
Birth	Kicks legs and thrashes arms Moro response active; stepping and placing reflexes; grasp reflex active	Looks at objects or faces	Responds positively to feeding and comforting	Cries Started by loud sudden sounds/someone making loud noise	Alert: interested in sights and sounds
1 mo	Raises head and chest when lying on stomach	Follows moving objects with eyes	Social smile Becomes active when sees human face	Cries in a special way when hungry	Responds to voices: turns head toward voice
2 mo	Head sustained in plane of body on ventral suspension Holds head steady when held sitting Head lag on pull-to-sit position	Holds objects put in hand Hand regard; follows moving object 180 degrees	Recognizes mother/primary caregiver Listens to voice and coos	Makes sounds "ah," "eh," "ugh." Laughs	Reacts to sight of bottle or breast
3 mo	Lifts head and chest, arms extended Head above plane of body on ventral suspension Tonic neck posture predominant Head lag partially compensated on pull-to-sitting position Early head control with bobbing motion; back rounded	Shakes rattle Reaches toward and misses objects Waves at toy	Recognizes most familiar adults	Says "ahh", "ngah"	Increases activity when shown toy

	Gross Motor	Fine Motor	Social	Language	Cognitive/Adaptive
4 mo	Turns around when lying on stomach In prone position, lifts head and chest, head in approximate vertical axis; legs extended No head lag on pull to sitting position: head steady, held forward, enjoys sitting with full truncal support When held in standing/erect position, pushes with feet	Puts toys or other objects in mouth	Interested in own image in mirror, smiles, playful Laughs out loud May show displeasure if social contact is broken Excited at sight of food	Squeals, "Ah-goo" sounds	Reaches for larger objects Sees pellet, but makes no move to it
5 mo	Rolls over from stomach to back	Picks up objects with one hand	Reacts differently to strangers/stranger anxiety Reaches for familiar persons	Makes razzing sounds—gives "raspberries"	
6 mo	Rolls over from back to stomach	Transfers objects from one hand to another		Babbles Responds to name, turns and looks	Looks for object after it disappears from sight (i.e., looks for toy after it falls off tray)
7 mo	Sits without support May support most of weight when standing Bounces actively	Holds two objects, one in each hand, at same time Transfers object from hand to hand Grasps using radial palm Rakes at pellet	Gets upset and afraid if left alone	Makes sounds like "da," "ba," "ga," "ka," "ma." Turns to own name	Anticipates being lifted by raising arms

10

Continued.

Table 10-1 Emerging Patterns of Behaviour from Birth to Five Years—cont'd

	Gross motor	Fine motor	Social	Language	Self-help
8 mo	Crawls on hands and knees	Uses forefinger to poke, push, or roll small objects	Plays "peek-a-boo"	Makes sounds like "ma-ma," "da-da," "ba-ba" (two-syllable babbling)	Feeds self cracker or cookie
9 mo	Pulls self to standing position	Picks up small objects using only finger and thumb	Resists having toy taken away	Imitates speech sounds	
10 mo	Sidesteps around playpen or furniture while holding on or walks	Picks up two small objects in one hand	Plays "patty-cake"	Imitates speech sounds	
11 mo	Stands alone well	Puts small objects in cup or other container	Shows or offers toy to adult	Uses "Mama" or "Dada" specifically for parent	Picks up spoon by handle
12 mo	Climbs up on chairs or other furniture Walks with one hand held "Cruises"	Turns pages of books a few at a time	Imitates simple acts such as hugging or loving doll Plays simple ball game Makes postural adjustment to dressing	Says one word clearly Points in response to word	Removes socks
13 mo	Walks without help	Builds tower of two or more blocks	Plays with other children	Shakes head to express "No" Hands object to you when asked	Lifts cup to mouth and drinks
14 mo	Stoops and recovers	Marks with pencil or crayon	Gives kisses	Asks for food or drink with sounds or words	Insists on feeding self

Age					
15 mo	Runs	Scribbles with pencil or crayon	Greets people with "Hi" or similar Hugs parents	Says two words besides Mama or Dada Makes sounds in sequences that sound like sentences	Feeds self with a spoon
18 mo	Sits on small chair Walks up stairs with one hand held Kicks a ball, good balance and coordination Explores drawers and waste baskets Puts toys into and takes toys out of container	Builds tower of four or more blocks Imitates scribbling Imitates vertical stroke Dumps pellet from bottle	Sometimes says "No" when interfered with Kisses parent with pucker Shared attention (points to share interesting observation with another)	Uses five or more words as names of things (i.e., water, cookie, clock) Follows a few simple instructions Understands phrases such as "Give me that" when gestures are used Recognizes names of common objects such as ball, table, bed, car Identifies one or more parts of body Follows a two-step command	Feeds self Eats with a fork Seeks help when in trouble May complain when wet or soiled Knows use of toothbrush and comb
24 mo	Runs well Walks up and down stairs, one step at a time Opens doors Climbs on furniture Throws ball Kicks ball	Tower of six cubes Circular scribbling Imitates horizontal stroke Folds paper once imitatively	Often tells immediate experiences Listens to stories with pictures	Puts three words together (subject, verb, object); knows "I" Points to appropriate picture when someone says "Show me that dog" (hat, man, etc.) Has expressive vocabulary of 50-250 words	Handles spoon well Helps to undress

10

Continued.

Table 10-1 Emerging Patterns of Behaviour from Birth to Five Years—cont'd

	Gross motor	Fine motor	Social	Language	Self-help
30 mo	Jumps	Tower of eight cubes Makes horizontal and vertical strokes, but generally will not join them to make a cross Imitates circular stroke, forming closed figure	Pretends in play	Refers to self by pronoun "I" Knows full name	Helps put things away
36 mo	Goes up stairs alternating feet; rides tricycle; stands momentarily on one foot	Tower of nine cubes Imitates construction of "bridge" of three cubes Copies circle Imitates cross	Plays simple games (in "parallel" with other children)	Knows age and sex; counts three objects correctly; repeats three numbers or sentence of six syllables, expressive vocabulary of over 1000 words Remembers some recent past events	Toilet trained Helps in dressing (unbuttons clothing, puts on shoes) Washes hands

48 mo	Hops on one foot Throws ball overhand Uses scissors to cut out pictures Climbs well	Imitates construction of "gate" of five cubes Copies cross and square Draws a man with two to four parts besides head Names longer of two lines	Plays with several children, with beginning of social interaction and role-playing	Counts four pennies accurately Tells story Asks many questions Uses four-to-five word sentences Uses plurals Can repeat three or four numbers Knows four colors	Goes to toilet alone
60 mo	Skips	Draws triangle from copy Names heavier of two weights	Asks questions about meaning of words Domestic role-playing	Repeats sentence of 10 syllables Counts 10 pennies correctly Follows three-part instructions Can name penny, nickel and dime Is understood in 80%-90% of what he or she says by people outside family Uses "I," "me," "you," "he," "she," "her," and "him" properly	Dresses and undresses

10

Adapted from Parker S, Zuckerman B, eds: *Behavioral and developmental pediatrics: a handbook for primary care*, Boston, 1995, Little, Brown.

Table 10-2 Clinical Guide to Commonly Encountered Psychodiagnostic Tests

Type of test	Age range	Uses	Limitations
Tests to Evaluate General Intelligence			
Stanford-Binet Intelligence Scale (Revised)	2 yr-adult	Yields mental age and IQ Used frequently for preschool children and preferred by some professionals over WISC-III up to 8 yr Can be used with children considered mentally retarded	Provides one global score No differentiation of strengths and weaknesses through test construction Is heavily weighted with verbal items Requires normal sensory and motor skills Biased re: language, culture
Wechsler Intelligence Scale for Children, Revised (WISC-III)	6-16 yr	Yields verbal IQ, performance IQ, and full-scale IQ Tests constructed according to skills areas permitting delineation of child's strengths and weaknesses	Caution indicated in interpretation of individual subtest scores at certain ages owing to lower reliability Biased re: language, culture
Wechsler Preschool and Primary Scale of Intelligence (WPPSI)	4-6 ½ yr	May use one of verbal or performance scales alone to estimate overall level of intelligence if administration of full scale precluded by child's handicap	Biased re: language, culture
Peabody Picture Vocabulary Test	2-18 yr	Effective test of receptive language Particularly useful for testing children with severe speech or motor impairment, since test requires only pointing response	Measures only one area of functioning (listening vocabulary) Can be misleading to generalize from this to other areas of intellectual or language ability Biased re: language, culture

Leiter International Performance Test	2-18 yr	Designed for use with deaf children and useful in assessment of speech-language handicapped children Measures nonverbal intelligence Test administration allows observation of learning ability (nonverbal reasoning) Less cultural bias	Limited range of abilities sampled Manipulation of materials can be difficult for motor-handicapped children
Hiskey-Nebraska Test of Learning Aptitudes	4-12 yr	Designed and standardized for deaf/aphasic children	Does not evaluate language skills
Tests to Evaluate Perception			
Bender Visual-Motor Gestalt test	5 yr-adult	Assesses visual-motor functioning in relation to maturation Nonthreatening, easy to administer, well researched	Open to overinterpretation in terms of IQ estimate and emotional status Requires functional graphomotor skills to provide useful information See limitation below (Beery)
Beery and Buktenica Development Test of Visual-Motor Integration	2-16 yr	Assesses visual motor performance Useful in evaluation of younger children compared to Bender Gestalt Not used to gauge IQ or emotional status	Like Bender, measures visual motor copying of shapes and designs, which may or may not correlate with ability to copy (print or write) letters or words
Wepran Auditory Discrimination Test	5-8 yr	Examines ability to detect likeness and difference between sounds in pairs of words presented aurally	Requires mastery of concepts of "same" versus "different" to respond to test items

10

Continued.

Table 10-2 Clinical Guide to Commonly Encountered Psychodiagnostic Tests

Type of test	Age range	Uses	Limitations
Tests to Evaluate Academic Achievement			
Wide Range Achievement Test (WRAT)	Kindergarten–12th grade	Used to quickly assess level of academic skills and improvement from one evaluation to next	Has been normed several times with different inaccuracies associated with each set of norms Reading subtest taps only word identification, not comprehension Math subtest tests computational skills, not problem-solving ability
Peabody Individual Achievement Test (PIAT)	Kindergarten–high school	Provides overview of mathematics, reading, spelling, and general information Requirement of only pointing response and use of large, clear response choices makes it useful in evaluation of handicapped children	Considered by authors to be screening instrument Manual suggests use of alternate instruments when more intensive study required
Social/Adaptive Scales			
Vineland Social Maturity Scale*	Infant–adult	Questionnaire type instrument for measurement of general social competences as reflected in eight different areas Constructed as age scale and yields social age equivalent and social quotient comparable to a mental age and IQ	Tends to have some cultural and socioeconomic bias Data obtained through interview with an informant who may not provide reliable information
Emotional and Projective Assessment Tests			
Children's Apperception Test (CAT) and Thematic Apperception Test (TAT)	3-10 yr > 10 yr	Assess child's adjustment patterns and social relationships	Marked controversy exists concerning reliability and validity data

Rorschach Inkblot Test	3 yr-adult	Evaluates personality structure, including ego strengths, reality testing, and defense mechanisms	Same as CAT Requires freedom from significant perceptual problems
Figure drawings (e.g. draw a person, house-tree-person, kinetic family drawing)	4 yr-adult	Reveal self-image and perception of interpersonal relationships, in addition to providing estimate of level of development or intelligence Appealing task for most children	Requires good graphomotor ability to interpret for emotional factors
Self-report Inventories	Varied	Assess perception of individual regarding own functioning level	Subject to intentional distortion
Tests for Infants			
Gesell Developmental Schedules	4 wk-6 yr	Forerunner in systematic observation of infant development Useful standardized procedure for evaluating and observing behavior in four major areas of functioning, including adaptive, gross and fine motor, language, and personal-social skills	Note: For all infant tests, scales are most useful for providing indication of current developmental levels and not for prediction; scales can be weighted with other items, which limit predictive accuracy for physically handicapped children; in children with language delays, their true cognitive potential may be masked by their verbal inadequacy
Bayley Scales of Infant Development	2-30 mo	Provides separate mental and motor scales and index for reporting quality of infant's behavior during evaluation	

10

Continued.

Table 10-2   Clinical Guide to Commonly Encountered Psychodiagnostic Tests—cont'd

Type of test	Age range	Uses	Limitations
Cattell Infant Intelligence Scale	2-30 mo	Yields mental age For 18-30 mo age children provides transition from infant scale to preschool Stanford-Binet Assesses level of sensorimotor and problem-solving skills and taps emerging language abilities	
Neurodevelopmental Diagnostic Tools			
PEER = Pediatric Examination of Educational Readiness	4-6 yr	Developed for pediatricians to review areas of cognitive, language, and motor function	No standardization No predictive validity established
PEEX = Pediatric Early Elementary Examination	7-9 yr	Goals: 1. Describes child's current function 2. Selects children who need in-depth assessment of specific skills area	
PEERAMID = Pediatric Examination of Educational Readiness at Middle Childhood	9-14 yr		

Developmental Screening Profiles

DISC	0–5 yr	Overview of different developmental areas Separates gross motor, fine motor, and receptive versus expressive language problems Predictive of learning and attention problems with its visual and auditory memory subscales Norms are for Canadian children	Longest screening measure (approx. 45 min to administer by skilled person)
Alpern-ell developmental profile	0–8 yr	Historical questionnaire to be done by parents Well-standardized when done by reliable parents and caregivers	
DISC screen	0–5 yr	Based on 12 items that have been deemed most predictive of development on the full DISC	Does not separate the different areas of development
Denver 11	0–6 yr	Separates the different areas of development	Personal-social scale is not sufficient to diagnose autism/PDD

Adapted from Molnar GE, ed: *Pediatric rehabilitation*, Baltimore, 1985, Williams & Wilkins.

*Note: A revised edition (1984) involves conducting semistructured interview with caregiver and provides data regarding adaptive skills in such areas as communication, daily living, socialization, and motor behavior, as well as the assessment of maladaptive behavior; covers birth to 18 yr.

10

Table 10-3 Stretched Penile Length

		Mean ± S.D.*	Mean − 2½ S.D.*
Newborn:	30 wk	2.5 ± 0.4	1.5
	34 wk	3.0 ± 0.4	2.0
	term	3.5 ± 0.4	2.5-2.4
0-5 mo		3.9 ± 0.8	1.9
6-12 mo		4.3 ± 0.8	2.3
1-2 yr		4.7 ± 0.8	2.6
2-3 yr		5.1 ± 0.9	2.9
3-4 yr		5.5 ± 0.9	3.3
4-5 yr		5.7 ± 0.9	3.5
5-6 yr		6.0 ± 0.9	3.8
6-7 yr		6.1 ± 0.9	3.9
7-8 yr		6.2 ± 1.0	3.7
8-9 yr		6.3 ± 1.0	3.8
9-10 yr		6.3 ± 1.0	3.8
10-11		6.4 ± 1.1	3.7
Adult		13.3 ± 1.6	9.3

Adapted from Lee PA, Mazur T, Danish R, et al: Micropenis I: criteria, etiologies and classification, *John Hopkins Med J* 146:158, 1980.
*Stretched penile length (cm) in normal males.

use, recurrent ear infections (± myringotomy tubes), endocrine conditions, celiac disease, neural tube disorders
- Physical examination (Table 10-6)
- Common predictors of school success obtainable from developmental history (see Box 10-2)

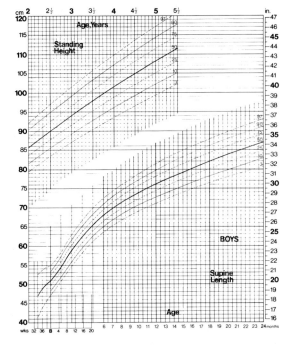

Fig. 10-1 Boys: birth through 5 yr: height. Note: Age scale divided into mo. (From Tanner JM, Whitehouse RH: *Growth and development record,* Swains Mill, Herts, England, 1984, Castlemead Publications, Ward's Publishing Services.)

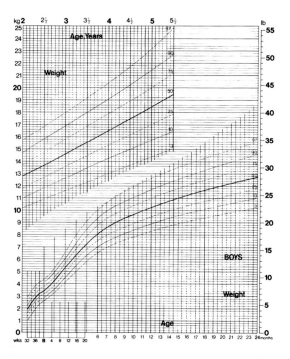

Fig. 10-2 Boys: birth through 5 yr: weight. Note: Age scale divided into mo. (From Tanner JM, Whitehouse RH: *Growth and development record*, Swains Mill, Herts, England, 1984, Castlemead Publications, Ward's Publishing Services.)

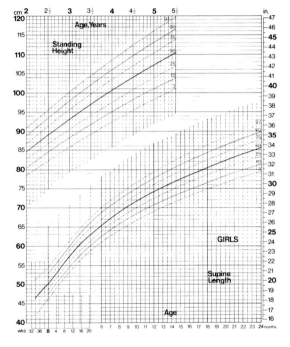

Fig. 10-3 Girls: birth through 5 yr: height. Note: Age scale divided into mo. (From Tanner JM, Whitehouse RH: *Growth and development record*, Swains Mill, Herts, England, 1984, Castlemead Publications, Ward's Publishing Services.)

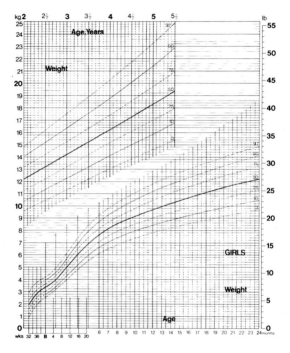

Fig. 10-4   Girls: birth through 5 yr: weight. Note: Age scale divided into mo. (From Tanner JM, Whitehouse RH: *Growth and development record*, Swains Mill, Herts, England, 1984, Castlemead Publications, Ward's Publishing Services.)

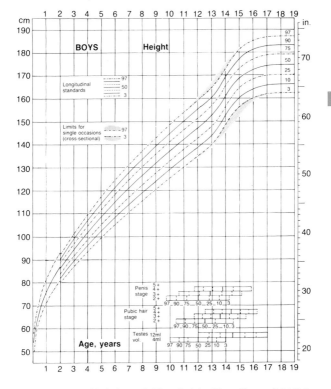

Fig. 10-5 Boys: birth through 19 yr: height. (From Tanner JM, White-house RH: *Growth and development record,* London, 1966, University of London, Institute of Child Health.)

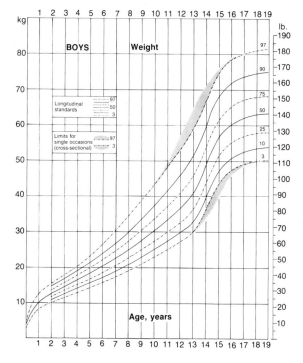

Fig. 10-6 Boys: birth through 19 yr: weight. (From Tanner JM, White-house RH: *Growth and development record,* London, 1966, University of London, Institute of Child Health.)

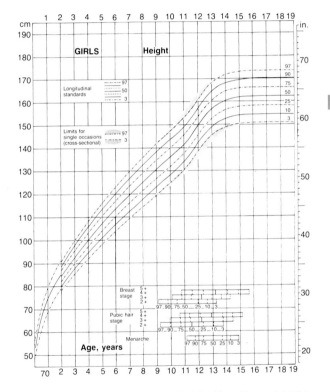

Fig. 10-7 Girls: birth through 19 yr: height. (From Tanner JM, White-house RH: *Growth and development record,* London, 1966, University of London, Institute of Child Health.)

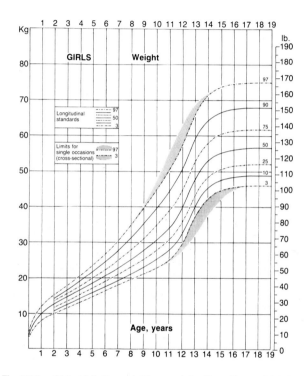

Fig. 10-8   Girls: birth through 19 yr: weight. (From Tanner JM, White-house RH: *Growth and development record,* London, 1966, University of London, Institute of Child Health.)

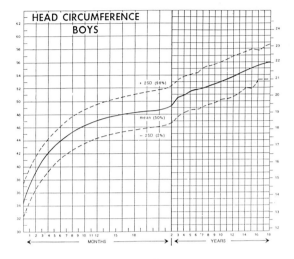

Fig. 10-9 Boys: birth through 18 yr: head circumference. (From Neihaus G: *Pediatrics* 41:106, 1968.)

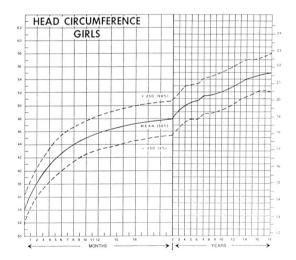

Fig. 10-10 Girls: birth through 18 yr: head circumference. (From Neihaus G: *Pediatrics* 41:106, 1968.)

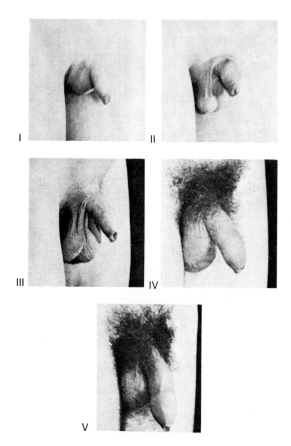

Fig. 10-11   Male genital and pubic hair development. *Stage I,* Prepubertal. *Stage II,* Enlargement of testes, appearance of scrotal reddening, and increase in scrotal rugations. *Stage III,* Increase in length and, to lesser extent, breadth of penis, with further growth of testes. *Stage IV,* Further increase in size of penis and testes and darkening of scrotal skin. *Stage V,* Adult. (Modified from Van Wieringen, Wafelbakker F, Verbrugge HP, et al: *Growth in diagrams,* Netherlands, 1971, Wolters-Noordhoof.)

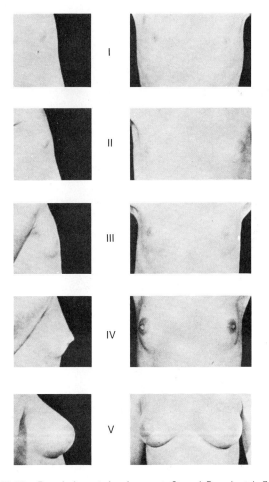

Fig. 10-12 Female breast development. *Stage I,* Prepubertal. *Stage II,* Budding. *Stage III,* Appearance of small adult breasts. *Stage IV,* Areola and papilla form a secondary mound. *Stage V,* Adult. (Modified from Van Wieringen, Wafelbakker F, Verbrugge HP, et al: *Growth in diagrams,* Netherlands, 1971, Wolters-Noordhoof.)

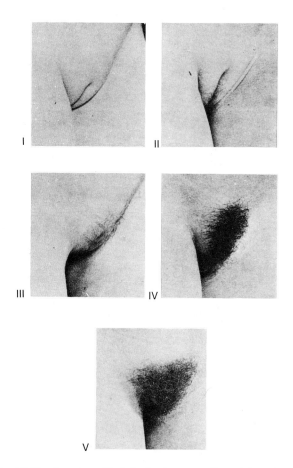

Fig. 10-13 Female pubic hair development. *Stage I,* Prepubertal. *Stage II,* Sparse growth of long, slightly pigmented hair. *Stage III,* Hair darker, coarser, and curlier and beginning to spread over symphysis pubis. *Stage IV,* Hair is adult in character but not distribution, without spread to medial surface of thigh. *Stage V,* Adult. (Modified from Van Wieringen, Wafelbakker F, Verbrugge HP, et al: *Growth in diagrams,* Netherlands, 1971, Wolters-Noordhoof.)

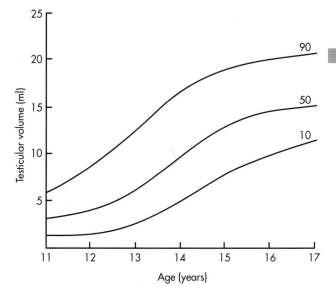

Fig. 10-14 10th, 50th, and 90th percentiles of testicular size in boys at different ages. (Modified from Zachmann M et al: In Brook CGD, ed: *Clinical pediatric endocrinology*, ed 2, London 1989, Blackwell Scientific.)

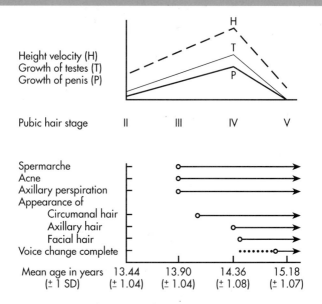

Fig. 10-15 Sequence of Maturational Events in Males (Adapted from Marshall WA, Tanner JM: Variations in the pattern of pubertal changes in boys, *Arch Dis Child* 45:13, 1970. From Behrman RE, Kliegman RM, Arvin AM: Nelson textbook of pediatrics, ed 15, Philadelphia, 1996, WB Saunders.)

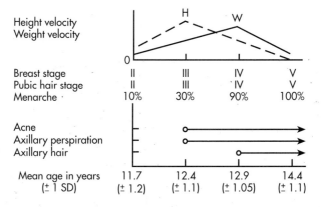

Fig. 10-16 Sequence of Maturational Events in Females. (Adapted from Marshall WA, Tanner JM: Variations in the pattern of pubertal changes in girls, *Arch Dis Child* 44:291, 1969. From Behrman RE, Kliegman RM, Arvin AM: Nelson textbook of pediatrics, ed 15, Philadelphia, 1996, WB Saunders.)

Table 10-4   Clinical Manifestations of Autism

Any two of the following	Examples
Social Interaction	
Marked lack of awareness of existence or feelings of others	Ignores emotions of others
No or abnormal seeking of comfort at times of distress	Does not show pain when hurt
No or impaired imitation	Does not imitate adaptive behavior
No or abnormal social play	Does not show cooperative play
Gross impairment in ability to make peer friendships	Does not engage in age-appropriate social activities
Language	
No mode of communication	No gestures or words
Markedly abnormal nonverbal communication	Lack of appropriate eye contact
Absence of imaginative activity	No dramatic role-playing
Marked abnormalities in production of speech	Monotonous tone
Marked abnormalities in form or content of speech	Repetitive "echolalia" of phrases
Marked impairment in ability to initiate or sustain conversation	Preoccupation with given subject out of context of conversation
Restricted Repertoire	
Stereotyped body movements	Repetitive hand-flapping
Persistent preoccupation with parts of objects	Gazing at moving lights
Marked distress over changes in trivial aspects of environment	Tantrums when light turned on
Unreasonable insistence on following routines in precise detail	Tantrums when different route taken
Markedly restricted range of interests	Repeatedly aligns objects

From Levine MD, Carey WB, Crocker AC: Developmental-behavioural pediatrics, 1992, WB Saunders. Adapted from American Psychiatric Association: Diagnostic and statistical manual of mental disorders, ed 3, Washington, DC, 1987, American Psychiatric Association.

10

Table 10-5   Stimulant Medication: Dosage and Techniques of Administration

Pharmacologic agent	Form of medication and duration of effect	Initial dose and incremental increase	Frequency of administration	Effects and how to respond	Side effects
Methylphenidate (Ritalin)	Short acting: 10-mg tablets; duration: 2½-4 hr Long acting: 20-mg Sustained release (SR); duration: 4-8 hr	0.3 mg/kg/dose; increase by 0.15 mg/kg/dose Use only when AM plus noon dose in tablet form reaches or exceeds 20 mg	tid dosing, AM, noon and 4 PM dose In AM only; may add 4 PM dose as needed	No effect: Increase dosage Wear-off effects: (1) add 4 PM dose; (2) switch to long-acting form Slow onset: Add tablet to AM dose Wear off in early PM: add 4 PM tablet	Anorexia, insomnia, irritability, crying, tics
Dextroamphetamine (Dexedrine)	Short acting: 5-mg tablets; duration: 4 hr Long acting: 5-mg, and 15-mg capsules; duration: 8 hr	0.15 mg/kg/dose; increase by 0.15 mg/kg/dose Add up total daily dosage in tablet form and give this as one dose in AM	Twice daily (AM and noon); add 4 PM dose as needed In AM only; also combined with tablets in AM or PM	Same as for methylphenidate Slow onset: Add tablet to AM dose	As above
Pemoline (Cylert)	Tablets: 37.5-mg, and 75-mg; chewable tablets 37.5 mg; duration: 8 hr	< Age 8 yr: 37.5 mg in AM > Age 8 yr: 37.5 mg plus 18.75 mg in AM Increase by 18.75 mg/dose	AM only at first; add 4 PM dose as needed	At any one dose, effects may not be seen for 1-2 wk No effect: Increase AM dose Wear off in early P.M.: add noon dose prn Monitor LFT q3 mo	As above, potential liver dysfunction

From Parker S, Zuckerman B, eds: *Behavioral and developmental pediatrics: a handbook for primary care*, Boston, 1995, Little, Brown.

BOX 10-1 Diagnostic Criteria for Attention-Deficit/Hyperactivity Disorder

I. Either A or B:
   A. Six (or more) of following symptoms of **inattention** have persisted for at least 6 mo to degree that is maladaptive and inconsistent with developmental level:

Inattention
     1. Often fails to give close attention to details or makes careless mistakes in schoolwork, work, or other activities
     2. Often has difficulty sustaining attention in tasks or play activities
     3. Often does not seem to listen when spoken to directly
     4. Often does not follow through on instructions and fails to finish schoolwork, chores, or duties in workplace (not caused by oppositional behavior or failure to understand instructions)
     5. Often has difficulty organizing tasks and activities
     6. Often avoids, dislikes, or is reluctant to engage in tasks that require sustained mental effort (such as schoolwork or homework)
     7. Often loses things necessary for tasks or activities (e.g., toys, school assignments, pencils, books, or tools)
     8. Is often easily distracted by extraneous stimuli
     9. Is often forgetful in daily activities
   B. Six (or more) of following symptoms of **hyperactivity-impulsivity** have persisted for at least 6 mo to degree that is maladaptive and inconsistent with developmental level:

Hyperactivity
     1. Often fidgets with hands or feet or squirms in seat
     2. Often leaves seat in classroom or in other situations in which remaining seated is expected
     3. Often runs about or climbs excessively in situations in which it is inappropriate (in adolescents or adults may be limited to subjective feelings of restlessness)
     4. Often has difficulty playing or engaging in leisure activities quietly
     5. Is often "on the go" or often acts as if "driven by motor"
     6. Often talks excessively

Impulsivity
     7. Often blurts out answers before questions have been completed
     8. Often has difficulty awaiting turn
     9. Often interrupts or intrudes on others (e.g., butts into conversations or games)
II. Some hyperactive-impulsive or inattentive symptoms that caused impairment were present before age 7 yr
III. Some impairment from symptoms is present in two or more settings (e.g., at school [or work] and at home)
IV. There must be clear evidence of clinically significant impairment in social, academic, or occupational functioning
V. Symptoms do not occur exclusively during course of pervasive developmental disorder, schizophrenia, or other psychotic disorder and are not better accounted for by another mental disorder (e.g., mood disorder, anxiety disorder, dissociative disorder, or a personality disorder)

American Psychiatric Association: *Diagnostic and statistic manual of mental disorders*, ed 4, Washington, DC, 1994, American Psychiatric Association.

BOX 10-2 Predictors of Academic Success from Developmental
History

Infancy
Temperament
Easy with regard to feeding, sleeping, routines (versus slow to warm up or difficult)
Enjoys social interaction
Preschool
Language
Mimicks sounds in reciprocal interaction
Phrases by age 2, sentences by age 3
Easily understood by strangers by age 3-4
Repeats nursery rhymes by age 3-4
Says address, phone number, singsong alphabet by age 5
Enjoys wordplay by age 4 or 5
Tells puns/jokes by age 6
Motor
Rides tricycle by age 3
Shows interest in drawing by age 4
Draws person with '5 parts', prints own first name, rides bicycle, ties shoelaces by
    age 5
Social
Plays in group and listens to group stories in nursery school
Cooperates with group activities in kindergarten
One or two preferred playmates in kindergarten
Same-age playmates at home
Emotional
Separates from parent readily
Not excessively anxious
Appreciates fantasy and magical play without excessive fear or preoccupation
School Age
Academic
Interest in being read to throughout
Reads for pleasure alone by 9 yr (8-10)
Social
Has same-age friends
Understands nonverbal communication
Experiences successful group activities
Understands causality; understands need for rules and social conventions
Cognitive
Possesses directionality/right-left concepts
Secure on self by age 8, on others by 10
Visuospatial: has adequate drawing ability, understands maps
Understands time and money concepts by 8-10 yr
Emotional
Copes with reality-based fears (e.g., accident, illness, separation, or death of parent)
Has positive self-esteem
Internalizes control of behavior
Adolescent
Cognitive
Draws inferences/appreciates abstract concepts
Tests hypotheses; understands probability, speed, simultaneous perspective, higher
    moral principle

Continued.

BOX 10-2 Predictors of Academic Success from Developmental
History—cont'd

Emotional

Struggles with issue of ongoing dependence on family support reconciled by acquisition
of independence

Mourns loss of perfect self, family, and world while maintaining self-esteem and confidence

Academic

Achieves goals through own effort

Roberts W, Humphries, T: School problems: a current perspective on assessment, *Can J Paediat* Dec. 21, 1990.

10

Table 10-6 Aspects of Physical Examination in Evaluation of Child
with Learning Problems

Aspect	Examples of findings with possible implication for school failure
General well-being and behavior	Limited alertness, stamina; moodiness; sadness; anxiety; tics; short attention span; impulsivity, overactivity
Phenotypic features	"Cluster" of minor congenital anomalies; stigmata of genetic syndromes (e.g., sex-chromosome abnormalities, fetal alcohol syndrome)
Skin	Multiple café au lait spots; adenoma sebaceum, "ash-leaf" spots
Tympanic membranes	Evidence of recurrent/chronic otitis media
Genitalia	Delayed sexual maturation (especially boys)
Measurements	Short stature; microcephaly; macrocephaly
Sensory	Hearing impairment; vision defect

From Dworkin PH: School failure *Pediat Rev* 10 (10): 301-312, 1989.

CHAPTER 11

GYNECOLOGY

GILLIAN OLIVER

VAGINAL BLEEDING

NEONATAL

- Usually occurs between 5-10 days of age
- Difficult to distinguish from hematuria
- Must do thorough search for other signs of bleeding diathesis
- Look for other supportive evidence of estrogen effect (e.g., breast buds)
- Major differential diagnoses include maternal estrogen effects (most common), gynecologic disease (infection, tumor), bleeding diathesis, urethral prolapse, sexual assault
- Investigations may include CBC, PT, PTT, bleeding time, platelets; vaginal swab for culture; vaginal cytology for hormonal effect (maturation index), urinalysis, and culture

Treatment

- If physical and laboratory data consistent, diagnosis is likely maternal estrogen effects causing withdrawal bleed; observe; follow-up in 6-8 wk; sooner if repetitive bleeding
- In absence of bleeding diathesis, all other causes need gynecology referral and assessment

PREMENARCHAL: EARLY AND LATE CHILDHOOD
Differential Diagnosis

- Trauma: careful perineal examination for trauma or discharge; generally limited to external examination of vagina and vulva; always do rectal examination to rule out perforating trauma
- Foreign body vaginitis
- Sexual abuse: observe patient's behavior (suggestive of sexual abuse); is history consistent with injury?
- Precocious puberty: assess height, weight, signs of pubertal change
- Vaginitis (uncommon; consider sexual abuse and sexually transmitted disease): group A β-hemolytic, nonspecific vaginitis
- Hormone withdrawal: history of estrogen ingestion or topical exposure (must ask if mother or adolescent in home is using these medications)
- Urethral prolapse: history of excessive valsalva (e.g., constipation)
- Uterine, vaginal, urethral pathology (uncommon): assess for evidence of systemic illness
- Bleeding diathesis (rare)

Investigations

- CBC
- Vaginal culture

- Vaginal cell maturation index
- Bone age
- Gonadostropin releasing hormone (GnRH) stimulation test

Treatment

- Gynecology referral for vaginoscopy and management (unless obviously only superficial trauma or foreign body can be easily removed)
- Vaginitis: perineal hygiene; antibiotic only for specific positive culture

PERIMENARCHAL

- Similar in pattern to those of premenarchal group
- Perform accurate pubertal staging (Tanner stage, see pp. 154 to 156)

Differential Diagnosis

- Menarche
- Trauma
- Sexual abuse
- Bleeding diathesis (presents as heavy flow at menarche)
- Uterine, vaginal disease (uncommon)
- Pregnancy complication (conception can occur prior to menarche)

Investigations

- CBC
- Platelets, PT, PTT, and bleeding time (if bleeding considered excessive for normal menarche)
- Urine or plasma β-hCG

Treatment

- Gynecology referral if trauma requiring examination under anesthesia (EUA) or sutures, pregnancy complication, or uterine and vaginal disease suspected; bleeding disorder may also require hematologic consultation
- Child protection services referral if sexual abuse (see p. 28)

POSTMENARCHAL

- Always consider patient sexually active until proven otherwise (e.g., pregnancy or complication thereof a strong possibility)
- Dysfunctional uterine bleeding (DUB) is diagnosis of exclusion
- Complete menstrual and sexual history is mandatory, but may not be completely reliable
- Determine contraceptive use, compliance, and need
- Do as complete a pelvic examination as possible

Differential Diagnosis

- Dysfunctional uterine bleeding (DUB) (75%): anovulatory cycles, common in first 2 yr postmenarche but consider thyroid disease, prolactinoma
- Bleeding diathesis (5%-20%)
- Gynecologic disease
  1. Ovarian cyst
  2. Infections: endometritis, cervicitis, vaginitis

3. Oral contraceptive misuse
4. Cervical disease

Investigations

- CBC, differential, platelets
- PT, PTT, bleeding time
- Thyroid function, prolactin
- Cervical swabs for gonorrhea and *Chlamydia*
- Pap smear
- β-hCG
- Urinalysis

Treatment

- Mild bleeding (DUB)
  1. Usually chronic erratic menses with normal hemoglobin
  2. Chemical curetage with medroxyprogesterone 5-10 mg/day × 10 days followed by "rescue regime"
  3. Rescue regime: medroxyprogesterone 5 mg/day × 5 days q40day if no spontaneous menses before that time
- Moderate bleeding (DUB)
  1. Usually Hb < 100 g/L and stable
  2. Oral contraceptive pill (OCP) × 3 cycles to improve Hb and give psychologic break from bleeding followed by progesterone rescue regime (see earlier discussion)
- Severe acute bleeding (DUB ± coagulation disorder)
  1. Hb < 100 g/L
  2. Admit to hospital: urgent gynecology referral
  3. IV fluid resuscitation and blood transfusion as necessary (see p. 6)
  4. Replace clotting factors as needed (fresh frozen plasma, cryoprecipitate, or platelets, see p. 197)
  5. Premarin (conjugated estrogens), 25 mg IV q4h prn, for maximum of 24 hr to stop bleeding
  6. Simultaneously Ovral, 2 tabs initially and then 1 tab tid-qid until bleeding stops (5 days maximum); when bleeding stops, continue 1-2 tablets PO daily for total of 21 days; then withdraw for 7 days; cycle with OCP for 2 mo until Hb normalized
  7. Give antinauseants with IV Premarin and Ovral
  8. Hematology consult for bleeding disorders

VULVOVAGINITIS

- Infection with gonorrhea, *Chlamydia, Trichomonas,* herpes, and condylomata generally means venereal transmission (nonvenereal possible but rare); must rule out sexual assault/abuse

PREPUBERTAL

- Nonbloody discharge and pruritus common in children because of poor hygiene, proximity to anus, and susceptibility of thin vaginal mucosa to infection

Differential Diagnosis

- Noninfectious
  1. Poor hygiene
  2. Foreign body
  3. Chemical irritant
  4. Trauma or sexual abuse
  5. Generalized skin disease
- Infectious
  1. Nonspecific bacterial (usually coliforms from bowel, not *Gardnerella* as in adults)
  2. Pinworms
  3. Group A β-hemolytic *Streptococcus*
  4. STD (e.g., *Trichomonas,* gonorrhea); latter causes vaginitis in prepubertal, not in postpubertal children; prepubertal girls do not develop cervicitis
  5. *Candida* vaginitis uncommon before hormonal changes of perimenarchal stage

Investigations

- Perineal examination; whiff test
- If discharge present, culture vagina for gonorrhea and β-hemolytic *streptococci* (use soft plastic eyedropper or moistened urethral swab to collect specimen if needed)
- Wet prep for *Trichomonas* if profuse purulent discharge or sexual assault suspected
- *Do not restrain child*
- Referral to gynecology for vaginoscopy if
  1. Bloody discharge
  2. Foreign body suspected and unable to remove by gentle irrigation with normal saline and Foley catheter (one attempt)
  3. Symptoms recurrent or not resolving

Treatment

- Hygiene education (cotton underwear, no underwear to bed)
- Sitz baths tid with oatmeal powder
- Avoid soaps
- Remove foreign bodies (see previous discussion)
- Treat specific organisms

POSTPUBERTAL
Differential Diagnosis

- Physiologic leukorrhea
- Noninfectious: generalized dermatitis, poor hygiene, retained tampon
- Infectious
  1. Nonspecific vaginitis ("*Gardnerella* vaginitis")
     - Synergistic infection caused by *Gardnerella* and anaerobes together
     - *Gardnerella* may be normal vaginal flora
     - Gray malodorous discharge with "clue cells"
  2. *Candidiasis* ("yeast"): cheesy white discharge, pruritic; common after antibiotics, in diabetics, pregnancy, immunosuppression

3. *Trichomonas:* green, frothy, foul discharge; often pruritic
4. Gonorrhea: often asymptomatic; may have cervicitis with purulent cervical discharge
5. *Chlamydia:* often asymptomatic; may be cervicitis; may be concomitant with or present after treatment of gonorrhea
6. Herpes: Primary: 50% asymptomatic, but can be bilateral with systemic fever; look for history of recurrence; usually painful, vesicles ulcerate, inguinal adenopathy
7. *Condylomata acuminata:* nonplanar perineal warts
8. Parasites: scabies, pediculosis pubis

Investigations

- Perineal examination
- Maturation index helpful in physiologic leukorrhea
- Vaginal swab: potassium hydroxide (KOH) prep for *Candida;* wet prep for *Trichomonas* and "clue cells" (*Gardnerella;* organisms on epithelial cell surface)
- Cervical swabs for *gonococcus* (Gram stain, culture) and *Chlamydia* cultures
- *Herpes:* viral culture of lesion; scrapings with Wright's stain: multinucleated giant cells
- Bimanual pelvic examination necessary in all sexually active girls to assess for pelvic inflammatory disease

Treatment

- No treatment for physiologic leukorrhea
- Hygiene education
- Nonspecific (*Gardnerella*) vaginitis: metronidazole 500 mg bid × 7 days
- *Trichomonas:* metronidazole 500 mg bid × 7 days or 2 g PO × one dose (adult); must treat partner; advise to avoid alcohol while taking metronidazole
- *Candida:* miconazole nitrate, clotrimasole cream or ovules intravaginally × 3-7 nights, terconazole for resistant strains
- *Chlamydia:* see Box 11-1
- *Gonococcus:* see Box 11-2
- *Herpes:* acyclovir 200 mg PO 5 ×daily × 7-10 day, symptomatic treatment if recurrent
- *Condylomata:* gynecology referral for chemical treatment, cryotherapy, cautery, or laser
- Scabies, pediculosis: see p. 84

LABIAL FUSION

- Generally asymptomatic benign condition, seen from age 2 mo to menarche; presents because of parental concern; resolves when endogenous estrogen produced; may be corrected by application of exogenous estrogen bid × 14 days to vulva and meticulous hygiene; treat if:
  1. Urethral meatus (and urinary output) obstructed (uncommon)
  2. Recurrent vaginitis, asymptomatic bacteria

3. Confusion with other diagnoses (e.g., vaginal agenesis, excessive virilization)
4. Strong parental anxiety
- Surgical intervention if acute urinary retention

SEXUALLY TRANSMITTED DISEASES (Table 11-1, Boxes 11-1 to 11-3)

- Always include in differential diagnosis of abdominal pain and urethral and/or vaginal discharge in adolescence
- Upper genitourinary tract infection in females often associated with pain and systemic symptoms
- *Chlamydia* and *N. gonorrheoa* often occur together (20%-30%) and along with genital herpes may be asymptomatic at any age
- Suspect child abuse in all prepubescent and nonsexually active postpubescent children with these infections

IMPORTANT MANAGEMENT TASKS

11

- Contact tracing and treatment
- Reporting to Public Health Department

Table 11-1 Causes of Major STD Syndromes*

Syndrome	Cause	
	Sexually transmitted	Other
Urethritis and PID	*Chlamydia trachomatis*	
	Neisseria gonorrhoeae	
Cervicitis	*C. trachomatis*	
	N. gonorrhoeae	
	Herpes simplex virus (HSV)	
Epididymitis	*C. trachomatis*	Urinary tract pathogens
	N. gonorrhoeae	
Prepubertal vaginitis	*C. trachomatis*	Group A streptococci
	N. gonorrhoeae	Nonspecific
Postpubertal vaginitis	*Trichomonas vaginalis*	Yeasts
	Bacterial vaginosis	
	(*Gardnerella vaginalis*)	
	Yeast	
Genital ulcer disease	*Treponema pallidum* (painless)	
	Herpes simplex	
	Haemophilus ducreyi	
Genital and anal warts	Human papillomavirus	
Proctitis	*C. trachomatis*	*E. histolytica*
	N. gonorrhoeae	*Campylobacter*
	Herpes simplex	*Shigella*
	T. pallidum	*C. difficile*

Note: Vaginitis rather than cervicitis occurs in prepubertal girls.
*See Canada Diseases Weekly Reports, 1988 Canadian guidelines for treatment of sexually transmitted diseases in neonates, children, adolescents, and adults. Health and Welfare Canada. Vol. 14 S2(April 1988) and vol. 15 S1(March 1989) for detailed diagnosis and treatment guidelines.

BOX 11-1 Treatment of Genital *Chlamydia trachomatis**

Uncomplicated Urethritis, Cervicitis, Proctitis
Tetracycline 500 mg PO qid × 7 days
or
Erythromycin 500 mg PO qid × 7 days
or
Doxycycline 100 mg PO bid × 7 days
Epididymo-Orchitis
Tetracycline 500 mg PO qid × 10 days
or
Doxycycline 100 mg PO bid × 10 days

---

*Children < 9 yr: Erythromycin, 10 mg/kg PO qid × 7 days (10 days for epididymitis)
Children > 9 yr: Tetracycline, 10 mg/kg PO qid × 7 days (10 days for epididymitis)

- Optimizing compliance
- Follow-up *essential* but may be difficult in some social situations
- Counseling regarding pregnancy, birth control, other STDs, HIV, safe sex
- Screening of high-risk groups for HIV, with consent
- Awareness of long-term risks for infertility, ectopic pregnancy, chronic pelvic pain

CLINICAL FEATURES OF PELVIC INFLAMMATORY DISEASE (PID) IN FEMALES

- Fever, abdominal pain
- Vaginal discharge or bleeding
- Often occurs following menses
- Pain worse with movement, intercourse
- Acute and subacute clinical courses
- Physical signs include lower quadrant tenderness, cervical excitation pain and adnexal tenderness, perihepatic pain (Fitz-Hugh–Curtis syndrome), fever, elevated WBC, and ESR
- Rarely unilateral pain unless IUD present
- Consider ectopic pregnancy, ovarian cyst or torsion, and appendicitis in differential diagnosis of PID

Chlamydia Trachomatis

- Inclusion conjunctivitis (neonates), pneumonia (1-4 mo), urethritis, cervicitis, epididymitis, lymphogranuloma venereum
- Often asymptomatic; may coexist with gonorrhea (must rule out) or present after gonorrhea treated
- Swab for *Chlamydia* cultures
- Treatment shown in Box 11-1

Neisseria Gonorrhoeae

- Urethritis, epididymitis, vaginitis (prepubertal); cervicitis, salpingitis (postpubertal)

BOX 11-2 Antibiotic Therapy for *Neisseria Gonorrhoeae*

Uncomplicated Urethritis, Cervicitis in Adults

Aqueous procaine penicillin G 4.8 million U injected IM at 2 separate sites, with probenecid 1 g PO

or

Ampicillin 3.5 g or amoxicillin 3 g with probenecid 1 g PO in single dose

or

Ceftriaxone 250 mg IM in single dose

All followed by

Tetracycline* 500 mg PO qid × 7 days

or

Doxycycline* 100 mg PO bid × 7 days

Pharyngeal Gonococcal Infection

Aqueous procaine penicillin G with probenecid plus tetracycline or doxycycline, as above, is preferred regimen

Anorectal Gonococcal Infection

Females: Treat as above for uncomplicated gonococcal disease

Males: Aqueous procaine penicillin G with probenecid plus tetracycline* or doxycycline,* as above, is preferred regimen

Penicillin-Resistant Gonorrhea

Ceftriaxone 250 mg IM in single dose

or

Spectinomycin hydrochloride 2 g IM

Both followed by

Tetracycline* or doxycycline* as above

Penicillin-Allergic Patients

Spectinomycin 2 g IM in single dose

or

Ceftriaxone 250 mg IM in single dose

Both followed by

Tetracycline* or doxycycline* as above

Pregnancy

All of above regimens are safe during pregnancy except tetracycline and doxycycline, which should be replaced by erythromycin 500 mg PO qid × 7 days

or

Erythromycin 250 mg PO qid × 14 days

Children < 45 kg

Recommended Dosages

Amoxicillin 50 mg/kg PO in single dose

Probenecid 25 mg/kg PO in single dose

Aqueous procaine penicillin G 100,000 IU/kg IM in single dose

Erythromycin 10 mg/kg PO qid

Ceftriaxone 125 mg IM in single dose

Spectinomycin 40 mg/kg IM in single dose

---

*In children age <9 yr, replace tetracycline and doxycycline with erythromycin 10 mg/kg PO qid.

- Gram stain and culture:
  In females: endocervical, vaginal, rectal, ± pharyngeal swabs
  In heterosexual males: urethral
  In homosexual males: urethral, pharyngeal, rectal
  Other: neonates: conjunctiva; joint, blood as indicated

BOX 11-3   Treatment of Pelvic Inflammatory Disease

Whenever possible, patients should be admitted and treated in hospital to have impact on long-term fertility

Hospitalized Patients

IV antibiotics for at least 4 days or 48 hr after patient defervesces

- Clindamycin 600 mg IV q6h
  plus
  Gentamycin/tobramycin 2 mg/kg IV followed by 1.5 mg/kg IV q8h
  followed by
  Clindamycin 450 mg PO q6h × 10-14 days
  or
- Metronidazole 1 g IV q12h
  plus
  Doxycycline 100 mg IV q12h
  followed by
  Metronidazole 500 mg PO bid and doxycycline 100 mg PO bid × 10-14 days
  or
- Cefoxitin 2 g IV q6h
  plus
  Doxycycline 100 mg IV q12h
  followed by
  Doxycycline 100 mg PO bid × 10-14 days

Nonhospitalized Patients

- Aqueous procaine penicillin G 4.8 million U IM at two separate sites with probenecid 1 g PO
  or
- Amoxicillin 3 g or ampicillin 3.5 g with probenecid 1 g PO in single dose
  or
- Cefoxitin 2 g IM with probenecid 1 g PO
  or
- Ceftriaxone 250 mg IM in single dose*

All followed by

- Doxycycline 100 mg PO bid for 10-14 days†

---

*Ceftriaxone is only regimen effective against PID associated with resistant *N. gonorrhoeae;* should be used if resistant strain is cultured or if sensitivity unknown; *Chlamydia* needs to be treated as well.

†Tetracycline hydrochloride, 500 mg PO qid × 10-14 days may also be used but is less active against certain infections.

Note: Follow-up: Clinical reevaluation of ambulatory patients treated for PID must be done in 48-72 hr; nonresponders should be hospitalized.

- Swabs should be plated promptly on to Thayer-Martin agar plates or placed in transport medium
- Include urethral (male), vaginal, and cervical cultures for *Chlamydia*
- Baseline VDRL for syphilis screen with follow-up at 8 wk
- Offer HIV screening and follow-up surveillance at 3, 6, and 12 mo

Treatment (see Box 11-2)

- Asymptomatic infant born to mother with gonorrhea
  1. Gastric and rectal cultures (for gonorrhea and *Chlamydia*)

2. Routine eye prophylaxis (erythromycin ointment)
3. Penicillin G 100,000 U IM/IV × one dose
4. If resistance suspected, use ceftriaxone 125 mg IM × one dose

- Gonococcal ophthalmitis: ceftriaxone or penicillin IV; consult ophthalmology (see p. 385)
- Uncomplicated gonorrhea: see Box 11-2
- If penicillin allergy or if organism is penicillin resistant or if sensitivity unknown, use ceftriaxone (Note: 15% cross-reactivity between penicillin and cephalosporins) IM × one dose or spectinomycin IM × one dose
- Pharyngeal or anorectal gonorrhea: amoxicillin and spectinomycin not effective; all females should have rectal cultures if gonorrhea suspected (see Box 11-2)
- Note: Everyone should receive in addition to above treatment simultaneous treatment for *C. trachomatis* with either tetracycline, doxycycline, or erythromycin
- Treat sexual partners
- Disseminated infection (sepsis, arthritis): Penicillin G IV × 7-10 days; ceftriaxone IV may be used for penicillin-resistant organisms
- All patients should return 3-7 days after completion of therapy for clinical evaluation and follow-up cultures
- Pelvic inflammatory disease (PID) (see Box 11-3)

11

Treponema Pallidum (Syphilis)

- Microscopic dark-field examination to identify spirochetes in material obtained from primary chancre and skin and mucocutaneous lesions
- Serology
  1. Screening test: VDRL; if negative, repeat in 8 wk
  2. Serology may be negative early (i.e., in contacts or in patients with primary lesion)
- Confirmatory specific tests: FTA-ABS (fluorescent treponemal antibody absorption), MHA-TP (microhemagglutination test for *T. pallidum*)
- Antibiotic therapy (treat contacts of positive cases as if they have disease) (Table 11-2)
- Follow-up
  1. Report to Public Health Department for contact tracing
  2. Repeat VDRL at 3, 6, and 12 mo to follow response to treatment

CONTRACEPTION (Tables 11-3 to 11-6 and Boxes 11-4 and 11-5)

METHODS OF CONTRACEPTION

- See Table 11-3 for list of methods of contraception that should be discussed when counseling an adolescent about contraception

BIRTH CONTROL PILLS

- Work up before use of birth control pills
  1. Complete history, including menstrual and sexual history and physical examination with blood pressure and pelvic examination if sexually active
  2. History of smoking (relative indication > 30 yr)

Table 11-2   Antibiotic Therapy for Syphilis

	Without penicillin allergy	With penicillin allergy
Congenital: proven or suspected (VDRL-positive baby with inadequate or unknown history of treatment in mother)		
Symptomatic or asymptomatic (regardless of baseline CSF)	Penicillin G 50,000 U/kg/day IM/IV ÷ q12h for minimum of 10 days, or procaine penicillin G 50,000 U/kg/day IM once daily for minimum of 10 days	
Acquired*		
1. Primary, secondary, or early latent (duration < 1 yr)	Benzathine penicillin G 50,000 U/kg IM (maximum 2.4 million U: 1.2 million U in each buttock)	Tetracycline (if >8 yr) or erythromycin† 40 mg/kg/day PO ÷ q6h (maximum 2 g/day) × 15 days
2. Latent (duration > 1 yr)		
Normal CSF	Benzathine penicillin G 50,000 U/kg (maximum 2.4 million U) IM once weekly × 3 wk	Tetracycline (if >8 yr) or erythromycin† 40 mg/kg/day PO ÷ q6h (maximum 2 g/day) × 30 days
Abnormal CSF	Penicillin G 200,000 U/kg/day (maximum 12-18 million U/day) IV ÷ q4h × 10 days; then benzathine penicillin G 50,000 U/kg (maximum 2.4 million U) IM once weekly × 3 doses	
	or	
	Procaine penicillin G 50,000 U/kg (maximum 2.4 million U) IM daily + probenecid 500 mg PO qid × 10 days: then benzathine penicillin G 50,000 U/kg (maximum 2.4 million U) IM once weekly × 3 doses	

*CSF should be examined for cells, protein, and VDRL if neurosyphilis suspected or if patient is symptomatic; CSF should be examined in any case of syphilis of >1-yr duration when patient has not been treated with penicillin G.

†Erythromycin has not been proved to be effective; careful follow-up required.

Note: Jarisch-Herxheimer reaction: Febrile reaction may occur 8-12 hr post Rx: most commonly in early syphilis; reaction often accompanied by malaise and not related to drug allergy, usually lasts few hours and can be treated with antipyretics.

Table 11-3 Contraceptive Methods and Efficacy with Full Compliance

Method	Efficacy* (per 100 woman yr)
Injectable Contraceptive (Depo-Provera)	99.7
Subcutaneous implant (Norplant®)	99.2
Oral contraceptives	98+
Intrauterine devices (IUDs)†	96-98
Diaphragm and spermicide‡	85-95
Condom and spermicide‡	85-95
Condom alone‡	70-95
Spermicide alone‡	70-75
Rhythm‡	65-70
Withdrawal	<65-70
Postcoital interception (Ovral, 2 tabs q12h × 2 doses)§	~98
Abstinence‡	100

From Special Advisory Committee on Reproductive Physiology to the Health Protection Branch, Health and Welfare, Canada: *Report on oral contraceptives,* 1985.

*Efficacy is lower in adolescents.

†IUDs not recommended in nulliparous women or if history of PID, but may be method of choice in individualized cases.

‡These methods notoriously poorly used in adolescents.

§"Morning After Pill."

11

   3. Pap smear within 1 year of coitarche
   4. Pregnancy test
   5. Urinalysis
   6. Check rubella immune status (potential for pregnancy)
   7. Offer screening for gonorrhea, chlamydia, HIV, and syphilis
   8. Opportunity for patient sexual education and health prevention
- In healthy adolescent, risks to health from pregnancy outweigh those of low-dose birth control pills

Major Side Effects

- Estrogen excess: nausea, vomiting, diarrhea, edema, chloasma, hypertension, breast tenderness
- Progesterone excess: acne, hirsutism, alopecia, depression, increased appetite, amenorrhea

DEPO-PROVERA

- Depo medroxyprogesterone acetate
- 150 mg IM q12wk
- Not Health-Protection-Branch (HPB)–approved, but HPB-approved for menstrual suppression
- WHO-endorsed for contraception
- Most widely used and safest hormonal contraception in world (>80 countries)

Indications

- Contraindication/intolerance of OCP
- Need for menstrual suppression

Text continued on p. 181

Table 11-4   Oral Contraceptives with Similar Endometrial, Progestational, and Androgenic Activities*

Group	Oral contraceptives	Estrogen-dose	Activity
#1	Micronor	No estrogen	Endometrial: Low Progestational: Low Androgenic: Low
#2	MinEstrin 1/20 LoEstrin 1.5/30	20 μg ethinyl estradiol 30 μg ethinyl estradiol	Endometrial: Low Progestational: Intermediate Androgenic: Intermediate/High
#3	Marvelon Ortho-Cept	30 μg ethinyl estradiol	Endometrial: Intermediate Progestational: High Androgenic: Low
#4	Min-Ovral	30 μg ethinyl estradiol	Endometrial: Intermediate Progestational: Intermediate Androgenic: Intermediate
#5	Triquilar† Triphaisl†	32 μg ethinyl estradiol (average)	Endometrial: Intermediate/High Progestational: Low Androgenic: Intermediate
#6	Cyclen	35 μg ethinyl estradiol	Endometrial: Low Progestational: Low Androgenic: Low
#7	Ortho 7/7/7† Ortho 10/11† Synphasic	35 μg ethinyl estradiol	Endometrial: Intermediate Progestational: Low/Intermediate Androgenic: Low/Intermediate
#8	Brevicon 0.5/35 Ortho 0.5/35	35 μg ethinyl estradiol	Endometrial: Intermediate Progestational: Low Androgenic: Low
#9	Brevicon 1/35 Ortho 1/35	35 μg ethinyl estradiol	Endometrial: Intermediate Progestational: Intermediate Androgenic: Intermediate
#10	Norinyl/50 Ortho-Novum 1/50	50 μg mestranol	Endometrial: Intermediate Progestational: Intermediate Androgenic: Intermediate
#11	Norlestrin 1/50	50 μg ethinyl estradiol	Endometrial: Intermediate Progestational: Intermediate Androgenic: Intermediate
#12	Demulen 30 Demulen 50	50 μg ethinyl estradiol	Endometrial: Low/Intermediate Progestational: High Androgenic: Low
#13	Ovral	50 μg ethinyl estradiol	Endometrial: High Progestational: High Androgenic: High

From Dickey RP, Yuzpee AA, eds: *Managing contraceptive pill patients,* ed 7, 1993, Emis-Canada.
*Arranged by estrogen type and dose.
†Multiphasic.

Table 11-5 Drugs that May Reduce Efficacy of Oral Contraceptives

Class of compound	Drug	Proposed method of action	Suggested management
Anticonvulsant drugs	Barbiturates: phenytoin, mephenytoin, ethotoin	Induction of liver microsomal enzymes; rapid metabolism of estrogen and increased binding of progestin and ethinyl estradiol to sex-hormone-binding globulin	Use another method, another drug, or high dose OC (50 µg ethinyl estradiol)
Cholesterol-lowering agent	Clofibrate	Reduces elevated serum triglycerides and cholesterol	Use another method
Antituberculosis antibiotics and antifungals	Rifampin Penicillin Ampicillin Cotrimoxazole Griseofulvin	Rifampin increases metabolism of progestins Enterohepatic circulation disturbance, intestinal hurry	For short course, use additional method or use another drug
	Metronidazole Tetracycline Neomycin Chloramphenicol Sulfonamide Nitrofurantoin	Induction of microsomal liver enzymes; see above	For long course, use another method
Sedatives and hypnotics	Benzodiazepines Barbiturates: phenobarbital, carbamazepin, primidone, ethosuximide Chloral hydrate Antimigraine preparations	Increased microsomal liver enzymes; see above	For short course, use additional method or another drug For long course, use another method or higher dose OCs

From Dickey RP, Yuzpee AA, eds: *Managing contraceptive pill patients*, ed 7, 1993, Emis-Canada.

Table 11-6 Modification of Other Drug Activity by Oral Contraceptives

Class of compound	Drug	Modification of drug action	Suggested management
Anticoagulants	All	OCs increase clotting factors, decrease efficacy	Do not use OC with anticoagulant
Antidiabetic agents	Insulin and oral hypoglycemic agents	High-dose OCs cause impaired glucose tolerance	Use low-dose estrogen and progestin OC or use another method
Antihypertensive agents	Guanethidine methyldopa	Estrogen component causes Na retention; progestin has no effect	Use low-estrogen OC or another method Possible need for dosage increase
Anticonvulsants	All	Fluid retention, increases seizures	Use another method
Corticosteroids	Prednisone	Markedly increases serum levels	Possible need for dosage decrease
Antipyretics and analgesics	Acetaminophen	Increases renal clearance	Increase dosage
	Aspirin		Increase dosage
	Antipyrine	Impairs metabolism	Decrease dosage
	Meperidine		Decrease dosage
Antibiotics	Troleandomycin	Possibly damages liver	Do not use OC with antibiotics

Tricyclic antidepressants	Clomipramine, imipramine	Increases side effects, depression	Decrease dosage by one third or use another method
Betamimetics	Isoproterenol agents	Estrogen causes decreased response to these drugs	Adjust dose of drug as necessary; discontinuing OCs can result in excessive drug activity
Beta blocking agents	Metoprolol	Increases drug effect (decreases metabolism)	Decrease dosage if necessary
Phenothiazine tranquilizers	All phenothiazines, reserpine, and similar drugs	Estrogen potentiates hyperprolactinemia effect of these drugs	Use other drugs or lower dose OCs; if galactorrhea or hyperprolactinemia occurs, use another method
Sedatives and hypnotics	Chlordiazepoxide Lorazepam Oxazepam Diazepam	Increases effect (increases metabolism)	Use with caution
Bronchodilators	All	Decreases oxidation, leading to possible toxicity	Use with caution
Alpha-II adrenoreceptor agents	Clonidine	Increases sedation effect	Use with caution

From Dickey RP, Yuzpee AA, eds: *Managing contraceptive pill patients*, ed 7, 1993, Emis-Canada.

11

BOX 11-4   Contraindications to Use of Birth Control Pill

Absolute Contraindications
Thromboembolic disorders
Cerebrovascular accident
Coronary artery disease
Breast or gynecologic estrogen-dependent malignancy
Pregnancy
Undiagnosed genital bleeding
Active liver disease
Relative Contraindications
Hypertension
Diabetes mellitus
Sickle cell disease
Impaired liver function within last year
Acute phase mononucleosis
Cardiac or renal disease
Depression
Epilepsy (pill may not be as effective if patient is taking anticonvulsants concurrently)
Lipid disorders
Migraine
Smoking

BOX 11-5   Noncontraceptive Benefits and Uses of OCP

Menstrual
↑ Regularity of cycles
↓ Flow
↓ Dysmenorrhea
↓ PMS
↓ Anemia
Endometrial
↓ Risk of endometrial cancer
Ovarian
↓ Ovarian cysts
↓ Androgen effects
Tubal
↓ Ectopic pregnancy
↓ Pelvic inflammatory disease
Breast
↓ Fibroadenoma
↓ Fibrocystic breast disease
Skin
↓ Acne
↓ Hirsutism

- Demonstrated noncompliance with oral contraceptives
- Menstrual-related anemia
- Need for privacy of contraception
- Lactating women

Contraindications

- Pregnancy

Side Effects

- Irregular bleeding pattern
- Amenorrhea
- Delayed return to fertility (50% conception within 9 mo of use)
- Weight gain (1-3 kg)
- Depression (<5%)
- Possible reduced bone density

LONG-ACTING IMPLANTS (NORPLANT)

- Levonorgestrel (36 mg/capsule) in 6 sialastic capsules implanted sub-dermally
- Effective for 5 yr, but may be removed at any time with return to fertility (40% by 3 mo, 70% by 1 year)

Indications

- Noncompliant with OCP
- Unable to tolerate other forms of contraception (e.g. IUD, diaphragm, Depo-Provera)

Contraindications

- Pregnancy
- Unexplained vaginal bleeding
- Breast cancer
- History of thromboembolic disease
- Bleeding disorder/anticoagulant use
- Sensitivity to progestational agents

Side Effects

- Irregular menstrual pattern (50%)
- Amenorrhea (10%)
- Headache (5%-20%)
- Weight change (<1.2 kg) (5%-20%)

CHAPTER 12

HEMATOLOGY

GIANNOULA KLEMENT

ANEMIA

- Definition: blood hemoglobin (Hb) concentration that is more than two standard deviations below mean for normal population (see p. 507 for normal values)
- Etiology: Caused by inadequate production, abnormal production or increased destruction; distinction between these can be made on basis of reticulocyte count and peripheral blood smear (see Table 12-1 and Figs. 12-1 and 12-2)
- If patient must receive transfusion before diagnosis is made, obtain blood for Hb electrophoresis, HbH prep, Heinz body prep, red cell enzymes, vitamin B_{12}, folate

IRON-DEFICIENCY ANEMIA (see Table 12-1)

- Most common
- Widespread when rapid growth results in large iron requirements
- Recommended iron intake: 1 mg/kg/day for full-term infants (0.5-3 yr), 2 mg/kg/day low birth weight infants (starting no later than 2 mo)
- Evidence that children who were iron deficient in infancy have lower scores on psychomotor function testing

Pathogenesis

- Iron is absorbed from gut and transported in plasma by specialized proteins (transferrin) and stored in cells as ferritin or its degradation product (hemosiderin)
- TIBC (percentage saturation of plasma transferrin) gives measure of iron supply to tissues (TIBC < 16% cannot support erythropoiesis)
- Iron depletion occurs because of inadequate absorption from gut or because of blood loss

Treatment

- Treat underlying cause (e.g., diet), identify source of blood loss (e.g., milk-induced microscopic blood loss)
- 6 mg elemental iron/kg/day PO divided into three doses on empty stomach ½ hr before meals (ferrous sulphate, ferrous fumarate, ferrous gluconate can be used equally)
- Expect reticulocyte response at 7-10 days, check Hb in 1 month; after Hb becomes normal, treat for 2-3 more mo to replenish iron stores
- *Therapeutic trial of iron*: In infants 12-24 mo old with hypochromic microcytic anemia, give iron for 4 wk without further investigation; if anemia responds, continue iron therapy; failure of response to therapy should prompt investigations for other causes of microcytic anemias (chronic inflammatory diseases, thalassemias, sideroblastic anemias).

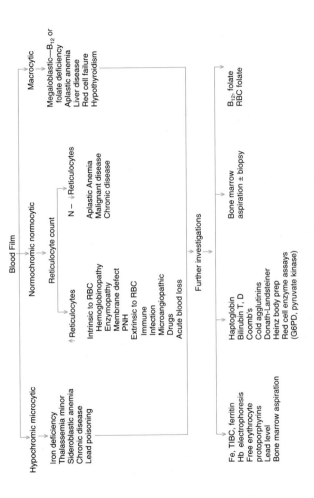

Blood Film

Hypochromic microcytic

Iron deficiency
Thalassemia minor
Sideroblastic anemia
Chronic disease
Lead poisoning

Normochromic normocytic

Reticulocyte count

↑ Reticulocytes

Intrinsic to RBC
Hemoglobinopathy
Enzymopathy
Membrane defect
PNH
Extrinsic to RBC
Immune
Infection
Microangiopathic
Drugs
Acute blood loss

N – ↓ Reticulocytes

Aplastic Anemia
Malignant disease
Chronic disease

Macrocytic

Megaloblastic—B$_{12}$ or
folate deficiency
Aplastic anemia
Liver disease
Red cell failure
Hypothyroidism

Further investigations

Fe, TIBC, ferritin
Hb electrophoresis
Free erythrocyte
protoporphyrins
Lead level
Bone marrow aspiration

Haptoglobin
Bilirubin T, D
Coomb's
Cold agglutinins
Donath-Landsteiner
Heinz body prep
Red cell enzyme assays
(G6PD, pyruvate kinase)

Bone marrow
aspiration ± biopsy

B$_{12}$, folate
RBC folate

Fig. 12-1 Approach to anemia.

HEMOLYTIC ANEMIA

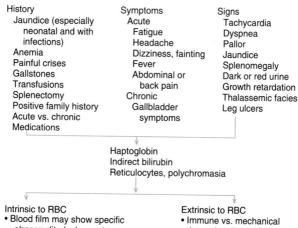

History
- Jaundice (especially neonatal and with infections)
- Anemia
- Painful crises
- Gallstones
- Transfusions
- Splenectomy
- Positive family history
- Acute vs. chronic
- Medications

Symptoms
- Acute
  - Fatigue
  - Headache
  - Dizziness, fainting
  - Fever
  - Abdominal or back pain
- Chronic
  - Gallbladder symptoms

Signs
- Tachycardia
- Dyspnea
- Pallor
- Jaundice
- Splenomegaly
- Dark or red urine
- Growth retardation
- Thalassemic facies
- Leg ulcers

↓

Haptoglobin
Indirect bilirubin
Reticulocytes, polychromasia

Intrinsic to RBC
- Blood film may show specific abnormality (spherocytes, stomatocytes)
- Osmotic fragility test
- G6PD, pyruvate kinase assay
- Hb electrophoresis

Extrinsic to RBC
- Immune vs. mechanical (occasionally direct membrane toxicity
- Warm immune: Coomb's test rule out malignancy, viral (EBV), collagen vascular disease
- Cold immune: mycoplasma, malignancy
- Mechanical: PT, PTT, fibrinogen, fibrin split products (DIC); consider HUS, hemangioma
- Sepsis, drugs

Fig. 12-2 Approach to hemolytic anemia.

ANEMIA OF CHRONIC DISORDERS (Table 12-1)

- Chronic inflammatory states (e.g., JRA), or chronic infections
- Multifactorial in origin: inflammatory mediators (i.e., interleukin 1), blunted response to erythropoietin, and other factors
- Iron stores variable and ferritin unreliable because of inflammatory state; bone marrow may be most efficient assessment of iron
- Treatment: erythropoietin being studied

ANEMIA OF CHRONIC RENAL FAILURE (see Table 12-1)

- Predominant mechanism is reduced erythropoietin production
- Regular monitoring of serum ferritin necessary as iron stores and availability vary because of blood loss with hemodialysis, reduced transferrin saturation

Table 12-1   Hematologic Parameters in Various Types of Anemia

Test	Aplastic anemia	Thalassemia major	Thalassemia minor	Iron deficiency	Anemia of chronic disease
Hemoglobin	↓	↓	↓	↓	↓
MCV	↑	↓	↓	↓	N or ↓
MCH	N	↓	↓	↓	N
Iron	N	↑	N or ↑	↓	N or ↓
TIBC	N	↓	N	↑	↓
Ferritin	N	↑	N or ↑	↓	↑
Transferrin	N	↓	N	↑	↓
Bone marrow stainable iron	N	↑	↑	Absent	N or ↑
Reticulocyte count	↓	N	N	↓	N

N, Normal; ↑, increased; ↓, decreased. Additional parameters may be helpful, i.e., ↑ RBC count in thalassemia, ↑ free erythrocyte protoporphyrins in iron-deficiency anemia and lead poisoning.

12

- Relative iron lack may be overcome by iron supplements, but reducing dose of erythropoietin may be more appropriate
- Treatment: erythropoietin

SIDEROBLASTIC ANEMIAS

- Primary: X-linked or acquired (myelodysplasias)
- Secondary: drug induced (pyridoxine agonists such as isoniazide or cycloserine, chloramphenicol), alcohol induced, or lead poisoning
- Treatment: trial of oral pyridoxine (25-100 mg tid) should be given, but clinically meaningful response is rare; folic acid if deficient; blood transfusions as necessary (iron overload will develop even without transfusions because of excessive iron absorption from diet); desferrioxamine required early on
- For lead poisoning only children with lead encephalopathy need chelation with dimercaprol (BAL) and calcium EDTA

THALASSEMIA SYNDROMES

- Most frequent single gene defects (4% of world population); result of impaired synthesis of one or more globin chains; manifested by microcytic hypochromic anemia; along with reduction of either α or β chain there is production of other chains
- Classified according to globin chain produced at reduced rate: alpha, beta, delta-beta and gamma-delta-beta types; if no α or β chains are produced, thalassemias are described as alpha^0 or beta^0

α-THALASSEMIAS:

- HbH (β$_4$, tetramer of β chains) prep positive
- For most, α-thals, no treatment required; if present in both parents, prenatal screening may be offered
- (α−/αα) heterozygous genotype, produces silent carrier or thal minor,

with none or only mild red cell changes; Hb variants are Hb Bart's (1%-2% γ_4) at birth but no variants in later life

- ($\alpha-/\alpha-$) homozygous or ($--/\alpha\alpha$) heterozygous genotypes produce thal minor with mild hypochromic microcytic anemia and high red cell count; at birth these have 2%-10% Hb Bart's; in later life HbH prep can be positive, making diagnosis difficult
- ($-\alpha/--$) produce HbH disease and chronic hemolytic anemia. At birth HbH Bart's (γ_4 β_4) 10%-40%, later 5%-40%

β-THALASSEMIAS

- Individuals usually normal in utero, anemia only after first months of life when β chain synthesis starts; clinical expression ranges from minor, intermedia to major depending whether one or two β-thal genes inherited
- Increased HbA_2 on electrophoresis
- β-Thalassemia Minor: Heterozygotes for β^0, β^+ (HbA_2 increased to 4%-7%), δβ (HbF 5%-15%) or γδβ; typically asymptomatic and no therapy required; diagnosis important for genetic counseling and to avoid unnecessary iron replacement
- β-Thalassemia Major: Usually diagnosed in first year of life (as γ-chain synthesis decreases): pallor, fatigue, failure to thrive, hepatosplenomegaly

Investigations

- CBC (decreased Hb, severe hypochromia, microcytosis), smear (target cells, bizarre poikilocytosis, basophilic stippling, nucleated red cells), bilirubin (increased because of ineffective erythropoiesis), Hb electrophoresis (decreased or absent HbA, increased HbF)

Treatment (Thal Major)

1. In absence of transfusions, death in first 2 yr of life
2. Blood transfusions (to Hb concentration sufficient to permit normal growth and development); use filtered and plasma-reduced blood (PRBCs) to avoid sensitization; RBC phenotype all new cases, because development of alloantibodies will make cross-matching difficult after numerous transfusions
3. Chelation therapy: Deferoxamine (desferrioxamine) infused subcutaneously overnight (12 hr) or through central venous line via indwelling subcutaneous port if chronic noncompliance with subcutaneous infusion; chelation should begin before age 3 yr, because effects on tissues start early; monitor neurotoxicity (audio and visual); Vitamin C (5-100 mg PO daily) enhances iron urinary excretion in response to deferoxamine and should be used concurrently; clinical trial of *L1* (hydroxypyridone), an oral chelator, is in progress
4. Surveillance for signs of iron overload: Hepatic, cardiac, and endocrine disturbances (delayed puberty, poor growth); monitor by ferritin concentrations
5. Splenectomy less common since transfusions, but indicated whenever transfusion requirements > 220 ml packed RBCs/kg/yr; give pneumococcal vaccine if splenectomy required, and continue child on penicillan V prophylaxis for life

6. Hormone replacement: Testosterone or estrogen when primary gonadal failure or secondary dysfunction resulting from hypothalamic-pituitary axis abnormality; insulin in pancreatic iron overload
7. Bone marrow transplantation from HLA identical siblings
8. Reactivation γ-globin gene: 5-azacytidine, hydroxyurea, or butyrates can reactivate fetal Hb production, but unclear whether this results in clinical elevations of Hb

SICKLE-CELL DISEASE

- Affects primarily persons of African, Afro-Caribbean, Middle Eastern, Indian, and Mediterranean descent; important sickling syndromes are homozygous (HbSS), double heterozygous (HbSC), and sickle β-thalassemia (Sβ thal) disease

DIAGNOSIS

- Smear (sickle cells, target cells polychromasia)
- Hb electrophoresis (see Table 12-2)

CLINICAL FEATURES
Infections

- Particularly with *Pneumococcus, Haemophilus influenzae,* and *Salmonella*
- Risk of *Pneumococcus* infection 600× that in a normal population and prophylactic Pen V can decrease this risk by 80%
- Pneumonia may be difficult to distinguish from chest crises (see the following discussion); osteomyelitis may be difficult to distinguish from vasocclusive crises (see the following discussion)
- Prevention:
  1. Pneumococcal vaccination (initially at 2 yr and booster 5 yr later)
  2. *H. influenzae* vaccine
  3. Influenza virus vaccination
  4. Antibiotic prophylaxis: < 35 mo: Pen VK 150 mg PO bid; > 35 mo: Pen VK 300 mg PO bid (infants ages 3-36 mo at greatest risk and prophylaxis should be started by age of 4 mo)

Table 12-2 Hemoglobin Electrophoresis Patterns in Sickle-Cell Disorders

	Major hemoglobins				
	S	A	F	C	A$_2$
SA	30%-40%	60%	<2%	0	2%-3.2%
SS	80%-90%	0	2%-20%	0	2%-3.2%
SC	50%	0	2%	<50%	—*
SB⁺thal	55%-75%	10%-30%	1%-13%	0	>3.2%
SB°thal	80%-95%	0	1%-15%	0	>3.2%

*Not available because of difficulty in determining HbA$_2$ in presence of HbC.

- Management: Admit if < 3 yr, toxic, febrile, pain, or retic count below steady-state values; cover with IV ampicillin pending cultures unless evidence of chest crises/pneumonia (see the following); if not admitted, must reassess within 24 hr

Vasoocclusive (Painful) Crises

- Provoked by infection, dehydration, or cold; can occur anywhere (bones, muscles, or abdomen most frequent); "hand and foot" most common in infants (dactylitis)
- No specific treatment of painful crises; treatment is supportive:
  1. Fluids (1½ × maintenance initially)
  2. Pain relief: IV bolus of morphine 0.15 mg/kg, then start morphine infusion 40 µg/kg/hr and titrate up/down as needed (see p. 424 for more information about pain management)
  3. Careful surveillance for any evidence of osteomyelitis (increased risk of *Salmonella* osteomyelitis)

Splenic Sequestration

- Major cause of early mortality; degree of sudden anemia often requires urgent transfusion
- Clinical manifestations: pallor, breathlessness, abdo pain, and splenomegaly
- Sequestration episodes tend to recur and after recovering from episode, patient should undergo splenectomy or start on prophylactic transfusion regimen

Chest Crises

- Most common cause of death in sickle-cell disease; may deteriorate rapidly with minimal physical signs
- Treatment consists of supplemental O_2, broad-spectrum antibiotic coverage (IV cefuroxime and erythromycin), packed RBC transfusion (exchange transfusion in severe cases)

Abdominal Crises

- Should be differentiated from cholelithiasis (high incidence, 30% of children > 10 yr) or surgical abdomen
- Abdominal x-rays, ALP, liver function tests, amylase
- Supportive care as previously listed
- Elective cholecystectomy for recurrent episodes of pain and gallstones

Central Nervous System Crises

- 5% incidence of cerebral infarction (may be as high as 30%)
- High risk of recurrence and therefore should be started on regular transfusion program to maintain HbS < 30%, and continue transfusions for minimum of 3 yr (risk of recurrence low thereafter)

Aplastic Crises

- Usually associated with acute infection (parvovirus)
- Supportive care and transfusion

Priapism

- Early surgical consultation, supportive treatment as previously discussed

SURGERY

- Screen all children at risk before surgery and if sickle-cell test positive, confirm by Hb electrophoresis
- HbSA (sickle trait): No specific preparation
- HbSS, SC, S thal: Routine quantitation of HbS unnecessary; transfuse to a Hb > 100 g/L for routine or emergency surgery or radiologic procedures using contrast materials
- For high-risk conditions (cardiovascular, neurosurgical, tourniquets in orthopedic procedures, eye surgery, history of previous stroke): Preoperative exchange transfusion to reduce HbS $< 30\%$
- If status unknown, postpone all elective procedures
- For emergency procedures, consult hematology

LONG-TERM MANAGEMENT

- Folate supplementation
- Ophthalmology (nonproliferative and proliferative retinopathy)
- Renal: tubular function, nephrotic syndrome, hematuria secondary to papillary necrosis
- Hepatobiliary: Gallstones in 11%-12%; 50% by adulthood
- Pulmonary: Multiple chest crises lead to ventilation/perfusion (V/Q) mismatch; restrictive lung disease as early as age 12 yr

12

THROMBOCYTOPENIA

- Low platelet count, but function usually normal (see p. 507 for normal values)
- Conditions with increased production of young cells (ITP) carry fewer risks than those with impaired production (aplasia), even at same numeric levels
- Highest risk of hemorrhagic problems when counts $< 10 \times 10^9$/L
- Causes: ITP, neonatal isoimmune thrombocytopenia, infection, drugs, autoimmune disorder, malignancy, posttransfusion purpura
- Investigations: CBC and differential, blood smear, cultures, and septic workup (exclude LP if Plts $< 50,000$), PL^{A1} antigen and antibody, Coombs' test and blood group, bone marrow examination
- If connective tissue disorder or immunodeficiency suspected: ESR, C_3, C_4 and total complement, immunoglobulins, ANA, ds-DNA

IDIOPATHIC THROMBOCYTOPENIC PURPURA (ITP)

- Immune-mediated thrombocytopenia unassociated with drugs or evidence of disease
- Incidence 4/100,000 children/yr
- Broadly divided into acute (80%-90%), relapsing, and chronic (10%-20%); unclear etiology, but suggestions that acute-phase antiviral IgM antibody cross-reacts with platelet antigens; chronic ITP resulting from IgG autoantibodies to platelet-specific antigens

Diagnosis

- Sudden onset of bruising and purpura in otherwise well child; sometimes history of upper respiratory tract infection (URTI); distinct peak at 2-4 yr of age
- No specific test available (platelet antibodies studies still unreliable)

Treatment

- Emergency (for life-threatening or CNS bleeding): ABCs (see p. 2), emergency splenectomy, ± craniotomy covered by massive platelet transfusion, IVIG and boluses of methylprednisolone (in that order)
- Acute
  1. Steroids: Prednisone 4 mg/kg/day × 3-7 days; taper over 3 wk
  2. 3-4 days pulse of prednisone or dexamethasone presently on trial
  3. IV gamma globulin (IVIG) 1 g/kg for 2 doses, infused over 12 hr each; 0.8 g/kg once appears as efficient in preliminary trials
  4. Observation only (when plt > 20,000)
- Both steroids and IVIG associated with fewer days of profound thrombocytopenia but do not differ significantly from each other (steroids avoid blood-product use or need for IV therapy, allowing for earlier discharge)
- Chronic: treat only if child symptomatic (menorrhagia, nosebleeds, significant purpura), as late remission possible; treatment usually consists of pulses of steroids, intermittent gamma globulin (often to cover elective surgery or other short-term problem), and splenectomy (75% effective, but used selectively because of associated morbidity)

NEONATAL THROMBOCYTOPENIA

- Results from transplacental passage of maternal antiplatelet antibodies
- Two groups:
  1. NAIT (neonatal alloimmune thrombocytopenia)
  2. Neonatal ITP (maternal autoimmune thrombocytopenia)

NAIT

- Results from fetomaternal incompatibility for platelet-specific antigens, most commonly PL^{A1} negative mother and PL^{A1} positive fetus
- Should be suspected whenever otherwise well newborn is profoundly thrombocytopenic but maternal platelets are normal and no history of maternal autoimmune disease or ITP
- Confirm diagnosis by demonstrating that maternal serum IgG reacts with father's/child's platelets
- Treatment options:
  - Benign problem with favorable outcome (observe)
  - If at risk of ICH (if plt count < 50,000), consider cesarean section for delivery
  - Maternal immunosuppression by weekly IVIG (1g/kg/wk for 6-7 wk before delivery)
  - For high-risk pregnancies: monitor plt count in utero and treat with in utero transfusions with washed, irradiated maternal platelets whenever plt <10,000; postnatally support with washed irradiated maternal platelets if necessary; should resolve in 2-3 wk

Neonatal ITP

- Clinically similar to NAIT but distinction important because treatment is different; in this case maternal platelets will be destroyed if transfused (passive ITP)
- Treatment options:
  - Steroids to mother 10-14 days before delivery may reduce need for cesarean section
  - Can also give IVIG to mother antepartum or to child postpartum
- Note: Mild asymptomatic maternal thrombocytopenia does not constitute ITP, and only 50% of children of mothers with ITP will be thrombocytopenic

DIAGNOSIS AND INVESTIGATIONS OF COAGULATION DISORDERS (Fig. 12-3)

HISTORY

- Infections or indwelling catheters, previous surgery or dental extractions (absence of bleeding is strong evidence against bleeding disorders), bleeding postcircumcision, delayed bleeding from umbilical stump (FXIII deficiency), hematomas following immunizations
- In older children, menorrhagia, trauma, etc.
- Sites of bleeding (skin and membranes = platelet disorders; deep hematomas = factor deficiencies)

LAB

- See Laboratory Reference Values, Table IV-4 (p. 510) for normal ranges
- Platelet count and smear
- BT: Bleeding time (abnormal in thrombocytopenia or abnormal platelet function)
- PT: Prothrombin time (extrinsic coagulation pathway: FII, FV, FVII, FX)
- INR: International normalized ratio (PT normalized to standard laboratory reference; used for follow-up of anticoagulated patients)
- APTT: activated partial thromboplastin time (tests intrinsic coagulation pathway: Fbg, FII, FVIII, FIX, FX, FXI, FXII, prekalikrein, and HMWK)
- Inhibitor test: Used whenever PTT prolonged without reason (repeat APTT with 1:1 mixture of patient's plasma and normal pool plasma; if circulating anticoagulant present, PTT remains prolonged)
- TT: Thrombin time (measures conversion of Fbg to fibrin and will be abnormal in hypofibrinogenemia or dysfibrinogenemia, heparin, or FDPs)
- FDPs and D-dimer (fibrinogen degradation products are generated by lysis of fibrinogen and noncross-linked fibrin and are therefore nonspecific; D-dimers generated by lysis of cross-linked fibrin in clots and therefore more specific)
- Factor assays screen: Order V, VII, VIII, and IX
  - VII is best indicator of liver disease (short half-life)
  - V is produced in liver, but is not Vitamin K dependent
  - IX and VII are K dependent

12

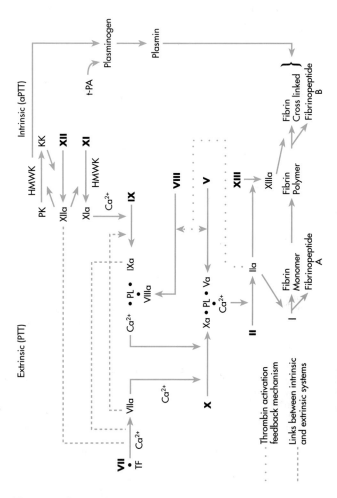

Fig. 12-3   Coagulation cascade. *HMWK,* High molecular weight kininogen; *PL,* phospholipid; *TF,* tissue factor; *t-PA,* tissue plasminogen activator. (Modified from Lilleyman JS, Hann IM, editors: *Pediatric hematology,* New York, 1992, Churchill Livingstone.)

- FVIII is produced by vascular epithelium, independently of liver or Vitamin K and should therefore be normal in liver disease, Vitamin K deficiency, but not in DIC
- Prothrombotic state workup: ATIII, Protein C and S, resistance to activated protein C, HCII (herapin cofactor II)

HEREDITARY COAGULATION DISORDERS

- Hemophilia A and B and von Willebrand disease account for 90%
- Diagnosis: prolonged APTT and reduction in specific factor levels; to exclude vWD need to include vWF:Ag and ristocetin cofactor activity

FACTOR VIII DEFICIENCY (CLASSIC HEMOPHILIA OR HEMOPHILIA A)

- X-linked recessive disorder, resulting from decreased plasma levels of procoagulant activity (FVIII:C) of FVIII molecule; gene coding for FVIII:C assigned to band q28 of X chromosome (DNA analysis most accurate in carrier detection and prenatal diagnosis)
- 30% of cases are spontaneous mutations, but diagnosis is easily made in bleeding newborn because FVIII:C levels should be at adult range at birth, and FVIII:C does not cross placenta
- Classified into mild (FVIII:C > 10%, bleed only with trauma or surgery)
  moderate (FVIII:C 2%-10%, bleed with minor trauma)
  severe (FVIII:C < 2%, bleed spontaneously)
- At least 50% of hemophiliacs are severely affected; these males will have recurrent bleeds into joints, muscles, and soft tissues
- Lab: ↑PTT, ↓FVIII:C; normal vWF and ristocetin cofactor activity

Long-Term Care

- Prevention of hemophiliac arthropathy in "target joint" by effective early replacement therapy (any time of day or night) and physiotherapy
- No IM injections (consult hemophilia nurse for vaccinations)
- No aspirin or antiplatelet drugs
- Prophylactic dental care and preparation for elective surgeries
- Surveillance for hepatitis and HIV even though products much safer today
- Patient education and psychosocial support

Treatment of Bleeding Episodes

- Avoid blood products if possible
- DDAVP (1-deamino-8-D-arginine-vasopressin) 0.3 μg/kg dissolved in 10-20 ml NS and infused over 20 min; should raise FVIII:C level 2-4 × its basal level and should be used preferentially whenever such a rise is sufficient to achieve hemostatic levels (30% FVIII:C); response will diminish if therapy needed for longer than 3-4 days; even mild hemophiliacs may require factor replacements for prolonged postsurgical hemostasis
- FVIII concentrates (Table 12-3): Hemophil-M, Koate HP or recombi-

12

Table 12-3   Factor VIII Concentrate Replacement Indications and Doses

Indications	Replacement	Desired FIII:C
Early hemarthrosis	15-20 U/kg once daily	30%
Mucous membrane bleed	Tranexamic acid or 15 U/kg once	30%
Established hemarthrosis, head injury without CNS deficit	25 U/kg once daily	50%
Life-threatening bleed (ICH, surgery, impending airway obstruction	70 U/kg loading dose, then 40-50 U/kg q12h or continuous infusion as long as symptoms persist	80%-100%

Table 12-4   Factor IX Concentrate Replacement Indications and Dose

Indications	Replacement	Desired FIX:C
Early hemarthrosis	20 U/kg once daily	20%
Established hemarthrosis, head injury without CNS deficit	40 U/kg once daily	40%
Life-threatening bleed (ICH, surgery, impending airway obstruction)	60 U/kg initially, then 40 U/kg till asymptomatic, then 20% FIX:C for total of 10 days	60%

nant Kogenate (1 U of FVIII/kg increases factor VIII:C activity by 2%, with a half-life of between 8-12 hr)
- Factor VIII inhibitors will develop in 6%-10% of patients regardless of frequency or type of replacement therapy; more common in specific family groups and blacks
- Treatment of bleeding in patient with inhibitors:
  1. For noncritical hemorrhage use activated prothrombin complex concentrates such as Feiba VH Immuno or Autoplex, to avoid anamnestic response in high responders
  2. For critical hemorrhage use human FVIII concentrate at doses 2-3 × higher (50 U/kg)
  3. Alternative approaches include
     - Porcine FVIII
     - Infusion of plasma-derived and recombinant FVIIa, which activates factor X directly, effectively bypassing FVIII-dependent step

FACTOR IX DEFICIENCY (CHRISTMAS DISEASE OR HEMOPHILIA B)

- Clinically indistinguishable from hemophilia A; also X-linked
- FIX is Vit K-dependent factor and is gestationally reduced at birth, making early diagnosis difficult
- Lab: ↑PTT, ↓FIX; normal FVIII:C, vWF and ristocetin cofactor activity
- Bleeds are treated with FIX concentrates (1 U/kg increases activity by

1% with half-life of 18-24 hr); longer half-life allows for less frequent replacement (Table 12-4)
- Avoid giving antifibrinolytic agents (epsilon-aminocaproic acid [EACA], tranexamic acid) concurrently with FIX concentrates; use heparin prophylaxis in patients receiving antifibrinolytics or FIX concentrates during surgery (increased risk of thromboembolic complications)

VON WILLEBRAND DISEASE (VWD)

- Von Willebrand factor (vWF) is large, highly complex molecule that (1) mediates platelet adhesion and (2) functions as carrier protein for FVIII:C
- vWF gene located on chromosome 12 (autosomal recessive)
- Incidence of vWD difficult to establish as some cases are very mild and go undetected
- Four main subtypes: I, IIa, IIb, and III; types I and II characterized by increased bruising and prolonged bleeding from cuts; type III associated with low level of VIII:C and will manifest by hemarthrosis and hematomas
- Lab: vWf: Ristocetin cofactor activity < 1

Treatment:

12

- Type-I vWD: 1-deamino-8-D-arginine-vasopressin (DDAVP, 0.3 μg/kg intravenously in normal saline at concentration of 0.5 μg/ml to a maximum of 24 μg over 20 min)
- Type-IIa vWD: Most of time DDAVP ineffective as mainly abnormal VIII-vWF complexes are released (subset will release large vWF multimers with some hemostatic activity)
- Type-IIb: DDAVP is *contraindicated,* because abnormal forms aggregate platelets and drop platelet counts
- Type-III vWD: unresponsive to DDAVP and should therefore be treated with FVIII concentrate rich in HMW multimers; if not available, may replace with cryoprecipitate (20-40 U factor VIII activity/kg daily)

DISSEMINATED INTRAVASCULAR COAGULATION (DIC)

- Always associated with underlying disorder (Box 12-1), which triggers coagulation via endothelial injury (intrinsic pathway) or via tissue factors (extrinsic pathway); main clinical problem is bleeding, even though thrombosis of small vessels occurs

Diagnosis

- PT, PTT, and thrombin time (TT) are prolonged; fibrinogen and platelet count are reduced; fibrin degradation products (FDP) and D-dimers are elevated
- Serial hematologic measurements necessary to rule out DIC, as consumption may be compensated

BOX 12-1 Disorders Associated with DIC

Children

Infection
  Bacterial (e.g., meningococcus)
  Parasitic (e.g., malaria)
  Mycotic
  Rickettsial
  Viral (e.g., disseminated varicella)
Neoplasms
  Leukemia, particularly M3 AML
  Metastatic solid tumors
Miscellaneous
  Giant hemangioma (Kasbach-Merritt syndrome)
  Purpura fulminans
  Hemolytic transfusion reaction
  Acute anaphylaxis
  Snakebite
  Burns
  Heatstroke
  Hypothermia
  Massive head injury or trauma
  Hemorrhagic shock

Neonatal

Hypoxia: acidosis (birth asphyxia, respiratory distress syndrome, polycythemia)
Infection (bacterial, viral)
Dead twin fetus
Small for gestational age
Abruptio placenta
Miscellaneous (erythroblastosis fetalis, necrotizing enterocolitis, brain injury)

Management:

- Most important to treat underlying disorder to remove trigger
- Replacement therapy: platelets (1 U/5 kg body weight)
    FFP (10-15 mg/kg body weight q8h)
    cryoprecipitate or FVIII as source of fibrinogen (1 bag/5 kg body weight)
    PRBCs as needed
- Use of heparin controversial

VITAMIN K DEFICIENCY

- Affects factors II, VII, IX, X and anticoagulants (proteins S and C)
- For urgent reversal use FFP 10 ml/kg body weight and vitamin K_1 1 mg SC or slow IV push (correction within few hours)
- To reverse therapeutic anticoagulation, larger doses of vitamin K_1 may be required (2.5-5 mg)
- For oral supplementation, vitamin K_3 is better absorbed

DEEP VENOUS THROMBOSIS

- Uncommon in children and mostly acquired (posttraumatic, SLE); rarely, inherited imbalance between activators and inhibitors of either coagulation or fibrinolysis will predispose to thrombosis

Table 12-5   Blood Products

Blood product	Indications	Dose/kg body weight	Source
Packed RBC's (250-300 ml/U)	Symptomatic anemia	10 ml/kg	Fractionated human blood
Fresh frozen plasma (200-250 ml/U)	Vit K def., liver dis., DIC	10 ml/kg	Fractionated human blood
Platelets (30-50 ml/U)	Thrombocytopenia	1 U/5 kg	Fractionated human blood
Albumin	Volume expansion	10-15 ml/kg	Human plasma
Cryoprecipitate	Factor replacement in DIC	1 bag/5 kg	Single human donor

- Latter are autosomally inherited and do not present until adolescence; heterozygotes have levels at half normal value
- Only homozygous protein C deficiency presents in newborn

Investigations

- Imaging: venogram (gold standard), ultrasonography or radionucleotide scans; impedance plethysmography (IPG): available, but not standardized for children
- Thrombotic workup (if no clearly identified precipitant): protein C, protein S, reptilase time, thrombin time, fibrinogen, plasminogen, antithrombin III, lupus anticoagulant, resistance to activated protein C (rAPC); baseline measurement of PT and PTT for monitoring of anticoagulant therapy
- If pulmonary embolism suspected: CXR and ventilation/perfusion scan

Management

- ABCs if pulmonary embolism suspected (see p. 2)
- Start anticoagulation before imaging if clinical suspicion of thrombosis high or life-/limb-threatening
- Initial bolus 75 U of standard heparin/kg IV, followed by maintenance dose of 28 U/kg/hr by continuous IV infusion for patients less than 1 year of age and 20 U/kg/hr for patients > than 1 year of age; titrate to maintain PTT 1.5-2.5 × normal; verify with heparin level
- If prolonged anticoagulation expected, start Coumadin from day 1 of anticoagulant therapy and continue heparin until INR 2-3; for Coumadin guidelines, see p. 612
- In small number of cases in which protein C deficiency is diagnosed early, initial treatment should be FFP (10-15 ml/kg); half-life of protein C is 7 hr, and concentrate should be obtained for acute cases (consult hematology)

TRANSFUSION REACTIONS

- Document any reaction and notify blood bank; return offending blood product to blood bank with 5 ml of patient's blood and first posttransfusional urine specimen

IMMEDIATE

- Fever (HLA antibodies against leucocyte and platelet antigens [Ag]); if multiple febrile reactions, give leukocyte-depleted blood (washed or filtered), and premedicate with acetaminophen
- Allergic manifestations:
  - Urticaria (foreign Ag from donor plasma reacts with corresponding IgE Ab in recipient), easily treated with diphenhydramine 1-2 mg/kg/dose IV q6h
  - Anaphylaxis (most commonly resulting from IgA Ab and may be fatal); see p. 17 for management of anaphylaxis
- Hemolysis:
  - Immune-mediated, intravascular, binding complement (e.g., ABO incompatibility); most serious in O individuals
  - Immune-mediated, extravascular, noncomplement binding (e.g., Rh incompatibility, but also Kell, Duffy, and Kidd), delay of 45 min before symptoms appear and peak at 4 hr
- Hemorrhagic state
  - Dilutional thrombocytopenia with massive transfusions or posttransfusion thrombocytopenia resulting from microaggregates (can be improved by filtering PRBCs)
  - Depletion of labile factors (V and VIII) with prolonged storage

DELAYED

- Hemolysis: When antibody (Ab) present in very low levels, blood screen will be negative and incompatible blood given; transfused blood will boost Ab production, and hemolysis will start 2-10 days later (whenever titers high); classically anti-Kidd Abs
- Sensitization to red cell antigens
- Infectious diseases (e.g., CMV, hepatitis, HIV)

CHAPTER 13

HEPATOLOGY

DAT J. TRAN

- See Box 13-1 for symptoms and signs of liver dysfunction
- See Table 13-1 for a guide to liver disorders
- See Fig. 13-1 for average values of liver spans
- See Fig. 13-2 for an approach to hepatosplenomegaly

LABORATORY EVALUATION

SERUM MARKERS OF HEPATOBILIARY DISEASE

- For normal values, see individual tests in Laboratory Reference Values section (p. 507)

Hepatocellular Necrosis

1. Aspartate aminotransferase (AST/SGOT)
   - Present in liver, skeletal muscle, heart, kidney, brain
   - Elevated in excess of ALT in alcoholic liver disease, typically by factor of ≥ 2
2. Alanine aminotransferase (ALT/SGPT)
   - Localized primarily in liver
   - More sensitive than AST for detecting liver damage

Cholestasis

1. Alkaline phosphatase (ALP)
   - Normal values vary with age (increase during pubertal growth spurt)
   - Present in liver, bone, intestine, placenta, kidney, leukocytes
   - Increased in cholestasis, hepatic carcinoma, bone disease
   - Decreased in Wilson's disease (presenting as acute liver failure with hemolysis), zinc deficiency, hypothyroidism, pernicious anemia, congenital hypophosphatasia
2. γ-Glutamyl transpeptidase (GGT)
   - Present in liver, kidney, seminal vesicles, pancreas, spleen, heart, brain, but not bone, unlike ALP
   - Normal values vary with age, sex
   - Most sensitive indicator of biliary tract disease
   - May be increased by hepatic microsomal enzyme-inducing drugs or substances (e.g., barbiturates, phenytoin, alcohol)
   - Used to confirm liver disease when ALP is raised if patient is not on inducer
3. 5′-Nucleotidase (5′NT)
   - Present in liver, intestine, brain, heart, blood vessels, pancreas
   - Elevated only in hepatobiliary disease (obstructive, cholestatic, infiltrative)

BOX 13-1 Symptoms and Signs of Liver Dysfunction

Constitutional
Fatigue, malaise, irritability, anorexia, weight loss, failure to thrive
Nausea, vomiting, diarrhea
Fever
Fetor hepaticus
Cutaneous
Jaundice (± dark urine and pale stools)
Pruritus, excoriations
Spider telangiectasias, palmar erythema
Xanthomas, xanthelasma
Vitiligo and acne (autoimmune hepatitis)
Finger clubbing
Leukonychia
Endocrine
Gynecomastia, testicular atrophy
Rickets
Puberty delay
Hypoglycemia
Gastrointestinal
Right upper quadrant abdominal pain
Abdominal swelling (hepatomegaly*, splenomegaly†, ascites)
Collateral abdominal circulation
Hepatic bruits
Varices, gastrointestinal bleeding
Hematologic
Anemia: pallor
Thrombocytopenia: petechiae, purpura
Coagulopathy: ecchymoses
Neurologic
Altered sleep pattern, somnolence
Subtle behavioral changes
Confusion, obtundation
Ataxia
Asterixis
Other
Pleural effusions
Arthritis

---

*See Fig. 13-1 for normal values for liver spans.
†Spleen tip may be palpable in children < 4 yr of age.

- Used to confirm liver disease when ALP raised if patient is on inducer
4. Bilirubin
    - Degradation product of heme
    - Serum concentration represents balance between bilirubin production and excretion
    - Elevated in hemolysis, parenchymal liver disease, extrahepatic bile duct obstruction, congenital disorders of bilirubin metabolism

Text continued on p. 205.

Table 13-1 Clinical Guide to Liver Disorders

Disorder	Investigations	Associated specific clinical features
Infectious		
Toxoplasmosis	Specific IgM antibody, rising IgG titers; detection by CF, IFA, ELISA; isolation of virus from CSF, liver	Chorioretinitis, diffuse intracranial calcifications
Rubella	Isolation of virus from pharyngeal secretions, urine, CSF, liver; IgM-specific antibody	Cataracts, hearing loss, patent ductus arteriosus
Cytomegalovirus	Typical inclusion bodies in exfoliated cells in urine, gastric contents, liver; identification of virus in buffy coat and tissue cultures; CF, IFA antibody tests	Chorioretinitis, hearing loss, periventricular intracerebral calcifications
Herpes simplex virus	Isolation of virus from vesicles, cell culture; rising antibody titers	Skin vesicles, signs and symptoms of sepsis
Syphilis	Bone x-rays, dark-field examination, VDRL, FTA-ABS, TPI test	Osteochondritis, periostitis, snuffles, rash
Hepatitis A	See Table 13-3	
Hepatitis B	See Table 13-3	
Hepatitis C	See Table 13-3	
Hepatitis D ("Delta AG")	See Table 13-3	
Coxsackievirus/echovirus	Isolation from respiratory tract, stool, liver, CSF, blood	Myocarditis, meningoencephalitis, hepatitis, fulminant liver failure
Adenovirus	Isolation from respiratory tract, stool; antibody titers	Pneumonitis, meningoencephalitis, hepatitis, myocarditis, fulminant hepatic failure in immunocompromised
Epstein-Barr virus	Heterophil antibody titer > 1:128; Anti-VCA, Anti-EA	Splenomegaly, lymphadenopathy, usually mild hepatic dysfunction; can be fulminant in Duncan Syndrome

Continued.

13

Table 13-1 Clinical Guide to Liver Disorders—cont'd

Disorder	Investigations	Associated specific clinical features
Varicella	Isolation from lesions, liver	Disseminated in immunocompromised hosts
Bacterial	Blood, urine, CSF cultures	Liver abscess: fever, weight loss, RUQ tenderness; nonspecific liver dysfunction; *E. coli, Klebsiella, Enterobacteriaceae, Staphylococcus, Pseudomonas, Proteus*
Listeria	Isolation of organism from blood culture, CSF, liver	Neonates: sepsis, meningitis, pneumonitis
Tuberculosis	CXR, gastric aspirates	Tender hepatomegaly, granulomatous hepatitis
Genetic and Metabolic		
Trisomy 13, 18, 21	Chromosomes	20%-30% have hepatitis
α-1-antitrypsin deficiency	Pi typing, α₁-antitrypsin levels	Autosomal codominant (chromosome 14) Pi ZZ, Znul, nul deficient; may present at any age, including neonatal hepatitis; 25%-50% develop cirrhosis
Cystic fibrosis	Sweat chloride, increased serum trypsinogen	Autosomal recessive (chromosome 7); neonates; inspissated bile; older children: focal biliary cirrhosis
Galactosemia	Nonglucose-reducing substances in urine, decreased galactose-1-phosphate uridyl transferase in RBCs	Autosomal recessive: vomiting, failure to thrive, cataracts; *E. coli* sepsis
Fructosemia	Fructose in urine, decreased or absent hepatic fructose-1-phosphate aldolase B	Autosomal recessive: vomiting, hypoglycemia, FTT; aversion to fructose-containing foods
Tyrosinemia	Increased urinary succinyl acetone, ↑alpha fetoprotein, abnormal serum amino acids	Autosomal recessive: FTT, hepatocellular failure, renal tubular dysfunction; 100% develop hepatomas
Glycogen storage disease	Liver biopsy for histology and enzyme assay	I: hepatomegaly, hypoglycemia, increased lactic acid, increased uric acid III: hepatomegaly, hypoglycemia, hepatic fibrosis IV: hepatosplenomegaly, cirrhosis, hypotonia VI, IX: hepatomegaly

Gaucher's disease	Gaucher cells in bone marrow; decreased glucosyl ceramide-β-glucosidase in liver, WBC, bone marrow
Niemann-Pick disease	Decreased sphingomyelinase in WBC, liver; sea-blue histiocytes in liver and BM
Wolman disease	Decreased acid esterase in WBC, liver
Cholesterol ester storage disease	Lipoprotein electrophoresis, partial deficiency of acid esterase
Zellweger disease	Increased iron, TIBC, decreased plasmalogens, absence of peroxisomes on liver biopsy
Perinatal hemochromatosis	Liver biopsy showing end-stage cirrhosis, increased ferritin, hemosiderin-laden macrophages from nasopharynx
Endocrinopathies	See section on *endocrinology*; increased suspicion if perinatal hypoglycemia
Wilson's disease	Increased basal 24-hr urine copper excretion; low serum copper, ceruloplasmin, haptoglobin; ophthalmologic examination for Kayser-Fleischer rings, low ALP with hemolysis; liver biopsy for copper content, specific EM changes
Nonalcoholic steato-hepatitis	Liver biopsy, lipoprotein electrophoresis
Byler's disease	Liver biopsy
Toxic	
Total parenteral nutrition	
Drugs	In vitro lymphocyte testing
Inspissated bile syndrome	Secondary to severe or prolonged hemolysis
Reye's syndrome	See section on Reye's syndrome

Hepatosplenomegaly, CNS involvement (neuronopathic) hemolytic anemia, bone pain
Hepatosplenomegaly, progressive dementia, blindness (Types A and C); may progress to cirrhosis; may present as neonatal hepatitis
Vomiting, hepatosplenomegaly, diarrhea, adrenal calcification, steatorrhea, developmental delay, onset in infancy
Hepatomegaly ± splenomegaly, hyperlipidemia type II, increased triglycerides, onset in late childhood
SGA, cataracts, severe hypotonia, microscopic renal cysts, stippled patella, abnormal facies
Hepatocellular failure, small liver, ascites
Hypopituitarism, diabetes insipidus, hypoadrenalism, hypothyroidism, hypoparathyroidism
Age of onset > 4 yr; may present as acute or chronic hepatitis, hepatic failure, hemolytic anemia, CNS or psychiatric symptoms
Obesity; no history of ingestion of alcohol or other toxins; mild aminotransferase elevation; exclude Wilson's disease
Progressive intrahepatic cholestasis, pruritis, jaundice, malabsorption, hepatomegaly, hepatic fibrosis
See p. 370
See Table 13-9
Prognosis good

13

Continued.

Table 13-1 Clinical Guide to Liver Disorders—cont'd

Disorder	Investigations	Associated specific clinical features
Vascular		
Congestive heart failure	CXR, ECG, 2-D echo	Hepatomegaly, increased respiratory and heart rate
Budd-Chiari syndrome	Abdominal US, venography	Oral contraceptive use
Shock	Liver biopsy	Associated with acute tubular necrosis, hypoxic-ischemic encephalopathy; liver dysfunction usually resolves
Venocclusive disease	Abdominal US, venography	Associated with antineoplastic drugs, bush tea
Portal vein thrombosis	Abdominal US and Doppler, venography	Hepatomegaly uncommon, associated with umbilical vein catheters; splenomegaly prominent
Structural		
Alagille syndrome	Liver biopsy: paucity of interlobular bile ducts	Butterfly vertebrae, posterior embryotoxin, peripheral pulmonic stenosis, abnormal facies, jaundice
Nonsyndromic bile duct paucity	Liver biopsy: paucity of interlobular bile ducts	Jaundice prominent; many causes, including cystic fibrosis, infections
Congenital hepatic fibrosis and Caroli's syndrome	Abdominal US, ERCP, PTC (percutaneous transhepatic cholangiography), liver biopsy	Hepatosplenomegaly with normal liver function tests, associated renal anomalies
Autoimmune		
Autoimmune chronic active hepatitis	ANA, ESR, antiliver/kidney microsomal antibody, increased IgG, antismooth muscle antibody, antimitochondrial antibody, decreased C_4, liver biopsy	Consider diagnosis after 1-2 mo liver dysfunction (vs. 6 mo in adults), associated with ulcerative colitis, polyserositis, polyarteritis nodosa, Coombs positive hemolytic anemia, thyroiditis, lupus, arthritis, glomerulonephritis
Primary sclerosing cholangitis	Increased ALP or GGT, IgG, ANA, antismooth muscle antibody, ERCP, PTC, liver biopsy	Associated with inflammatory bowel disease, often precedes onset of bowel symptoms

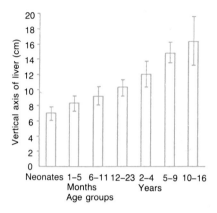

Fig. 13-1   Normal (average) values for liver spans in various age groups. (Adapted from Deligeorgis D, Yannakos D, Doxiadis S et al: Normal size of liver in infancy and childhood, *Arch Dis Child* 48:792, 1973.)

13

TESTS OF LIVER FUNCTION
Albumin

- Low serum level suggests poor hepatic synthetic function
- Not good indicator of hepatic protein synthesis in *acute* liver disease
- Also depressed with malnutrition and renal disease

Lipoproteins

- Cholesterol increased in chronic cholestasis
- Decreased levels of cholesterol esters and cholesterol-derived hormones (e.g., testosterone) in chronic liver failure

Globulins

- Gammaglobulins increased in viral hepatitis, autoimmune hepatitis, cirrhosis
- Absent α_1-globulin in α-1-antitrypsin deficiency

Clotting Factors

- Hepatocytes synthesize factors I, II, V, VII, IX, X
- Kupffer's cells synthesize factor VIII

Prothrombin time

- Prolonged because of decreased coagulation factor synthetic capacity (factors II, VII, IX, X)
- Also prolonged with vitamin K deficiency, consumptive coagulopathy

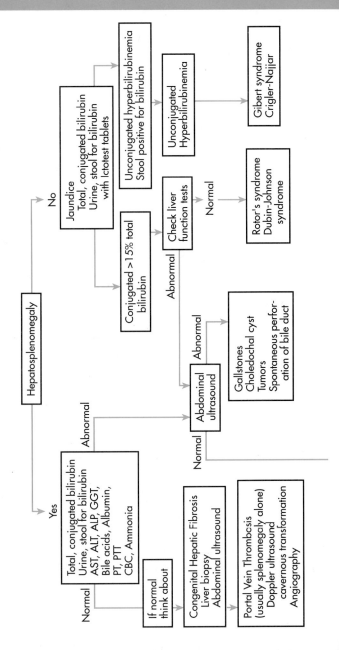

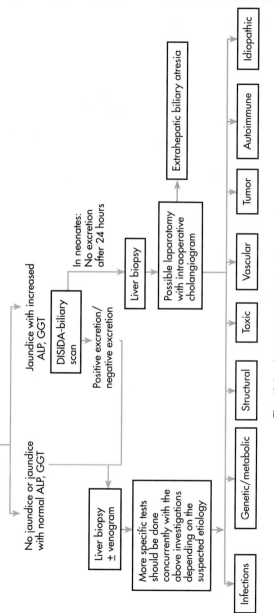

Fig. 13-2 Approach to hepatosplenomegaly.

13

Bilirubin

- See discussion in previous section
- Measure conjugated and unconjugated bilirubin

Bile Acids

- Major organic anions excreted by liver
- Required for lipid digestion and absorption
- Normally undergo enterohepatic recirculation
- Increased serum level is sensitive indicator of hepatic dysfunction
- May be increased in both acute and chronic liver disease

OTHER TESTS
Serum Ammonia

- Major source is bacterial production in large bowel
- Elevated with hepatic dysfunction because of disturbances in urea cycle
- Elevated in liver disease, hemodialysis, valproic acid therapy, Reye's
- syndrome, urea cycle enzyme deficiencies, organic acidemias, carnitine deficiency

Alpha-Fetoprotein (AFP)

- Elevated in hepatoblastoma and hepatocellular carcinoma
- Increased in tyrosinemia with or without hepatocellular carcinoma

RADIOLOGIC EVALUATION

Plain-Film Radiography

- Still provides useful information such as:
  - Major anomalies (e.g., transverse-lying liver seen in asplenic syndrome)
  - Air in hepatic portal system (e.g., NEC, patulous sphincter of Oddi)
  - Slightly radiolucent liver (e.g., fatty liver in malabsorption states or storage diseases)
  - Parenchymal calcifications (e.g., hemangiomas, TB, syphilis, CMV, tumors)
  - Liver size

Ultrasound ± Doppler

- Screening for biliary tree dilation, gallstones, parenchymal (focal and diffuse) disease
- Can assess patency of blood vessels and direction of flow with color-flow Doppler
- Can quantify ascites
- Major disadvantage: dependence on skilled operator

CT ± Intravenous Contrast

- Best for focal parenchymal liver disease, also biliary tract disease
- Contrast enhancement allows assessment of space-occupying lesions (e.g., abscess, tumor, vascular lesions)

Magnetic Resonance Imaging (MRI)

- Similar utility to CT
- Allows some visualization of vessels without contrast dye
- No radiation involved

Radionuclide Scans

- Older sulfur colloid scan ("liver/spleen scan") largely superseded by ultrasound (US)
- Hepatobiliary scan (e.g., DISIDA scan) most applicable in study of congenital biliary aberrations (e.g., biliary atresia)
- Premedication with phenobarbital 5 mg/kg/day $\times$ 3-5 days greatly enhances accuracy

Angiography

- Conventional method replaced by digital subtraction angiography for assessment of hepatobiliary vasculature

Cholangiography

- Percutaneous transhepatic cholangiography (PTC), percutaneous transhepatic transcholecystic cholangiography (PTTC), endoscopic retrograde cholangiopancreatography (ERCP)
- Most useful after abnormal preliminary screening by US, CT, or MRI for detailed imaging of biliary tree
- PTC has few age restrictions; must be > 4 yr of age for ERCP
- Consider risk after acute pancreatitis

REYE'S SYNDROME

- Acute sporadic encephalopathy of unknown cause, characterized by reversible abnormality of mitochondrial structure with decreased mitochondrial enzymatic activity
- Predominantly in patients aged 6 mo to 15 yr (range, 4 days-29 yr)
- 0.2-4.0/100,000 children
- 3-4 day prodromal viral illness (e.g., respiratory tract infection, gastroenteritis, varicella, influenza A and B)
- Vomiting: profuse, persistent
- Rapid appearance of neurologic changes, seizures in 30%
- Encephalopathy: five stages leading to brain death (Table 13-2)
- Onset may be atypical in rheumatologic patients
- Etiology unknown, associated with ASA, aflatoxin

LABORATORY

- Serum aminotransferases elevated 2-100 $\times$ normal
- Hyperammonemia may be transient
- Mildly prolonged prothrombin time; bilirubin usually normal
- Hypoglycemia in severe cases
- CSF normal, but glucose concentration may be low

Table 13-2 Stages of Encephalopathy in Reye's Syndrome

	I	II	III	IV	V
Level of consciousness	Quiet, responds to verbal commands	Lethargic, difficulty counting	Agitated, delirium, responds to pain	Coma, decerebrate posturing	Coma, spinal reflexes preserved
Muscle activity	Normal	Clumsy	Poorly controlled gross movements ± clonus	Opisthotonus, extensor spasms of arms, legs	Flaccid paralysis
Respiratory rate	Normal	Normal–increased	Normal–increased	Increased	None
Pupillary response	Normal	Normal	Dilated, responds rapidly	Dilated, responds slowly	Dilated, unresponsive
Fundi	Normal	Normal	Venous engorgement	Papilledema	Variable

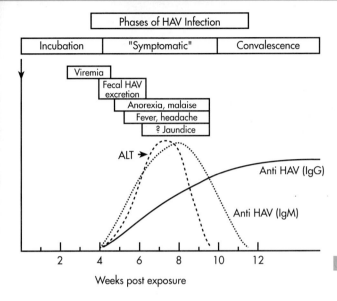

Fig. 13-3 Typical course of hepatitis A infection. (From Balistreri WF: Viral hepatitis, *Pediatr Clin North Am* 35:640, 1988.)

13

TREATMENT

- Intravenous glucose (D10W), fluid restriction (60% of maintenance)
- See management of ICP (p. 13) and fulminant hepatic failure (Fig. 13-5)
- Mortality 30%-60%

TOTAL PARENTERAL NUTRITION (TPN)— ASSOCIATED LIVER DISEASE

- Etiology unknown
- Frequency decreases with increasing gestational age
- Other associated factors: sepsis, hypoxia, blood transfusion, intraabdominal surgery, drugs
- Onset: 10-180 days (onset earlier in premature infants)
- Elevation of AST, GGT, or ALP appears first
- Conjugated hyperbilirubinemia
- Hepatosplenomegaly
- Elevated serum bile acids (may be difficult to measure in premature infants and newborns)
- Acute acalculous cholecystitis, biliary sludge, cholelithiasis
- Cholestasis, hepatocellular damage with multinucleated giant cell transformation, mild inflammation
- May progress to fibrosis and cirrhosis

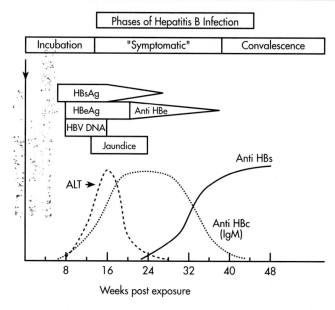

Fig. 13-4   Typical course of acute, resolving hepatitis B infection. (From Balistreri WF: Viral hepatitis, *Pediatr Clin North Am* 35:647, 1988.)

TREATMENT

- Withdrawal of TPN and start of oral feeds
- Liver function tests usually return to normal within 5 months
- Liver biopsy changes may persist for up to 1 yr
- If TPN continued, progressive liver disease with cirrhosis occurs

VIRAL HEPATITIS

- See Table 13-3 for comparison of major hepatotrophic viruses
- See also Tables 13-4 and 13-5, Figs. 13-3 and 13-4, and Box 13-2

LIVER FAILURE

- See Fig. 13-5 for definition, signs and symptoms, investigations, and management of fulminant liver failure
- See Table 13-6 for manifestations and management of chronic end-stage liver disease
- See also Tables 13-7 and 13-8

Table 13-3 Comparison of Major Hepatotropic Viruses

	Hepatitis A ("Infectious" hepatitis)	Hepatitis B ("Serum" hepatitis)	Hepatitis C ("Transfusion-related NANB" hepatitis)	Hepatitis D (Delta hepatitis)	Hepatitis E ("Epidemic or enterically transmitted NANB" hepatitis)
Causative Agent	HAV Picornavirus; 27 nm spherical, nonenveloped RNA virus	HBV Hepadnavirus; 42 nm double-enveloped DNA virus	HCV Flavivirus; 27-60 nm enveloped RNA viruses	HDV Deltavirus; Defective 35-37 nm hybrid RNA particle with HB-sAg coat*	HEV Calicivirus; 27-34 nm nonenveloped RNA virus
Age Group	First three decades in developed countries First decade in developing countries	Adolescents and adults in nonendemic areas Young children in endemic areas	All ages More frequent in children with transfusion history	Uncommon in children	More common in adults (peak = 15-40 yr)
Onset	Abrupt	Insidious (adolescent) More abrupt (toddler)	Insidious	Often abrupt	Abrupt
Incubation Period • Mean (Range)	25-30 days (15-50)	120 days (45-160)	7-9 wk (2-24)	Coinfection: same as HBV Superinfection: 2-8 wk	40 days (15-60)

*Replicates and causes hepatitis only in patients who concurrently are infected with HBV.

13

Continued.

Table 13-3 Comparison of Major Hepatotropic Viruses—cont'd

	Hepatitis A ("Infectious" hepatitis)	Hepatitis B ("Serum" hepatitis)	Hepatitis C ("Transfusion-related NANB" hepatitis)	Hepatitis D (Delta hepatitis)	Hepatitis E ("Epidemic or enterically transmitted NANB" hepatitis)
Transmission					
• Parenteral	± (Brief viremic phase)	+++++	Sporadic (no exposure history in 20% 40%) +++++ (40% IV drug use, 10% transfusion)	+++++ (In developed countries)	—
• Fecal-oral	+++++	—	—	—	+++++
• Sexual	—	+++	++ (Reported with multiple partners)	++ (In developing countries)	?
• Perinatal	—	++++ (Accounts for most of mother-infant transmission; horizontal maternal–child transmission high in first 5 yr; transplacental rare)	++ (Risks have not been defined)	+	? (↑ fetal deaths with hepatitis E in mother)
Symptomatology	Majority asymptomatic. If symptomatic, mild nonspecific signs and symptoms	Majority of young children asymptomatic. If symptomatic, more likely to be severe and to involve skin and joints	Majority asymptomatic or mildly symptomatic	Similar to HBV, often more severe	Similar to HAV, often more severe

Nonspecific					
• Fever	Common before jaundice	Uncommon	Uncommon	Uncommon	Common
• Malaise, anorexia	Common	Common	Common	Common	Common
• Nausea, vomiting	Common	Common	Common	Common	Common
• Diarrhea	Uncommon	Uncommon	Uncommon	Uncommon	Common
• Abdominal pain	Common	Common	Uncommon	Common	Common
Hepatic					
• Jaundice	Uncommon in children	Less common	Uncommon	Less common	Common
• Tender hepatomegaly	Common	Common	Uncommon	Common	Common
Extrahepatic					
• Lymphadenopathy	Common	Common	Common	Common	Common
• Splenomegaly	Uncommon	Common	Uncommon	Common	Less common
• Immune complex diseases (e.g., rash, arthritis, glomerulonephritis)	Rare	Less common	Uncommon	Uncommon	Less common
Infectious Period	Fecal excretion maximal 2 wk prior to onset of illness or jaundice, and minimal by 1 wk post	During HBsAg positivity (occasionally only with anti-HBc positivity)	? During anti-HCV positivity	During HDV RNA or anti-HDV positivity	Unknown

Continued.

13

Table 13-3 Comparison of Major Hepatotropic Viruses—cont'd

	Hepatitis A ("Infectious" hepatitis)	Hepatitis B ("Serum" hepatitis)	Hepatitis C ("Transfusion-related NANB" hepatitis)	Hepatitis D (Delta hepatitis)	Hepatitis E ("Epidemic or enterically transmitted NANB" hepatitis)
Serologic Diagnosis	(See also Figs. 13-3 and 13-4)				
• Acute infection	Anti-HAV-IgM Viral particles in stool (Anti-HAV-IgG signifies previous infection)	Anti-HBc-IgM (5 mo) HBsAg (1-3 mo)	Clinical and serologic exclusion (Anti-HCV negative in 60%-90%) (HCV RNA by PCR)	Anti-HDV-IgM Coinfection (2-4 wk): Anti-HBc-IgM Superinfection (10 wk): HBsAg *but* negative Anti-HBc-IgM	Clinical and serologic exclusion (Anti-HEV)
• Chronic infection	Not applicable	HBsAg (≥ 6 mo) Anti-HBc-IgG ± HBeAg (high infectivity) ± Anti-HBe	Anti-HCV	Anti-HDV persistence HBsAg	Clinical and serologic exclusion
• Immunity	Anti-HAV-IgG (5% reinfection)	Anti-HBs (Post infection or immunization)	Anti-HCV does not confer immunity	Anti-HBs	Unknown
Outcome					
• Severity	Mild	Mild to moderate	Mild to moderate	Moderate to severe	Mild to moderate
• Recovery	98% (children) >90% (adults)	80%-85% (children and adults)	Variable (50%-90%)	Unknown	Unknown
• Mortality†	Low (0.1%)	Low (1%-3%)	Low (1%-3%)	Low to moderate	Low (high in pregnant women)

• Fulminant disease	Rare (0.1%-0.2%) 40% survival	Uncommon (1%-2%) 17% survival	Uncommon (<5%) 10% survival	More common (5%-20%) (highest risk with superinfection)	Uncommon (1%-2%) 10%-30% in pregnant women, with high mortality
• Carrier state	No	Yes	Yes	Yes	No
• Chronic hepatic disease	No	Yes	Yes	Yes	?
• Chronic hepatitis	5%-10%	10%-50%	50%-70%	Similar to HBV (more common with superinfection)	?
• Cirrhosis	Low	1%-5%	10%	Worse prognosis than HBV infection alone	
• Hepatocellular carcinoma	No	High (accounts for 80% of HCC) (Risk of carrier, chronic disease, and carcinoma related inversely to age at time of infection)	Yes (less than HBV)	?	?
Treatment					
• Acute	Supportive	Supportive	Supportive	Supportive	Supportive
• Chronic		Interferon α-2b available for chronic hepatits B and C in adults with compensated liver disease	Supportive		
Prophylaxis	Hygiene IG before or within 2 wk of exposure HAV vaccine (see Box 13-2)	Universal precautions HBIG HBV vaccine (see Tables 13-2 and 13-3)	Universal precautions ?? IG (equivocal) No vaccine	Universal precautions HBV prophylaxis (see Table 13-3)	Hygiene ? IG (equivocal) No vaccine

13

†Aplastic anemia can complicate severe hepatitis from any of these viruses.

Table 13-4 Indications and Dosing Schedule for Hepatitis B Vaccine and Immunoglobulin

Group at risk	Vaccine			HBIG	
	Recombivax HB (µg)	Engerix-B (µg)	Schedule	Dose (ml)	Schedule
Neonates					
Infants of HBsAg-positive mothers[a]	5	10	Birth (within 7 days), 1 mo, 6 mo	0.5	Within 12 h of birth
Infants of HBsAg-negative mothers[b]	2.5	10	Birth, 1-2 mo, 6-18 mo[d]		None
Contact with Acute HBV					
Intimate					
<11 yr old	2.5	10	Exposure, 1 mo, 6 mo	0.06/kg	Exposure[f]
11-19 yr old	5	20	Exposure, 1 mo, 6 mo	0.06kg	Exposure[f]
≥20 yr old	10	20	Exposure, 1 mo, 6 mo	0.06/kg[e]	Exposure[f]
Household[c]	None	None	None		None
Casual	None	None	None		None
Contact with Chronic HBV					
Intimate and household					
<11 yr old (incl. neonates)	2.5	10	Exposure, 1 mo, 6 mo		None
11-19 yr old	5	20	Exposure, 1 mo, 6 mo		None
≥20 yr old	10	20	Exposure, 1 mo, 6 mo		None
Casual	None	None			None

| Dialysis and Other Immunosuppressed Patients | 40 | 40 | Exposure, 1-6 mo | None |

Adapted from Behrman RE, Kligman RM, Arvin AM: *Nelson textbook of pediatrics*, ed 15, Philadelphia, 1996, Saunders.

a Check infant's serology at 7 mo; if HBsAg and anti-HBs are negative, repeat dose of vaccine; if HBsAg is positive, prophylaxis has failed, follow as carrier; if anti-HBs is positive, vaccination was successful.

b AAP recommendation for universal vaccination of infants (USA); NACI recommendation for universal vaccination of all school-age children (Canada).

c Give HB vaccine and HBIG in infant (<12 mo) exposed to acutely infected primary caregiver.

d Infants in populations with high rates of childhood hepatitis B infection should complete the three-dose series by 6-9 mo.

e Maximum 5 ml.

f Exposure means within 14 days.

Note: High-risk groups for hepatitis B include:

1. Household and sexual contacts of HBsAg carriers
2. Healthcare workers frequently exposed to blood and blood products
3. Residents and staff of institutions for mentally handicapped
4. Hemodialysis patients, hemophiliacs, and other recipients of blood products
5. Active homosexuals
6. Users of illicit injectable drugs
7. Heterosexually active persons with multiple partners
8. Some experts recommend vaccination of children in group childcare

13

Table 13-5 Recommendations for Hepatitis B Prophylaxis after Percutaneous Exposure to HBsAg-Positive Blood

Exposed Person	HbsAg-Positive	Treatment when source found to be:	
		HbsAg-Negative	Unknown or Not Tested
Unvaccinated	Administer HBIG* × 1 and initiate HB vaccine series†	Initiate HB vaccine series	Initiate HB vaccine series (May give HBIG within 48 hr if high-risk source).
Previously vaccinated			
Known responder	Test exposed person for anti-HBs‡ 1. If adequate, no treatment 2. If inadequate, one HB vaccine booster dose	No treatment	No treatment
Known nonresponder	HBIG × 2 or HBIG × 1 and HB vaccine × 1	No treatment	If known high-risk source, treat as if source were HBsAg-positive
Response unknown	Test exposed person for anti-HBs 1. If adequate, no treatment 2. If inadequate, HBIG × 1 and one HB vaccine booster dose	No treatment	Test exposed person for anti-HBs 1. If adequate, no treatment 2. If inadequate, one HB vaccine booster dose

From American Academy of Pediatrics: Hepatitis B. In Peter G, ed: *1994 Red book: report of the committee on infectious diseases*, ed 23, Elk Grove Village, IL, 1994, American Academy of Pediatrics.

*HBIG dose is 0.06 ml/kg IM: Administer within 48 hr; should double-check that HBIG is clear of HCV.

†HB vaccine dose: see Table 13-4.

‡Adequate anti-HBs ≥ 10 mIU.

Table 13-6 Management of Chronic/End-Stage Liver Disease

Problem	Approach
Malnutrition*	
1. Fat malabsorption	Administer:
• Multifactorial origins (one is decreased intestinal bile salts)	• Medium-chain triglyceride or MCT–containing formulas (e.g., Pregestimil), or supplemental MCT oil
2. Protein and caloric malnutrition	Ensure:
a. Abnormal amino acid metabolism (elevated total free amino acids, aromatic acids, and methionine)	• Adequate (preferably ≥ 1.5 g/kg) and appropriate protein (vegetable source, branched-chain amino acid supplement)
b. Failure to thrive	• Adequate calories (glucose polymers such as Caloreen)
3. Fat-soluble vitamin deficiency (A, D, E, K)	At least twice recommended daily allowance
a. Vitamin A deficiency	• Vit A (Aquasol A) 5000-25000 IU PO daily
• Xerophthalmia	
• Dermatitis	
b. Vitamin D deficiency	• Vit D₂ 5000-10000 IU PO daily or 25-OH-D 3-5µg/kg PO daily
• Bone changes: rickets (young child), osteomalacia (adolescent)	• Follow Ca, P, ALP, ± vit D level
c. Vitamin E deficiency	• TPGS (tocophenyl polyethylene glycol succinate) 15-25 IU/kg/day
• Anemia	• Follow vitamin E levels, may require megadoses
• Ataxic neurodegenerative syndrome	
d. Vitamin K deficiency	• Vit K₁ 2.5/wk-5 mg/day PO or 2-5 mg SC prn (dose variable)
• Abnormal coagulation	• Follow PT
• Abnormal calcium and phosphorus utilization (osteocalcin: vitamin K–dependent protein in osteoblasts that contributes to bone calcification)	

Continued.

13

Table 13-6 Management of Chronic/End-Stage Liver Disease—cont'd

Problem	Approach
Malnutrition—cont'd	
4. Water-soluble vitamin deficiency	Twice recommended daily allowance
5. Mineral deficits	Supplementation not routine
a. Calcium deficiency	• Calcium 25-100 mg/kg PO daily
b. Phosphorus deficiency	• Phosphorus 25-50 mg/kg PO daily
c. Zinc deficiency	• Zinc 1 mg/kg PO daily
• From intestinal and urinary loss	
d. Iron deficiency	• Iron 1 mg/kg/day
Cholestasis	
Jaundice, pruritus, xanthomas, xanthelasma	Low-cholesterol diet
• From bile acids and cholesterol	Choleretic agent
	• Cholestyramine 100-300 mg/kg/day PO
	Symptomatic control:
	• Nocturnal antihistamines
Bleeding	
Etiologies	Management
a. Esophageal varices resulting from portal hypertension	a. Endoscopic sclerotherapy or variceal ligaton vs. portosystemic shunting
b. Hypersplenism (thrombocytopenia)	b. Avoid antiplatelet drugs (e.g., ASA, NSAIDS)
c. Coagulopathy	c. Vitamin K
• Prolonged PT (prolonged PTT in very advanced disease)	d. Fresh frozen plasma
• Pathogenesis	e. H$_2$ blocker, vasopressin, and transfusion prn
• Vitamin K malabsorption	
• Inadequate hepatic production of nonvitamin K–dependent factors	

Anemia

Normocytic anemia

Etiologies

a. Fe deficiency secondary to
   - Gastrointestinal blood loss
   - Fe malabsorption
   - Low transferrin levels
b. Hypersplenism
c. Hemolysis
d. Folic acid deficiency
e. Increased concentration of bile acids
f. Vitamin E deficiency
g. Hypoproteinemia

Management

a. Monitor Hb periodically
b. Control/treat varcies
c. Often refractory; consider:
   - Iron only if ↓ serum Fe and ↑ TIBC; (TIBC often normal and Fe supplementation not helpful)
   - Vit E
   - Folic acid
   - Steroids if hemolytic anemia

Ascites (± Edema/Pleural Effusions)

Fluid is transudative† (see Table 13-7)

Pathogenesis

a. Increased renal sodium retention
b. Portal hypertension (increased hydrostatic pressure)
c. Hypoalbuminemia (decreased oncotic pressure)
d. Impaired free water excretion

Complications

a. Increased variceal hemorrhage
b. Hepatorenal syndrome
c. Spontaneous bacterial peritonitis
d. Anorexia
e. Hernia
f. Pleural effusion
g. Pulmonary insufficiency, atelectasis, pneumonia
h. Iatrogenic (azotemia, hypokalemia, hyponatremia)

Management

a. Sodium restriction (25 mg/kg/day)
b. Bedrest occasionally helpful
c. Diuretics
   - Spironolactone 1-4 mg/kg/d (diuretic of choice, monitor for ↓ [Na$^+$], occasionally ↑ [K$^+$], and metabolic acidosis)
   - Furosemide 1-2 mg/kg/d (monitor for ↓ [K$^+$])
d. Water restriction (insensibles + losses)
   - Only if dilutional hyponatremia prominent
e. Salt-poor albumin (0.5-1 g/kg/day) ± furosemide
   - In cases of azotemia and intravascular volume depletion

Surgical management
   - Paracentesis for distress

Vigilance for spontaneous bacterial peritonitis

13

Continued.

Table 13-6 Management of Chronic/End-Stage Liver Disease—cont'd

Problem	Approach
Increased Susceptibility to Infections	Diagnosis
Sites: Pulmonary infections	a. High index of suspicion
SBP (see below)	b. Fever may be inconspicuous and may be little leukocytosis
Septicemia	Management
UTI	• Appropriate antibiotic course
Pathogenesis: Defective neutrophilic chemotaxis	
Decreased complement	
Spontaneous Bacterial Peritonitis	Diagnosis
Incidence	a. Confirmatory = PMN count $> 250/mm^3$ ± positive culture;
• 20% of patients with cirrhosis	(inoculate 5-10 ml sample into blood culture bottle at bedside)
Pathogenesis	b. Highly suggestive = PMN count $> 250/mm^3$, pH < 7.31, low protein
a. Route: most likely hematogenous (concomitant bacteremia in 40%-60%)	(<20 g/L)
b. Organisms: *E. coli*, 70%; *S. pneumoniae*, 10%-15%	Management
Presentation	• Third-generation cephalosporin (avoid aminoglycosides because of poor
a. Fever, chills	penetration into ascitic fluid, inactivation at acid pH, and nephrotoxicity)
b. Increasing abdominal distention and pain with rebound tenderness, decreased bowel sounds	
c. May have few abdominal signs	
d. Worsening of both mental status and renal function (i.e., hepatic encephalopathy)	

Renal Insufficiency

Etiologies
a. Prerenal failure
b. Acute tubular necrosis
c. Functional renal failure or hepatorenal syndrome (HRS)
   • Documented afferent arteriolar constriction from likely combination of
     –Increased false neutrotransmitters
     –Decreased circulating angiotensinogen
     –Circulating endotoxins
     –Decreased renal prostaglandins

Differential diagnosis
a. Infection (sepsis, UTI)
b. Urinary tract obstruction
c. Cardiac disease
d. Drug-induced nephrotoxicity
e. Hypotensive event

Impaired Drug Clearance

Pathogenesis
a. Hepatic failure
b. Renal failure (see above)
c. Portal-systemic shunting
d. Hypoalbuminemia

Diagnosis (See Table 13-8)

Management
a. Prerenal failure
   • Volume expansion
b. ATN
   • Can recover with dialysis
c. HRS
   • Treatment is expectant (no predictably effective therapy)
   • Therefore must rule out treatable causes of renal failure and treat appropriately before making diagnosis of HRS

General principles of drug usage
a. Reduce dosage
b. Follow closely for signs of toxicity and serum levels when available
c. Choose alternative agents not significantly metabolized by liver, not associated with chronic liver disease, and not nephrotoxic

Continued.

13

Table 13-6   Management of Chronic/End-Stage Liver Disease—cont'd

Problem	Approach

Chronic Portosystemic (Hepatic) Encephalopathy
 	
Early features
• Mood changes, behavior changes, deterioration of intellectual performance, altered sleep pattern
 	
Pathogenesis
a. Hypotheses
  • Ammonia (directly encephalopathic)
  • Synergistic neurotoxins (ammonia, mercaptans, short-chain fatty acids, phenols)
  • GABA (↑penetration through abnormal BBB and ↑GABA receptor density)
  • False neurotransmitters (aromatic acids, tryptophan, octopamine, and secretin precursors)
	Management:
	a. Identify, remove/correct, and avoid precipitants
	  • Tight fluid and electrolyte control
	b. Dietary
	  • Protein (vegetable) restriction (0.5-1 g/kg/day), increase to maximum tolerated
	c. Lactulose (PO/PR)
	  Reduces ammonia resorption by:
	  • Decreasing bacterial production of ammonia (by lowering colonic pH, which alters hydrolysis by colonic bacteria)
	  • Speeding colonic evacuation

b. Precipitating factors
  - Gastrointestinal hemorrhage
  - Hypokalemia (especially with alkalosis)
  - Sepsis, SBP
  - High-protein diet
  - Constipation
  - Sedative-hypnotic medications (safest is diazepam at 25%–50% of normal dose)
  - Azotemia
  - Development of hepatocellular carcinoma
  - Pancreatitis
  - Surgery (especially portosystemic shunts)

Inexorable Progression of All Above

d. Antibiotics (neomycin, metronidazole)
  - Reduces amount of bacterial urease available
  - No more efficacious than lactulose
  - Neomycin causes small bowel mucosal damage, is nephrotoxic and ototoxic (should be used for short courses only)
e. Combination therapy
  - Lactulose + antibiotic may be synergistic
  - Consider in cases refractory to either agent alone

Transplantation
1. Timely assessment and listing
2. Give all immunizations prior to transplant, if possible

13

---

*May require supplemental NG feeds or TPN to prevent catabolic state, rickets, ataxia syndrome, coagulopathy, xerophthalmia.

†Has a high albumin gradient (≥ 11 g/L). The serum-ascites albumin gradient (serum albumin concentration minus ascitic fluid albumin concentration) correlates directly with portal pressure, and is superior to the old exudate-transudate concept in differentiating ascites because of portal hypertension (albumin gradient ≥ 11 g/L) from those not resulting from portal hypertension (albumin gradient < 11 g/L)

Table 13-7 Comparison of "Typical" Findings in Transudates and Exudates

Findings	Transudates	Exudates
Specific gravity†	<1.016	>1.016
Protein (g/L)	<30	>30
Peritoneal fluid–serum ratio‡	<0.5	>0.5
LDH (IU/L)	<200	>200
Peritoneal fluid–serum ratio‡	<0.6	>0.6
Peritoneal fluid–upper limit normal serum ratio‡	<2/3	>2/3

Adapted from Wallach J: *Interpretation of diagnostic tests,* ed 5, Boston, 1992, Little, Brown.

*"Typical" means 67%-75% of patients.

†Long-standing transudates can produce high specific gravity.

‡*All* three of these criteria constitute best differential of exudate and transudate; transudates meet all of these criteria, and exudates meet at least one criterion.

Table 13-8 Diagnostic Approach to Renal Insufficiency in End-Stage Liver Disease

	Prerenal	Hepatorenal syndrome	ATN
Clinical	Signs of hypovolemia Resolves with volume expansion	No preceding hypovolemia No response to volume expansion Hypothermia Usually accompanied by hepatic encephalopathy and ascites	
Laboratory			
Na_u (mmol/L)	<10%	<10	>30
Fractional Na excretion*	< 1%	<1%	>3%
Cr_u/Cr_{Pl}	>30	>30	<20
$Osmol_u/Osmol_{Pl}$	>1.1	>1.1	1
Urine sediment	Normal ↑BUN> ↑CR	Normal BUN and CR ↑proportionally	Protein, casts, cellular debris

Adapted from Tanner S: *Pediatric hepatology,* Current Reviews in Paediatrics 4, New York, 1989, Churchill Livingstone.

$$*\frac{Na_u}{Na_{Pl}} \times \frac{Cr_{Pl}}{Cr_u} \times 100 \text{ } (u, \text{ urine}; Pl, \text{ plasma})$$

BOX 13-2 Hepatitis A Prophylaxis Before Exposure (Travelers to Endemic Regions)

< 3 mo trip	IG: 0.02 ml/kg once
	Vaccine*
≥ 3 mo trip	IG: 0.06 ml/kg every 4-6 mo
	Vaccine*

After Exposure

Household and intimate contacts	
Day care or custodial care	IG: 0.02 ml/kg within 2 wk once
Common-source outbreaks	
Casual contact	None

From Behrman RE, Kliegman RM, Arvin AM: *Nelson textbook of pediatrics,* ed 15, Philadelphia, 1996, Saunders.

*When available, vaccine will replace need for IG for travelers; HAV vaccine (HAVRIX) in the licensing process for children in Canada; in U.S., licensure includes use for children 2 to 18 yr of age in whom dosage of 360 ELU is recommended at schedule of 0, 1, and 6 to 12 months; likely that licensure in Canada will be updated to coincide with that of U.S.; in anticipation of approval, Canadian children who would benefit from vaccine when traveling should be offered it.

Definition: syndrome of severe impairment of hepatic function associated with progressive mental changes. Encephalopathy must develop within 8 wk of onset of liver disease, with no clinical evidence of previous liver disease.

Signs and Symptoms
Jaundice
Hepatic encephalopathy
Asterixis
Fetor hepaticus (sweetish, slightly fecal smell of exhaled breath)
Bleeding
Ascites
Vomiting
Hypoglycemia
Lethargy
Combativeness

Biochemical Parameters
Prolonged PT, PTT
Factors V, VII important in prognosis
Increased bilirubin, ammonia
Decreased fibrinogen, glucose
Follow BUN, creatinine, electrolytes, calcium, phosphorus, magnesium

Abdominal ultrasound
Diagnosis
Assessment of portal vein and flow in case transplantation required
Follow liver size

Neurologic status
Early stages assess with Trail test

Metabolic screen
Wilson's disease
Galactosemia
Tyrosinemia
Fructosemia

Viral tests
Hepatitis A
Hepatitis B
Hepatitis C

Transjugular liver biopsy
Contribute to diagnosis and prognosis
Liver tissue for virology, electron microscopy, antibody staining, histology, enzyme assay
Venogram and venous pressure
(Percutaneous biopsy contraindicated because of coagulopathy)

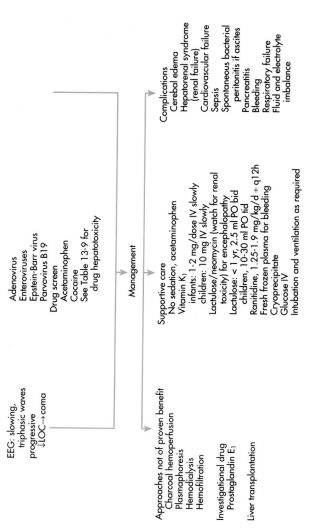

Adenovirus
Enteroviruses
Epstein-Barr virus
Parvovirus B19
Drug screen
  Acetaminophen
  Cocaine
  See Table 13-9 for
    drug hepatotoxicity

EEG: slowing,
  triphasic waves
  progressive
  ↓LOC→coma

Complications
  Cerebral edema
  Hepatorenal syndrome
    (renal failure)
  Cardiovascular failure
  Sepsis
  Spontaneous bacterial
    peritonitis if ascites
  Pancreatitis
  Bleeding
  Respiratory failure
  Fluid and electrolyte
    imbalance

Management

Supportive care
  No sedation, acetaminophen
  Vitamin K₁
    infants: 1-2 mg/dose IV slowly
    children: 10 mg IV slowly
  Lactulose/neomycin (watch for renal
    toxicity) for encephalopathy
  Lactulose: < 1 yr, 2.5 ml PO bid
    children, 10-30 ml PO tid
  Ranitidine, 1.25-1.9 mg/kg/d ÷ q12h
  Fresh frozen plasma for bleeding
  Cryoprecipitate
  Glucose IV
  Intubation and ventilation as required

Approaches not of proven benefit
  Charcoal hemoperfusion
  Plasmapheresis
  Hemodialysis
  Hemofiltration

Investigational drug
  Prostaglandin E₁

Liver transplantation

13

Fig. 13-5 Fulminant liver failure.

Table 13-9 Drug Hepatoxicity

Drug	Type of liver injury	Comments
Acetaminophen	Hepatocellular necrosis	Fatality usually because of drug overdose, but dose may be in therapeutic range; measure plasma concentrations; treatment with N-acetylcysteine preferably within 24 hr of ingestion; prognosis better than other etiologies of fulminant liver failure
Aspirin	Nonspecific focal hepatitis	Association with Reye's syndrome; usually mild-to-moderate dose-dependent rise in serum aminotransferases in patients on high doses of aspirin (e.g., rheumatic diseases, Kawasaki disease)
Carbamazepine	Hepatocellular necrosis	Rarely can develop hepatic failure; may be associated with cholangitis
Cocaine	Hepatocellular necrosis Steatosis	Hepatitis, fulminant hepatic failure, associated myoglobinuria, tachycardia, high fever, rapid increase in aminotransferases; look for cocaine metabolite in urine
Erythromycin	Focal hepatic necrosis Cholestatic reaction	<6%; onset usually within 1-4 wk; may be associated eosinophilia; prognosis excellent on withdrawal of drug
Halothane	Hepatocellular necrosis	Usually requires more than one exposure to halothane; asymptomatic hepatitis to fulminant liver failure; also reported with methoxyflurane and enflurane
Isoniazid	Hepatocellular necrosis	Mild hepatitis, chronic hepatitis, fulminant liver failure
Methotrexate	Steatosis, fibrosis	May lead to cirrhosis despite normal liver-function tests; total dose and duration of treatment important factors; biopsy may be recommended before institution of drug
Phenytoin	Hepatocellular necrosis Granulomatous hepatitis	May be associated rash, fever, lymphadenopathy, absolute eosinophilia; may develop fulminant liver failure
Rifampicin	Hepatocellular necrosis	Hepatitis, impairment of bilirubin uptake by liver
Sulfonamides	Hepatocellular necrosis	May have associated fever, arthralgia, rash, eosinophilia; chronic active hepatitis, granulomatous hepatitis, fulminant liver failure reported; reaction usually occurs within 2 wk of starting drug; in vitro lymphocyte testing
Valproic acid	Hepatocellular necrosis Microvesicular steatosis	10% will develop elevation of serum aminotransferases; this is usually asymptomatic and reverses spontaneously; raised ammonia levels may be present; fatal hepatitis usually in children under 10 yr, within 6 mo of start of therapy, males > females, usually on multianticonvulsant therapy; can also develop Reye's-like syndrome

CHAPTER 14

INFECTIOUS DISEASES

JANE KIM

IMMUNIZATION

- Canadian guidelines for immunization published regularly by National Advisory Committee on Immunization (NACI)
- Premature infants: normal schedule based on postnatal age
- Schedule interruptions: no need to restart from beginning
- Universal precautions: do not recap needles
- Site of injection: Infants: anterolateral thigh; all others: deltoid area
- IM injections: Use long needles (e.g., >7/8 in)
- Acetaminophen 15 mg/kg at 0 and 4 hr postvaccination and then q4h prn to decrease fever and fussiness
- All routine vaccines can be given safely and effectively at the same time using different sites
- Monitor all children for 15 min postvaccination and have epinephrine immediately available for possible anaphylaxis
- Report any significant adverse reaction to local Medical Officer of Health (Public Health Department)

Contraindications

- Anaphylactic reaction to previous dose of vaccine
- Anaphylactic reaction to constituent of vaccine
- Moderate to severe illnesses with or without fever (*not* simple colds)
- Oral egg allergies: avoid influenza and yellow fever vaccines
- Live vaccines (MMR, OPV, BCG, and yellow fever) contraindicated in:
  1. Pregnancy (mother's children still eligible)
  2. Immunodeficiency diseases such as hypogammaglobulinemia or combined immunodeficiency
  3. Altered immune status resulting from diseases such as leukemia or other generalized malignancy. (Note: MMR *should* be given to all HIV patients)
  4. Within 3 mo of chemotherapy or immunosuppressive therapy (vaccinations may not be effective until 3-12 mo posttreatment)

DIPHTHERIA, PERTUSSIS, TETANUS , POLIOMYELITIS AND HIB CONJUGATE VACCINE (Table 14-1)
Preparations

- For use under 7 yr: Pentavax (DPT-IPV-Hib), combined DPT-polio (inactivated polio virus, IPV) and Hib, or DPT and OPV (oral live polio virus) and Hib each separately; Pentavax (DPT-IPV-Hib) available in Canada (except Manitoba)
- DPT-Hib and DPT-IPV combinations currently licensed in United States

Table 14-1 Schedule of Immunizations

Age or timing	Vaccine
Infants Beginning Series in Early Infancy	
2 mo	DPT Polio + Hib
4 mo	DPT Polio + Hib
6 mo	DPT Polio + Hib[a]
After 1st birthday	MMR[b]
18 mo	DPT Polio + Hib
4-6 yr[c]	DPT Polio, MMR[b]
14-16 yr	Td[d] Polio[e]
For Children 1 through 6 yr of Age not Immunized in Early Infancy	
First visit	DPT Polio + Hib, MMR[b]
2 mo after 1st visit	DPT Polio + Hib[f]
2 mo after 2nd visit	DPT Polio[e]
12 mo after 3rd visit[g]	DPT Polio
4-6 yr of age[c]	DPT Polio, MMR[b]
14-16 yr of age	Td§ Polio[e]
For Unimmunized Children 7 yr of Age and Over	
First visit	Td[d] Polio + Hib, MMR[b]
2 mo after 1st visit	Td Polio
6-12 mo after 2nd visit	Td Polio
Every 10 yr thereafter	Td

Modified from the National Immunization Committee on Immunization (NACI): *Canadian immunization guide,* ed 4, Ottawa, 1993, Health Canada

[a]This dose may be omitted if PedVax HIB (PRP-OMP by Merck Frosst) is used for doses 1 and 2.

[b]MMR administered subcutaneously and must be given after 1st birthday; all school pupils in Ontario must have documented receipt of 2 doses of measles vaccine; rubella vaccine also indicated for all girls and women of child-bearing age who lack proof of immunity; at all medical visits opportunity should be taken to check whether such patients have received rubella vaccine.

[c]The 4-6 yr (5th) dose of DPT polio not necessary if preceding (4th) dose given after 4th birthday.

[d]Diphtheria and tetanus toxoid (Td), combined adsorbed "adult-type" preparation for use in persons 7 yr of age or more, contains less diphtheria toxoid than preparations given to younger children and is less likely to cause reactions in older persons.

[e]This dose may be omitted if live (oral) polio vaccine being used.

[f]This dose may be omitted if child >15 mo but recommended for higher-risk children (e.g., asplenia, sickle-cell disease, or immunosuppression).

[g]When last of above doses given before the 4th birthday, consideration should be given to administration of additional dose at school entry.

- For use above 7 yr: Combined Td-polio (IPV) or Td-OPV (pertussis vaccine not indicated)
- Acellular pertussis vaccine undergoing field trials in young infants and appears to have similar efficacy with lower rate of local and systemic adverse reactions in infants after 5 mo of age; not yet available for use in Canada

Administration

- Booster dose of Td should be given every 10 yr following primary immunization
- Majority of systemic side effects of DPT are due to pertussis vaccine
  - Minor: 50%-75% will have local pain, redness, swelling; fever; irritability

- Major: prolonged crying (1%), hypotonic unresponsive state (1:1750), seizure (1:1750)
- If child recovers from culture-proven pertussis, no further doses of pertussis vaccine required, although, for convenience, routine immunization, including pertussis, may be continued
- OPV may rarely produce paralytic illness in recipient (1 in 11.7 million doses); adults at greater risk
- OPV (not IPV) may be recommended for outbreak control because of fecal shedding and secondary "immunization"
- Inadequate or unknown status of polio immunity in household not contraindication to immunization of child with OPV; "household" adults may be given one dose of IPV at same time as first dose in infant (risk to unimmunized "household" contacts 1 in 5 million doses)
- Polio has been eradicated from Western Hemisphere

Contraindications Against DPT Vaccine

- Absolute: Anaphylactic reaction to previous dose of vaccine
- Precaution: Hypotonic-hyporesponsive state within 48 hr of previous dose of DPT
  Note: Deferral of pertussis vaccine may be considered in children with progressive, evolving, or unstable neurologic condition to prevent confusion of diagnosis of adverse reaction; continue vaccination with combined DT without pertussis component

Contraindications Against Polio Vaccine

- OPV: Children with HIV infection or immunodeficiency state
  Household contacts with HIV infection or immunodeficiency state
  May be used in pregnancy with precaution
- IPV: Anaphylactic reaction to streptomycin or neomycin
- Note: All inpatients in neonatal intensive care setting should receive IPV at scheduled times; if possible, routine polio immunization with OPV should be delayed until after discharge; OPV may be used in specific long-term situations

HAEMOPHILUS INFLUENZAE TYPE B (Tables 14-1, 14-2)

- Active immunization (*Haemophilus influenzae* type b conjugate vaccine)
- Side effects: local pain and erythema, mild fever (10%)

Table 14-2 Recommendations for Hib Conjugate Vaccine if Initial Vaccination Delayed until >7 Mo of Age

Age at initiation of vaccine (mo)	Number of doses	Timing of doses
7-11	3	2 doses separated by 2 mo, then 3rd dose at 12-18 mo, given at least 2 mo after 2nd dose
12-14	2	2 mo interval
>15	1	Some recommend 2 doses separated by 2 mo for higher-risk children (e.g., asplenia, sickle cell, immunosuppression)

Modified from the National Immunization Committee on Immunization (NACI): *Canadian immunization guide,* ed 4, Ottawa, 1993, Health Canada.

Postexposure Prophylaxis with Rifampin

- In cases of invasive *H. influenzae* type b disease (e.g., meningitis, arthritis, pneumonia), rifampin given to
  1. All household contacts and index case if there is immunocompromised child, child less than 12 mo, or unvaccinated child less than 48 mo of age at home
  2. Day care center attendees (controversial)
  3. If two or more cases are detected within 60 days
  4. In day care homes resembling households with children <2 yr old in which contact at least 25 hr/wk (same regimen as recommended for household contacts); not required when all contacts >2 yr old and fully immunized

MEASLES, MUMPS, AND RUBELLA (see Table 14-1)
Recommendations

- In Ontario: 2 doses recommended at 12-15 mo and 4-6 yr

Side Effects

- General: fever (day 6 or later), rash, hypersensitivity reactions in children allergic to eggs
- Measles and mumps
  1. Encephalitis (rare)
  2. TB skin test reactivity may be suppressed if administered 1-6 wk following measles vaccination
- Rubella: Arthralgia, arthritis

Contraindications

- Pregnancy: rubella vaccine contraindicated 3 mo before and during pregnancy; however, if vaccine inadvertently given to pregnant woman, termination of pregnancy not recommended
- Anaphylactic reactions to eggs or neomycin; administer measles and mumps vaccines only after skin testing, graded challenge, and with available treatment for anaphylaxis
- Administration of immune globulin preparations or blood products in preceding 3-10 mo, depending on product
- Immunodeficiency state, malignant disease, or immunosuppression (except HIV infection)

Postmeasles Exposure Prophylaxis

- Immune globulin to
  1. Infants <1 yr of age: Give 0.25 ml/kg IM within 6 days after exposure
  2. Susceptible persons in whom vaccine contraindicated (e.g., leukemics): give 0.5 ml/kg (maximum 15 ml) IM within 6 days after exposure
- Measles vaccine: might be protective if given to susceptible persons (in whom vaccine *not* contraindicated) up to 3 days following exposure

Postrubella Exposure Prophylaxis In Pregnant Women

- Serology immediately following exposure
  1. If rubella immune, no risk of congenital infection; reassure mother

2. If rubella susceptible, repeat serology in 2 wk; if repeat serology negative, no infection has occurred; reassure mother; vaccinate following delivery and before discharge from hospital; if seroconversion, rubella infection has occurred; individualized counseling of patient by obstetrician and consultant recommended

- If exposure occurs early in pregnancy in susceptible woman and termination of pregnancy not an option, immune globulin may be given (0.55 ml/kg; maximum 20 ml)

PROPHYLAXIS FOR SPECIFIC DISEASES

NEISSERIA MENINGITIDIS
Active Immunization

- Preparations: bivalent (A and C) and quadrivalent (A, C, Y and W-135); no vaccine available against Group B strains
- Indications
  1. Control of outbreaks (resulting from serogroups represented in vaccine) in closed population
  2. As adjunct to chemoprophylaxis in household contacts during epidemics
  3. Travel to endemic or epidemic areas
  4. May be helpful in children with complement deficiencies or asplenia, especially if administered before splenectomy
- Efficacy: adequate antibody levels achieved for group A vaccine in children 3 mo or older and with other vaccine groups in children 2 yr or older
- Side effects: local erythema and discomfort (rare), transient fever (2%)
- In Ontario, distribution arranged by local Medical Officer of Health

Postexposure Prophylaxis with Rifampin

1. Index case
2. Household contacts
3. Best friend
4. Day care contacts
5. Intimate contact (e.g., mouth-to-mouth resuscitation, intubation, or suctioning)
6. Dose: 20 mg/kg/day (maximum 1200 mg/day) PO ÷ q12h × 2 days
7. If organism known to be sensitive to sulfonamides, use sulfisoxazole instead of rifampin
   <1 yr: 500 mg PO once daily × 2 days
   1-12 yr: 500 mg PO q12h × 2 days
   >12 yr: 1 g PO q12h × 2 days

HEPATITIS A

- See Table 13-3, p. 216

HEPATITIS B

- See Tables 13-3 to 13-5, pp. 216 to 220

14

INFLUENZA
Influenza Vaccine

- Preparations
  1. Vaccine contains polyvalent killed flu strains (A and B); strains vary by location and year
  2. Only split product available now (fragments of virus envelope with attached hemagglutinin)
  3. Given annually in autumn; two doses separated by 4 wk in previously unimmunized children <6 yr of age; otherwise one dose only
  4. >3 yr: 0.5 ml split product SC or IM
  5. <3 yr: 0.25 ml split product SC or IM
- Indications
  1. Severe chronic disease (e.g., hemodynamically significant cardiac disease, chronic pulmonary disease such as cystic fibrosis or severe asthma, chronic renal disease, diabetes mellitus, sickle cell anemia, and other hemoglobinopathies)
  2. HIV infection or immunosuppression
  3. Long-term ASA therapy (e.g., rheumatoid arthritis, Kawasaki disease, stroke (increased risk of Reye's syndrome)
  4. Residents of chronic-care facilities
  5. Close contacts of high-risk individuals (e.g., hospital personnel, household contacts)
- Contraindications
  1. Age <6 mo
  2. Anaphylactic reactions to egg ingestion

Amantadine

- Postexposure prophylaxis and treatment for influenza A virus only
- Indications
  1. During outbreaks in custodial institutions
  2. High-risk groups, during influenza A epidemics, for those in whom vaccine contraindicated or those not expected to have good antibody response
- Administration
  1. <9 yr: 5 mg/kg/day (maximum 150 mg/day) PO divided bid
  2. ≥9 yr and >40 kg: 200 mg/day PO divided bid
  3. For *treatment,* start as soon as possible (preferably <48 hr) after symptoms begin and continue for 2 to 7 days or until asymptomatic × 48 hr
  4. For *prophylaxis,* give × 10-14 days (may be given throughout an epidemic up to 90 days)
- Precautions
  1. Not recommended for infants under 1 yr
  2. Children with impaired renal function
  3. Children with active seizure disorder
- Side effects: 5%-10% insomnia, light-headedness, irritability

STREPTOCOCCUS PNEUMONIAE ("PNEUMOCOCCUS")

- Purified capsular polysaccharides of 23 serotypes of *S. pneumoniae*
- Indicated in children ≥ age 2 yr with:
  1. Anatomic or functional asplenia

2. Sickle-cell disease
3. Nephrotic syndrome
4. Chronic CSF leak
5. HIV infection or immunosuppression

Administration

- 0.5 ml IM/SC single dose; if possible give 2 wk before splenectomy or immunosuppression
- Revaccination not recommended at present time (in children who were previously vaccinated at age 2, need for revaccination currently being reevaluated)
- 70%-80% of recipients will achieve adequate antibody levels to antigens in vaccine (partial response seen in Hodgkin's disease or renal transplant patients)
- Conjugate vaccine containing seven serotypes for use in children <2 yr is in preparation

Precautions

- Vaccine does not represent all pneumococcal serotypes; therefore antimicrobial coverage in certain patients (e.g., splenectomized children) still advised
- Side effects: soreness, erythema, fever, Arthus-type local reactions, anaphylactic reactions (rare)

RABIES

- For general treatment of animal bites see p. 241

Preparations

- Active: Human diploid cell vaccine (HDCV)
- Passive: Human rabies immune globulin (RIG)

Administration Following Bite (Table 14-3)

- Not previously immunized
  1. HDCV: 1 ml IM, days 0, 3, 7, 14 and 28 (5 doses)
  2. RIG: 20 IU/kg, half IM and half infiltrated around bite site
  3. Always give HDCV and RIG with different syringes at different sites
- Previously immunized (with HDCV or other vaccine with documented positive antibody response), HDCV: 1 ml IM days 0 and 3 (no RIG)
- Note: Follow-up serology recommended only in immunocompromised patients

Precautions

- Chloroquine interferes with development of active immunity
- Allergies (including anaphylaxis) can occur
- Pregnancy: HDCV and RIG may be given if substantial risk of rabies exists

Side Effects

- HDCV (common): pain, erythema, swelling, headache, nausea, abdominal pain, myalgias, dizziness, serum sicknesslike reactions following boosters
- RIG: local pain and low-grade fever

Table 14-3   Rabies Postexposure Prophylaxis Guide

Details of animal	Nature of exposure	Management of exposed person
Rabid Suspect rabid Wild animal* (particularly skunk, fox, coyote, raccoon) in endemic area	No skin or mucosal contact with animal saliva, or casual contact (e.g., petting with no possible contamination of broken skin or mucous membrane)	No treatment
Escaped dog or cat in endemic area (unless exposure was clearly provoked)	Bite or contamination of scratch, abrasion, open wound, or mucous membrane with saliva, body fluids or tissue (except blood, urine, or feces)	Local treatment of wound RIG† (local and intramuscular) Full course‡ of HDCV§
	Bite marks may or may not be observed	As above
Apparently healthy domestic dog or cat that can be held under observation for 10 days	Bite or contamination of scratch, abrasion, open wound or mucous membrane with saliva, body fluids, or tissue (except blood, urine, or feces)	Local treatment of wound At first sign of rabies in animal during holding period, give RIG (local and intramuscular) and start full course of HDCV

Modified from the National Immunization Committee on Immunization (NACI): *Canadian immunization guide*, ed 4, Ottawa, 1993, Health Canada.

*If possible, animal should be killed and brain tested as soon as possible; holding for observation not recommended. Bites of squirrels, chipmunks, rats, mice, other rodents, rabbits, and hares are seldom, if ever, indication for rabies prophylaxis.

†*RIG*, Rabies immune globulin (human).

‡Vaccine may be discontinued if fluorescent antibody test of animal killed at time of attack is negative.

§*HDCV*, Human diploid cell vaccine.

TETANUS

- See Table 25-1, p. 434

VARICELLA

- Varicella vaccine: universal vaccination recommended in United States for all healthy children without history of varicella infection; vaccine stability continues to pose problems; no immediate plans for licensure in Canada
- Immunocompromised patients should be tested for varicella antibody titers

Varicella-Zoster Immune Globulin (VZIG)

- Prepared from plasma of outdated blood with high V-Z antibody titers
- Indications
  1. Immunocompromised susceptible patients exposed to V-Z infection (exposure to household contact, indoor playmate contact >1 hr, or hospital contact: same room or prolonged face-to-face contact)
  2. Neonates whose mothers have developed varicella ≤ 5 days before or within 2 days after delivery
  3. Exposed premature infants < 28 wk gestation or ≤ 1 kg
  4. Exposed premature infant ≥ 28 wk gestation whose mother lacks history of chicken pox
- Dose
  - To be given within 96 hr after exposure (preferably sooner)
  - <10 kg = 125 U (one vial)
  - >10 kg = 12.5 U/kg; maximum 625 U (five vials)
- Precautions
  - Strict isolation of exposed patient necessary between days 10 and 21 following exposure
  - If VZIG given, isolate until 35 days following exposure

DISEASES AND SYNDROMES

BITES
Animal Bites

- Organisms: anaerobes, aerobes including *Grp A streptococci, S. aureus, Pasteurella multocida*
- Document type and health status of animal; also circumstances surrounding delivery of bite
- Note location and severity of wound and any signs of infection
- High-pressure irrigation with copious amounts of sterile saline using syringe
- Debridement of dead tissues
- Leave unsutured if wound involves hand or if more than 6-8 hr have elapsed since injury (consult plastic surgeon)
- Prophylactic antibiotics (controversial): use in major facial or hand injuries or injuries presenting >12 hr
  1. Amoxicillin-clavulanic acid × 5 days
  2. Penicillin allergy: tetracycline (if over 8 yr) or erythromycin (but 50% of *P. multocida* are resistant)

- Tetanus prophylaxis (see p. 434)
- Rabies prophylaxis (see p. 240)
- Instruct parents to return if fever develops, wound becomes infected, or infection spreads

Human Bites

- Organisms: *S. aureus, streptococci,* anaerobes; more virulent than cat or dog bites
- Document: location, severity of wound (involvement of deep structures), and any signs of infection
- Irrigation, debridement as for animal bites
- Leave unsutured
- Elevate extremity
- Tetanus prophylaxis (see p. 434)
- Antibiotic prophylaxis
  1. Amoxicillin-clavulanic acid
  2. Penicillin allergy: Clindamycin
- Infection: Generally requires admission to hospital, early surgical exploration and debridement; Gram stain, culture wound, elevate and immobilize affected part; IV antibiotics (penicillin and cloxacillin; clindamycin)
- Joint involvement requires *urgent* referral for surgical exploration and debridement

CELLULITIS

- Nonfacial cellulitis: group A *streptococci, S. aureus;* neonates: group B *streptococci*
- Buccal cellulitis: above plus *S. pneumoniae, H. influenzae*
- If patient toxic and lesion spreads very quickly and extremely tender or anesthetic, consider necrotizing fasciitis; although rare, this requires immediate surgical debridement and IV antibiotics (to cover *streptococci, staphylococci,* gram-negative organisms, and anaerobes)

Management

- CBC, blood culture
- Needle aspiration of advancing edge for culture
- If etiology unclear:
  1. No local or remote trauma, no break in skin: IV cefuroxime or cloxacillin; PO cefazolin or cephalexin for minor cases
  2. Secondary to break in skin (e.g., VZV, trauma) with marked erythema: IV penicillin and clindamycin
     Duration of antibiotics: 7-10 days

PRESEPTAL AND ORBITAL CELLULITIS

- Etiologic organisms:
  - Nontraumatic: *S. pneumoniae,* group A *streptococci, S. aureus, H. influenzae*
  - Traumatic: *S. aureus*
- Often associated with sinusitis, minor skin trauma, or dental abscess
- Preseptal cellulitis should be differentiated from orbital cellulitis by ab-

sence of proptosis, chemosis, and presence of full ocular movement and normal vision
- Blood culture
- Sinus x-rays
- CT scan if orbital cellulitis a possibility
- Orbital cellulitis may require urgent surgical drainage in addition to IV antibiotics (along with orbital damage, untreated orbital cellulitis can lead to cavernous sinus thrombosis); consult ophthalmology on admission
- Treatment
  - Traumatic periorbital cellulitis: cloxacillin or cefazolin
  - Nontraumatic in <5 yr age: cefotaxime
  - Nontraumatic periorbital cellulitis in >5 yr age: cloxacillin or cefazolin

CERVICAL ADENITIS

- Acute: Group A *streptococci, S. aureus,* Group B *streptococci* (neonates), anaerobes, adenovirus, enterovirus less common
- Subacute and chronic (1-3 wk): Cat-scratch fever, anaerobes, EBV, CMV, atypical mycobacteria, *M. tuberculosis,* toxoplasmosis, histoplasmosis, HIV
- Rule out malignancy, drugs (phenytoin, isoniazid), Kawasaki disease, neck anomalies (cystic hygroma, branchial cleft cyst, thyroglossal duct cyst)

14

Management

- Cultures (skin, throat, blood)
- If node fluctuant, consider incision and drainage (send sample for Gram stain and culture)
- In mild infection, cloxacillin or amoxicillin-clavulanic acid PO × 10 days
- If dental source suspected, use penicillin V or clindamycin PO
- Neonatal infections and more severe infections may need IV therapy and surgical drainage
- If no improvement or chronic infection, investigate for mycobacterial (atypical or TB), viral, cat scratch, HIV, or malignant disease

CLOSTRIDIUM DIFFICILE

Investigations

- History of current or recent antibiotic therapy
- Stool for
  1. Anaerobic culture on selective media
  2. Filtration and detection of cytotoxin B
- Sigmoidoscopy-colonoscopy if pseudomembranous colitis suspected

Treatment

- Supportive care: institute fluid and electrolyte replacement
- Asymptomatic patients do not require treatment; neutropenic patients should be treated even if asymptomatic, since they may be at higher risk for severe infections

- Empiric therapy of diarrhea recommended for children with hematologic malignancy
- Avoid antidiarrheal drugs
- If symptomatic:
  1. Enteric isolation
  2. Discontinue antibiotics if feasible (mildly symptomatic patients may benefit by stopping antibiotics alone)
  3. Metronidazole PO or IV
- Relapses are common (10%-20%); may require additional course of treatment

CONGENITAL INFECTIONS (Box 14-1)

- Infection occurs in utero (by transplacental transmission) or perinatally (by passage through birth canal)
- Most are asymptomatic at birth but may still have late sequelae
- CMV most common (0.1%-1% of liveborn infants)

ENCEPHALITIS
Etiology

- Direct viral invasion such as HSV, enterovirus, mumps
- Postinfectious immune-mediated disease (acute disseminated encephalomyelitis or ADEM); may follow childhood exanthem, immunization, EBV, HSV, influenza, group A *streptococci,* probably mycoplasma or unknown infection

Investigations

- Lumbar puncture
  - CSF usually has normal or increased protein, normal glucose, polymorphic or lymphocytic pleocytosis
  - Increase in RBC suggestive of HSV
  - If focal signs or signs of increased ICP present on history or physical exam, lumbar puncture should not be done until CT scan has ruled out space-occupying lesion
- Viral detection
  - CSF culture (rarely positive for HSV)
  - Polymerase chain reaction (PCR) for viral DNA in CSF
  - Throat, stool; other tissue, if applicable
- CT scan or MRI: may be normal early in illness
- Paired blood serology (acute and 2-4 wk later): rise seen one to several wk later
- EEG: Often focal findings (poor prognostic sign if bilateral)
- Brain biopsy: most definitive way of making diagnosis (used for pathology, EM, IF, viral culture, PCR); may be useful to confirm diagnosis of HSV encephalitis or identify other causes of encephalitis

Treatment

- Supportive care, including treatment of seizures, treatment of increased ICP, and monitoring for SIADH
- For HSV or VZV resulting from direct viral invasion, treat with acyclovir 45 mg/kg/day IV ÷ tid × 14-21 days

---

BOX 14-1 Congenital and Perinatal Infections

Causes (CHEAP TORCHES)
C Chickenpox and shingles
H Hepatitis B,C,D,E
E Enteroviruses
A AIDS
P Parvovirus B19

T Toxoplasmosis
O Other (gr B *strep, Listeria, Candida,* Lyme)
R Rubella
H Herpes simplex virus
E Everything else sexually transmitted (gonorrhea, *Chlamydia, Ureaplasma,* papillomavirus)
S Syphilis

Obstetric History
Serologic results (HBV, VDRL, rubella): early and if positive, late
Rash, arthritis, profound fatigue, other illness; health of partner
Employment in day care center, elementary school
Travel, country of origin
Raw meat ingestion
Sexually transmitted disease risk of mother and father of infant

Findings Suggestive of Congenital Infection
Cerebral calcifications, microcephaly, hydrocephaly
Cataracts, chorioretinitis, glaucoma, keratoconjunctivitis, microphthalmia
Congenital heart disease
Purpura, vesicles, maculopapular exanthem, jaundice
Hepatosplenomegaly
Anemia with or without hydrops
Bone lesions
Paralysis

Investigations
CT head
Opthalmologic exam
Audiologic exam
Large bone x-rays (for syphilis, rubella, CMV)
Maternal and infant blood (not cord blood) for pertinent serologic tests
Infant urine for CMV
Follow-up infant sera at 4-6 wk

14

- Empiric acylovir advised in febrile encephalopathic patients, especially if focal disease; await results of CT or MRI, CSF exam, EEG, and clinical course before deciding on duration of therapy
- If MRI supports ADEM, treat with corticosteroids

HIV INFECTION AND AIDS (Tables 14-4 to 14-7)

- Most children with perinatally acquired HIV-infection will become ill in first 2 yr of life; small number may remain asymptomatic for several yr

Text continued on p. 250.

Table 14-4 Determining HIV Status in a Child According to Age

Age	Testing technique	Result	HIV status
Newborn to 18 mos	Following tests at separate times: polymerase chain reaction (PCR) or viral cultures	2 positives of either test	Infected
		1 negative, 1 positive	Consider infected; repeat testing immediately
		2 negatives	Repeat at four separate times; if negative, uninfected
	p24 Ag (very specific, poor sensitivity)	Positive	Consider infected; repeat
		Negative	Repeat wih PCR, viral culture
	2 ELISA and confirmatory tests	Negative, negative	Negative
If child is breast-feeding, repeat test 3 mo after stopping breast-feeding			
>18 mos	2 ELISA tests	Negative	Uninfected
	ELISA and confirmatory tests separated by 1 mo	Positive	Infected

Table 14-5 The 1994 Revised Classification for HIV in Children <13 Yr of Age*

Immunologic categories‡	Clinical categories†			
	N: No signs/symptoms	A: Mild signs/symptoms	B: Moderate signs/symptoms§	C: Severe signs signs/symptoms§
1: No evidence of suppression	N1	A1	B1	C1
2: Evidence of moderate suppression	N2	A2	B2	C2
3: Severe suppression	N3	A3	B3	C3

From Center for Disease Control: Morbidity and Mortality Weekly Review (MMWR), 43, NO RR-12, pp. 1-10, Atlanta, 1994, CDC.

*Children whose HIV status not confirmed are classified using above grid with letter E (for perinatally exposed) placed before appropriate classification code (e.g., EN2).

†For clinical categories, see Table 14-7.

‡For immunologic categories, see Table 14-6.

§Both category C and lymphoid interstitial pneumonitis in category B are reportable to state and local health departments as acquired immunodeficiency syndrome.

14

Table 14-6   Immunologic Categories Based on Age-Specific CD4+ T-Lymphocyte Counts and Percentage of Total Lymphocytes

Immunologic category	Age of the child					
	<12 mo		1-6 yr		6-12 yr	
	Cells/mm³	%	Cells/mm³	%	Cells/mm³	%
No evidence of suppression	≥1500	≥25	≥1000	≥25	≥500	≥25
Evidence of moderate suppression	750-1499	15-24	500-999	15-24	200-499	15-24
Severe suppression	<750	<15	<500	<15	<200	<15

Table 14-7 Clinical Categories for Children with HIV Infection

Category	Description
N: Not symptomatic	Children who have no signs or symptoms considered to be result of HIV infection or who have only one of conditions listed in category A
A: Mildly symptomatic	Children with ≥2 or more of following conditions, but none of conditions listed in categories B and C: lymphadenopathy; hepatomegaly; splenomegaly; dermatitis; parotitis; recurrent or persistent upper respiratory infection, sinusitis, or otitis media
B: Moderately symptomatic	Children who have symptomatic conditions other than those listed for categories A or C that are attributed to HIV infection; examples of conditions listed in category B include but are not limited to: • Anemia (<80 g/L), neutropenia (<1 × 10^9/L), or thrombocytopenia (<150 × 10^9/L) persisting ≥30 days • Bacterial meningitis, pneumonia, or sepsis • Candidiasis, oropharyngeal, persisting >2 mo in children >6 mo • Cardiomyopathy • CMV infection with onset <1 mo of age • Diarrhea, acute or chronic • HSV stomatis, recurrent (>2 episodes in 1 yr) • Lymphoid interstitial pneumonia (LIP) • Persistent fever (>1 mo) • Varicella, disseminated (complicated chicken pox)
C: Severely symptomatic	Examples of conditions listed in category C include but are not limited to: • Serious bacterial infections, multiple or recurrent of the following types: septicemia, pneumonia, meningitis, bone/joint infection, abscess of internal organ or body cavity • Candidiasis, esophageal or pulmonary • Coccidioidomycosis, disseminated • Cryptococcus, extrapulmonary • Cryptosporidiosis or isosporiasis with diarrhea >1 mo • CMV infection with onset >1 mo of age • Histoplasmosis, disseminated • Kaposi's sarcoma • Lymphoma (primary, in brain; B-cell non-Hodgkin's) • Mycobacterial infection (extrapulmonary, disseminated) • *Pneumocystis carinii* pneumonia (PCP) • Progressive multifocal leukoencephalopathy (PML) • Wasting syndrome

14

Adapted from Centers for Disease Control: Revised classification system for human immunodeficiency virus (HIV) infection in children less than 13 years of age, Atlanta, 1994, MMWR 43. No. RR-12.

Pediatric Risk Groups for AIDS

1. Children who have received blood or blood products (e.g., hemophiliacs) before screening for HIV antibodies (begun in Canada in November 1985)
2. Infant of mother with HIV infection or mother belonging to high-risk group such as IV drug users, someone with multiple sexual partners, someone from community with high prevalence of HIV infection; risk of vertical transmission with HIV-positive mother in Canada approximately 14% to 25%; use of zidovudine (ZDV, AZT) antenatally reduces this risk to about 8%
3. High-risk behaviors such as intravenous drug use, unprotected sex with known HIV partner, multiple sexual partners, homosexual/bisexual men or street youth
4. Sexual abuse

Management

- Infants of infected mothers are treated with AZT for 6 wk, then placed on Septra PCP prophylaxis from 2-8 mos (period of high PCP risk) until infection either confirmed or excluded
- Often difficult to distinguish seropositive children <18 mo with true HIV infection from those with only passively acquired maternal antibodies
- Consent with pretest and posttest counseling must be obtained; *pediatric diagnosis may lead to parental diagnosis*
- Breast-feeding by HIV-infected mothers (or mothers at significant risk of acquiring infection postpartum) discouraged in North America because of possible transmission risk; in countries where safe, alternative sources of nutrition not available, breast-feeding still recommended

Therapeutic Considerations

- Antiretroviral therapy such as AZT or DDI
- PCP prophylaxis (trimethoprim-sulfamethoxazole)
- IV immune globulin
- All routine vaccinations, including MMR, recommended (avoid BCG and OPV)
- Prompt evaluation and treatment of acute infections
- Immune globulin after measles or varicella exposures
- Additional immunizations: influenza (annually), pneumococcal vaccine
- CMV negative blood transfusions
- Universal blood and body-fluid precautions

INFECTIOUS MONONUCLEOSIS
Investigations

- WBC and differential (increased atypical lymphocytes)
- Multiple specific serologic antibody tests available
- Most commonly used: (see p. 554 for interpretation)
  1. Heterophil Abs (Monospot test, Paul-Bunnel test)
  2. IgG against viral capsid Ag (VCA)
  3. Anti-EA (early Ag)
  4. EBV IgM

Treatment

- Isolation not required
- Symptomatic: bed rest, encourage fluids, warm saline gargles for sore throat, acetaminophen
- Admission and steroids indicated in airway obstruction (start with equivalent of 1-2 mg/kg/day of prednisone; give PO in divided doses and taper over 1-2 wk)

Follow-Up

- Usually resolves over 2-3 wk period, although fatigue may persist for weeks
- Contact sports should be avoided if splenomegaly resulting from risk of splenic rupture

INTRAVASCULAR LINE-RELATED SEPSIS

- Spectrum includes occult bacteremia (most common; positive blood cultured at tip but site appears normal), cellulitis, septic thrombus or phlebitis
- Absolute indications for line removal:
  1. Life-threatening disease
  2. Persistent bacteremia/sepsis at 48 hr
  3. Fungus
  4. Tunnel infection

BACTERIAL MENINGITIS
Etiology

- Neonates: Group B *streptococci, E. coli, Listeria,* Group D *streptococci*
  Infants and children: *S. pneumoniae, N. meningitidis, H. influenzae*
  Compromised hosts: in addition to preceding, *S. aureus,* gram-negative bacilli, *Listeria*

Investigations

- CSF examination (Table 14-8): lumbar puncture should be done as soon as possibility of meningitis raised (for procedure and precautions, see p. 501); if fundoscopic exam not possible in child with closed fontanelle, or if focal neurologic signs of increased intracranial pressure, CT should be performed, and LP done only if CT rules out intracranial space-occupying lesion; CSF studies include cell count and differential, Gram stain, culture and sensitivity, protein, glucose, antigen detection testing (e.g., latex agglutination even if patient has been taking antibiotics); save one tube for other investigations (e.g., virology, TB)
- CBC, differential, platelet count
- Blood glucose, electrolytes, urea, creatinine, urine electrolytes
- Blood cultures
- PT, PTT, fibrin split products (if indicated)
- Urine: latex agglutination, specific gravity, electrolytes, and osmolality (if SIADH suspected)

Management

- ABCs (see p. 2)
- Vital signs, hydration, neurologic status, appropriate monitoring

14

Table 14-8 Interpretation of CSF Findings in Meningitis

	Bacterial	Viral	TB	Partially treated
Cell count*	Usually >1000	Usually <300	<1,000	>1000
Predominant cell	Polymorphs	Early polymorphs, then mononuclear	Lymphs	Polys or mononuclear
Gram stain	Usually positive (acid-fast stain may be positive)	Negative	Negative	May be negative
Glucose†	Low	Normal	Low or normal	Low or normal
Protein‡	High	Normal or high	Very high	High
Bacterial culture	Usually positive	Negative	Culture for TB may be positive	Often negative

*Units: $\times 10^6$/L. The WBC count in normal spinal fluid should be at most 5×10^6/L (5/mm^3); neonates may have higher WBC numbers, especially low birth weight; even though WBC usually quite high, in bacterial meningitis, any count above normal must be viewed suspiciously; RBC to WBC ratios in CSF specimens contaminated with blood must be interpreted with caution; treatment should not be withheld if clinical picture suggestive of meningitis; seizures alone do not increase CSF WBC count.

†CSF glucose: <50% of blood glucose.

‡Increased protein seen in meningitis, encephalitis, abscess, leukemia, or other intracranial malignancy.

- IV at 60% daily maintenance, oral intake, depending on level of consciousness
- Early management of shock, seizures, raised ICP as necessary (see p. 6)
- Careful assessment (daily): head circumference, skull transillumination (infants), metastatic foci
- Follow hydration, weight, serum, and urine electrolytes (for SIADH)
- Family and index case prophylaxis with rifampin (see p. 236)
- Give one dose steroid (dexamethasone IV 0.15 mg/kg/dose) before antibiotic in children and infants >6 wk of age; if *H. influenza* type b or *S. pneumoniae,* then continue dexamethasone 0.6 mg/kg/day ÷ q6h × 2 days
- Never delay treatment because LP cannot be done or while awaiting CT
- For empiric antibiotic selection, see Table 14-9
- Switch to appropriate antibiotic once organism identified and sensitivities known
- Duration:
  1. Neonates: 2 wk (3 wk in gram-negative meningitis)
  2. *H. influenzae, S. pneumoniae, N. meningitidis:* 7 days in uncomplicated cases
  3. *S. aureus:* minimum 3 wk
  4. Gram-negative bacilli: minimum 3 wk
- Prolonged or recurrent pyrexia (more than 5 days) may be resulting from:
  1. Nosocomial illness (e.g., URI, gastroenteritis)
  2. Phlebitis
  3. Secondary focus: arthritis, pneumonia, pleural effusion, pericarditis
  4. Subdural effusions (common; in most cases medical intervention not needed; neurosurgical consultation and aspiration if increasing head circumference, vomiting, seizures, or focal neurologic findings)

14

Table 14-9   Empiric Antibiotic Selection for Meningitis*

Patient	Organism	Antibiotic
Neonate	Gr B *strep,* gram-neg bacilli *Listeria*	Ampicillin + cefotaxime
1-3 mo	Neonatal and community-acquired organisms	Ampicillin + cefotaxime
>3 mo	*S. pneumonia, N. meningitidi H. influenzae*	Ceftriaxone or cefotaxime Add Vancomycin if *Pneumococcus* suspected (e.g., gram-pos cocci on LP)
		or
		Chloramphenicol + vancomycin (if penicillin allergy)
Immunocompromised		
Nonneutropenic		Vancomycin + cefotaxime
Neutropenic		Vancomycin + ceftazidine
Shunt related		Vancomycin + ceftazidine

*Empiric antibiotic recommendations are only a guide; antimicrobial selection should reflect pathogens and patterns of resistance in your institution or community.

5. Drug fever
6. Failure of conventional management

Follow-Up (All Patients)

- Hearing testing within 1 mo after discharge
- Psychologic assessment before starting school or before that if developmental delay suspected
- Neurologic assessment and follow-up if indicated

MUMPS (Epidemic Parotitis)
Confirmation of Diagnosis

- Saliva, urine, CSF (if indicated) for viral isolation
- Mumps serology (p. 555)

Treatment

- Respiratory isolation (may be contagious as long as 7 days before parotid swelling and 9 days after onset)
- Symptomatic treatment only (acetaminophen for pain; cold or warm packs to areas of swelling)

OTITIS MEDIA (OM)

- Child with acute OM (i.e., fever; pain; red, bulging tympanic membrane) requires antibiotic therapy
- In absence of *all* of these findings, it reasonable to withhold antibiotic therapy
- In uncomfortable, restrained child, tympanic membrane may be red in absence of acute otitis media; quiet, comfortable child can be examined fairly quickly
- Complete ear examination includes measure of fluid behind membrane (i.e., by pneumatic otoscopy, tympanogram)
- First-line therapy: Amoxicillin
- If child has received Amoxil in past 4 wk or there is no improvement in 48 hr (5%), select second-line antibiotic regimen (see Table 23-1)
- If pinna protrudes out and inferiorly, mastoiditis should be suspected, and ENT referral made
- See pp. 421 and 422 for recurrent and serous otitis media

OVA AND PARASITES (Table 14-10)

- No need to screen asymptomatic child
- Nonpathogenic parasites *not* requiring treatment include:

Chylomastix mesinii	*Endolimax nana*
Entamoeba coli	*Iadamoeba buetschlii*
Entamoeba hartmanni	*Retortamonas intestinalis*
Enteromonas hominis	*Trichomonas hominis*

PERTUSSIS

- WBC and differential (lymphocytosis)
- Nasopharyngeal swab or aspirate (Auger suction) for culture
- Admit if severe illness or apnea (seen most commonly in infants <12 mo)
- Supportive care: Clear airway secretions, O_2 for cyanotic episodes

Table 14-10 Selected Parasitic Diseases

Disease	Treatment
Helminth (worm)	
Ascaris lumbricoides	Pyrantel pamoate or mebendazole or albendazole
Hookworm (*Ancylostoma duodenale, Necator americanus*)	Mebendazole or pyrantel pamoate or albendazole
Pinworm (*Enterobius vermicularis*)	Pyrantel pamoate or mebendazole or albendazole
Protozoa	
Entamoeba histolytica	Iodoquinol or paromomycin or diloxanide furoate
Blastocystis hominis (symptomatic)*	Metronidazole
Dientamoeba fragilis (symptomatic)*	Iodoquinol or paromomycin or tetracycline
Giardia lamblia (symptomatic)*	Metronidazole or furazolidone
Malaria	
Plasmodium vivax, ovale, malariae, and chloroquine-sensitive *falciparum*†	Oral drug of choice: Chloroquine phosphate or Parenteral drug of choice: Quinidine gluconate or quinine hydrochloride IV
To prevent relapses (*P. vivax* and *P. ovale* only)	Primaquine phosphate PO × 14 days (test for G6PD deficiency before Rx)
P. falciparum malaria† acquired in areas of known chloroquine resistance	Oral drug of choice: Quinine sulphate × 3 days plus Clindamycin or pyrimethamine-sulfadoxine Alternative: single-dose mefloquine Parenteral drug of choice: Quinidine gluconate IV

See formulary for dosages and methods of administration.

*Pathogenicity of this parasite has not yet been proven; rule out presence of other known pathogens; efficacy of therapeutic agents is questionable.

†*P. falciparum* is only species of plasmodium causing human malaria that develops resistance and is frequently lethal; suggest urgent infectious disease referral.

- Antibiotics
  1. Erythromycin estolate may prevent paroxysmal stage if started in catarrhal stage and may shorten period of communicability
  2. Treat secondary bacterial infections

Prevention

- Chemoprophylaxis
  - Indications: household or close contacts if <1 yr regardless of immunization status, or <7 yr and not fully immunized; some authorities believe that all contacts should receive chemoprophylaxis
  - Erythromycin estolate (dose as for infection); alternatively trimethoprim-sulfamethoxazole
- Active immunization of contacts: give DPT if <7 yr and either
  - Unimmunized or immunizations are not up to date or

- Partially immunized and third dose was ≥6 mo ago or
- No DPT in last 3 yr

STREPTOCOCCAL PHARYNGITIS ("Strep Throat")

- Diagnosis: throat culture or latex agglutination test for rapid detection of group A streptococcal antigen in pharyngeal secretions
- Rationale of therapy: prevents suppurative complications (e.g., peritonsillar abscess), prevents rheumatic fever, (see p. 73) and alleviates symptoms; role in prevention of nephritis uncertain
- Antibiotics
  1. Penicillin V PO × 10 days or benzathine penicillin G as single IM dose
  2. Penicillin allergy: Erythromycin estolate × 10 days
- Follow-up cultures not necessary except in rheumatic fever
- Carriers not treated unless family member has rheumatic fever
- Clindamycin or penicillin for 10 days given with rifampin concurrently for last 4 days more effective than oral penicillin therapy alone in eradicating carrier state

SEPTIC SHOCK
Management

- For monitoring and the acute mangement of shock and its complications, see p. 6
- Use of steroids controversial
- Obtain necessary specimens (blood, urine, appropriate swabs, CSF) for microscopy, Gram stain, cultures, latex agglutination
- Remove intravascular catheters; send tip for culture
- Radiologic (e.g., CXR, ECHO, CT scan) or nuclear scan studies if indicated
- Prompt institution of antibiotics (Table 14-11)

SINUSITIS

- Acute: *S. pneumoniae, H. influenzae, M. catarrhalis*
- Chronic: *Bacteroides,* anaerobic and aerobic *streptococci, S. aureus, H. influenzae,* fungus

Management

- Sinus x-rays: diagnostic specificity in children not proven
- Rule out dental abscess clinically or on Panorax
- Antimicrobials
  1. Acute: amoxicillin, trimethoprim-sulfamethoxazole, amoxicillin-clavulanic acid, or cefprozil × 10-21 days
     Chronic; clindamycin
  2. If severe and has associated preseptal cellulitis, see p. 242
  3. If persistent, may require ENT referral (sinus lavage, drainage)
- Antihistamines and decongestants: clinical efficacy not proven and also may reduce local resistance
- Complications: preseptal/orbital cellulitis, subdural or epidural effusion ± Pott's puffy tumor, brain abscess, parameningeal infection, cavernous sinus thrombosis

Table 14-11 Empiric Antibiotic Selection for Septicemia/Bacteremia* (excludes meningitis)

Patient	Organism	Antibiotic
Neonate	Gr B *strep*, *Listeria* gram neg enteric bacilli	Ampicillin + aminoglycoside; consider cloxacillin if risk of *S. aureus*
1-3 mos	Neonatal and community-acquired organisms	Ampicillin + cefotaxime
>3 mos	*S. pneumoniae*, *Meningococcus*, *S. aureus*, *H. influenzae*	Cefuroxime†
Febrile neutropenic	Coagulase-negative staphylococci, *S. Aureus*, gram-neg enteric bacilli	Extended spectrum penicillin (e.g., pipercillin) + aminoglycoside or vancomycin + ceftazidime
Sickle cell disease with fever	*S. pneumoniae*, *H. influenzae*	Ampicillin‡
Typhoid fever	*S. typhi*	Cefotaxime
Line related		Cloxacillin + aminoglycoside
Shunt related		Vancomycin + ceftazidine
Intraabdominal		Clindamycin or metronidazole aminoglycoside ± ampicillin†
Urinary tract		Ampicillin + aminoglycoside

*Empiric antibiotic recommendations are only a guide; antimicrobial selection should reflect pathogens and patterns of resistance in your institution or community.

†In patients whose condition is severe or deteriorating, consider cefotaxime ± vancomycin.

‡If evidence of chest crisis/pneumonia, use broad-spectrum antibiotic coverage (cefuroxime ± erythromycin).

TUBERCULOSIS (TB)

- Children are less likely to contain infection than adults and are more likely to develop extrapulmonary complications, such as miliary disease, meningitis, and osteomyelitis

Investigations

- History of exposure (Box 14-2)
- Tuberculin skin testing: Mantoux/PPD 5TU (0.1 cc) intradermally (Box 14-3)
- Chest x-ray
- Stains for acid-fast bacilli and TB cultures:
  1. Sputum if produced (usually >8yr, cavitary disease)
  2. Gastric aspirate × 2 (not recommended if no pulmonary symptoms and normal CXR)
  3. Urine (3 × 1st morning void) if signs of renal involvement
  4. CSF (if indicated)
- Histology and TB culture when indicated: lymph nodes, liver, pleura, bone marrow
- Treatment: see Table 14-12

VARICELLA (Chicken Pox)

- Incubation period: 10-21 days (35 days if patient has received varicella zoster immune globulin (VZIG)

BOX 14-2 Children at Risk for Increased TB in Canada

Contacts of confirmed or suspected cases

Children emigrating from endemic areas (Africa, Asia, Latin America, Middle East)

Children who travel to endemic areas or are close contacts of people who travel to endemic areas

Frequent exposure to high-risk people (e.g., homeless, IV drug users, HIV, incarcerated)

BOX 14-3 Criteria for Positive Mantoux Tuberculin Reaction in Children (5-unit PPD)

≥5 mm induration = positive if
  Close contact of infectious case
  Clinical and/or radiographic findings suggestive of TB
  Immunocompromised (disease or treatment including HIV)
≥10 mm induration = positive if
  Children at increased risk of dissemination
    Young age < 4 yr
    Other medical risk factor (e.g., chronic renal failure, diabetes, malnutrition)
  Increased environmental exposure to TB
≥15 mm = positive if
  Age ≥ 4 yr and no known risk factors

Note: Negative Mantoux does not rule out TB diagnosis; history of BCG does not alter interpretation of test.

- Contagious: 48 hr before appearance of rash until lesions are dried and scabbed, approximately 6 days after onset (immunosuppressed patients may be contagious for longer periods)

Management

- Isolation (strict)
- Symptomatic therapy: baking soda baths, calamine lotion, topical antipruritic, systemic antihistamines if severe itching
- IV acyclovir in neonates and immunosuppressed patients
- VZIG prophylaxis for specific contacts (see p. 241)

VIRAL HEPATITIS

- See p. 213

INFECTIONS IN IMMUNOCOMPROMISED HOST

PRINCIPLES

- Early consultation with infectious disease specialist advisable
- All isolated organisms in immunocompromised patients should be considered as potential pathogens

Table 14-12 Recommended Treatment Protocols for Tuberculosis

Site of tuberculosis	Length of therapy (mo)	Drug regimen	Remarks
Pulmonary	9	Daily INH	• For better compliance, twice weekly supervised • If INH-resistant, add RIF • If multiply resistant, expert consultation
Pulmonary	6	First 2 mo: Daily INH, RIF, and pyrazinamide Last 4 mos: Daily or twice weekly INH, RIF	• For better compliance, twice weekly supervised • If resistant, four drugs in expert consultation • Pyridoxine in teens, CNS disease, malnutrition, pregnancy • If from areas of high resistance (e.g., SE Asia, Somalia), four drugs may be used (i.e. addition of ethambutol)
Extrapulmonary	6-12		• Expert consultation

INH, Isoniazid; *RIF,* rifampin.

14

- Fever represents infection until proven otherwise (versus tumor lysis, transfusion or drug reactions)
- Start empiric therapy early against most common, serious pathogens; from beginning, keep in mind your clinical end points for changing or ending treatment

AGGRAVATING FACTORS

- Indwelling catheters (IV, Foley; remove/replace when possible)
- Malnutrition
- Skin and mucosal breakdown
- Prolonged broad-spectrum antibiotics (increased fungal risk)
- Prolonged hospitalization (resistant organisms, nosocomial infections)
- Graft versus host disease (increased CMV risk)

WORK-UP
All Patients

- Complete physical exam with special attention to fundi, oropharynx, chest, catheter sites, skin, and perianal area
- Central line and peripheral blood cultures (bacteria and fungi)
- Urine cultures (bacteria and fungi)
- Drainage cultures
- CXR
- Liver enzymes, creatinine

Selected Patients

- Bronchoalveolar lavage (BAL) if pulmonary focus suspected (cultures for bacteria, CMV, and respiratory viruses, fungi, and mycobacteria; stains for fungi, bacteria, mycobacteria, and *Pneumocystis*)
- Esophagoscopy (bacterial, CMV, HSV, and fungal cultures)
- CSF culture, Gram stain, cell count, chemistry, latex agglutination
- Buffy coat and urine cultures for CMV
- Ophthalmology consult (CMV, fungal retinitis)
- Abdominal/renal US (abscesses, fungal balls)
- Vesicular scrapings for EM and cultures (*varicella, herpes simplex*)

IMMIGRANTS AND REFUGEE CHILDREN IN CANADA

- Classification of population of children entering Canada:
  - Immigrant (permanent)
  - Immigrant (nonpermanent)
  - Refugee claimant
  - Nonstatus (illegal)
- These differences in circumstances mean differences in timing and nature of health assessment, as well as differences in socioeconomic status and available support

RECOMMENDED SCREENING OF CHILDREN NEW TO CANADA
History

- Personal exposures:
  - Food (unpasteurized milk, uncooked meat), water (purity)

Table 14-13	Common Risk Groups and Associated Infectious Disease Syndromes

At risk group	Infectious disease syndrome
Postchemotherapy neutropenia	Polymicrobial sepsis
	Fungi (late)
Immunosuppressive therapy (malignancies, posttransplant, collagen vascular disease, renal disease)	Polymicrobial sepsis
	CMV, varicella
	Pneumocystis pneumonia
Splenic dysfunction	Overwhelming encapsulated *(Pneumococcus)* bacterial sepsis
Hypogammaglobulinemia	Sinopulmonary bacteria
Low-birth–weight premature infants with CVLs plus broad-spectrum antibiotics	Fungi

- Insects, animals
- Blood transfusions, reused immunization syringes
- Worms or blood in stool; TB, leprosy
- Sexual activity
- Parental consanguinity
- Environmental exposures
  - Climate where born and raised (arid, tropical, temperate)
  - Rural or urban
  - Travel route to Canada
- Immunization
- Family relationships, plans to return, adaptation to immigration
- Psychologic well-being, unique cultural practice

Physical Exam

- Respiratory (TB)
- Lymphadenopathy and hepatosplenomegaly (portal hypertension, typhoid, HIV)
- Seizure (cystocercosis)
- Musculoskeletal (tropical myositis)
- Genitourinary (STD, female genital mutilation)
- Skin lesions, ulcers, hyper/hypopigmentation, hypoesthesia (leprosy), subcutaneous nodules (rheumatic fever), BCG scar, rose spots (typhoid)
- Nutritional assessment
- Dental assessment
- Any developmental delay, chorioretinitis, cerebral calcifications, hearing loss, or heart murmur (congenital toxoplasmosis, rubella, or syphilis)
- For adolescent girls, possible pregnancy

Investigations

- Mantoux testing if child from endemic area
- Consider following blood tests, depending on origin of child:
  - CBC + differential (anemia, eosinophilia)
  - HBsAg
  - Hepatitis C antibody (with counseling)

Table 14-14   Cephalosporins

1st generation	2nd generation	3rd generation
Excellent gram-pos coverage *(S. aureus,* group A strep, *S. pneumoniae)*	Good gram-pos coverage *(S. aureus,* group A strep, *S. pneumoniae)*	Ceftriaxone good gram-pos coverage; all others poor
Poor *Enterococcus*	Poor *Enterococcus*	Poor *Enterococcus*
Some resistant *Pneumococcus*	Some resistant *Pneumococcus*	Some resistant *Pneumococcus*
Poor gram-neg coverage	Active versus *H. influenzae*	Good gram-neg coverage
Sometimes used in UTIs	Spotty versus gram-neg enterics	Ceftazidime good *P. aeruginosa* coverage; all others poor
No CSF penetration	±CSF penetration	Good CSF penetration
Cefazolin, cephalexin	Cefuroxime, cefaclor	Cefotaxime, ceftriaxone, ceftazidime, cefixime

- HIV (with counseling and informed consent)
- VDRL (if sexually active, war victim, possible congenital syphilis)
- Sickle-cell prep (in children of African descent)
- G6PD screen or Hb electrophoresis (African, Asian, Mediterranean descent)
- Consider following microbiologic tests:
  - Throat swab for diphtheria (if signs and symptoms)
  - Genital, rectal, oral swabs for *Chlamydia,* gonorrhea, HSV (if sexually active)
  - Stool C+S, plus 2 bottles with fixative for O & P (if abdominal pain or diarrhea)
  - Urinalysis (hematuria, proteinuria)
- Immunization
  - Update all routine childhood immunizations

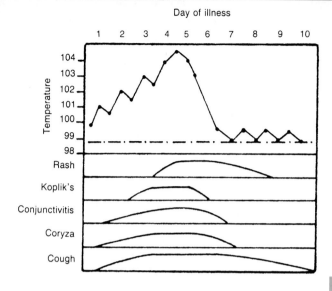

Day of illness

14

1. Measles

Rash
- Erythematous
- Maculopapular
- Starts at hairline, behind ears and upper neck
- Spreads to face and neck and then extends to trunk and extremities
- Fades in order of appearance
- Desquamates (except palms, soles)

Incubation period
- 8–13 days

Period of communicability
- 4 days before symptoms to 4 days after rash appears

Therapy
- See p 236 for post-exposure prophylaxis

Isolation
- Respiratory

Fig. 14-1   Common Childhood Exanthems. (From Krugman S, Katz S, Gershon AA, Wilfert C: *Infectious diseases of children,* ed 9, St Louis, 1992, Mosby.)   *Continued.*

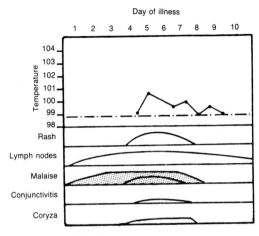

2. Rubella

Rash
• Pink
• Maculopapular
• Lesions on extremities may be
  discrete
• Starts on face, neck→trunk,
  extremities (spreads more quickly
  than measles)

Incubation period
• 14–21 days

Period of communicability
• 7 days pre-rash to 7 days after
  rash appears

Therapy
• None

Isolation
• Respiratory

Fig. 14-1, cont'd.   For legend see p. 263

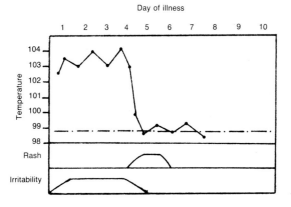

Day of illness

3. Roseola infantum

14

Rash
• Macular-maculopapular
• Neck-arms-trunk ± face
• Onset of rash accompanies
  disappearance of fever

Incubation period
• 5–15 days

Period of communicability
• Unknown

Therapy
• None

Isolation
• None

Fig. 14-1, cont'd.   For legend see p. 263

Continued.

**4. Erythema infectiosum
(a parvovirus infection)**

Rash
- Red flushed face, slapped-cheek
  appearance
- Maculopapular rash over trunk and
  extremities with lacelike
  appearance

Incubation period
- 4–14 days

Period of communicability
- Unknown

Therapy
- None

Isolation
- Respiratory (for 7 days following
  onset of illness)

Fig. 14-1, cont'd.   For legend see p. 263

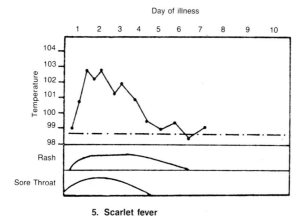

5. Scarlet fever

Rash
- Erythematous
- Blanches on pressure
- Starts in axillae, groin, and neck
  → generalized
- Circumoral pallor
- Desquamates (palms, soles involved)

Incubation period
- Occurs 2–5 days following streptococcal pharyngitis or impetigo

Period of communicability
- Maximum during the acute infection

Therapy
- Penicillin or erythromycin
  × 10 days

Isolation
- Barrier until on antibiotics for 24 hr

Fig. 14-1, cont'd. For legend see p. 263

CHAPTER 15
METABOLIC DISEASE

ANH DO

RECOGNITION AND MANAGEMENT OF INHERITED METABOLIC DISEASE

- See Fig. 15-1 for overview of major metabolic pathways
- Inherited metabolic disease generally manifests clinically as (Table 15-1):
  - Neurologic syndrome: acute and chronic encephalopathy
  - Hepatic syndrome
  - Acute metabolic acidosis

IN NEWBORNS

- Metabolic disease should be excluded in any newborn who becomes acutely ill after period of normal behavior and feeding
- Illness attributed to inborn errors of metabolism usually progresses rapidly; delay in recognition and initiation of appropriate management may lead to permanent neurologic impairment
- Acute metabolic disease in newborns generally "small molecule" in origin (i.e., involving carbohydrate, amino acid, organic acid, or ammonium metabolism)

IN INFANCY AND CHILDHOOD

- Any of inherited metabolic diseases presenting acutely in newborn period may present later in infancy or childhood as acute illnesses
- Conditions presenting in older infants and older children are generally milder variants and are often precipitated by infection or intercurrent illness
- Manifestations of metabolic disease may be superimposed on chronic history of failure to thrive or developmental delay.
- Metabolic diseases that cause slowly progressive encephalopathy generally affect degradation of macromolecules (i.e., storage diseases such as lysosomal hydrolase deficiencies)

INITIAL LABORATORY INVESTIGATIONS

- Electrolytes, ABG: Rule out congenital adrenal hyperplasia; calculate anion gap
- CBC, differential, smear: Neutropenia ± thrombocytopenia may be seen with organic acidemia; leukocyte inclusions may be suggestive of storage disease (may be reported as "atypical lymphocytes")
- Blood glucose: hypoglycemia may be seen in organic acidemia, fatty acid oxidation defects, and glycogen storage disease
- Blood lactate: may be falsely elevated with hemolysis or delay in separation of serum from RBC

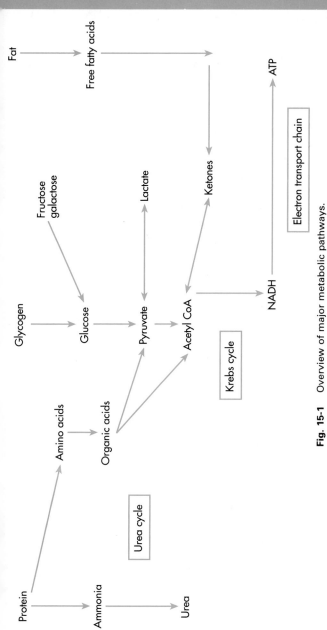

Fig. 15-1 Overview of major metabolic pathways.

15

Table 15-1 Clinical Presentation of Inherited Metabolic Disease—Other Recognizable Features

Feature	Description	Condition
Odor	Burnt sugar	MSUD*
	Sweaty feet	Isovaleric aciduria; glutaric aciduria, type II*
	Musty	PKU*
	Cabbagelike	Tyrosinemia
	Ammonia-like	MMA*, PA*, UCED*
Skin	Hypopigmentation	Albinism
	Hyperpigmentation	Gaucher's disease, Niemann-Pick, adrenoleukodystrophy
	Rash/eczema	PKU*, Hartnup disease, biotinidase deficiency, porphyria
	Icthyosis	Steroid sulfatase deficiency, multiple sulfatase deficiency, neutral lipid storage disease, Refsum's disease
	Xanthomas	Hyperlipoproteinemias I-III
Hair	Alopecia	Homocystinuria, Menkes' syndrome
	Hirsutism	Hunter's syndrome, Hurler's syndrome, Scheie's disease, porphyria
	Abnormal architecture	Homocystinuria, Menkes' syndrome, argininosuccinic aciduria
	Fair coloring	Albinism, PKU, homocystinuria, histidinemia, isovaleric acidemia, cystinosis, Menkes' syndrome
Eyes		
Cornea	Clouding	Mucopolysaccharidosis (Hurler's, Scheie's, Maroteaux-Lamy) (Note: not Hunter's)
	Crystals	Cystinosis
Lens	Cataracts	Galactosemia, mannosidosis, Refsum's disease, Wilson's disease
	Dislocation	Homocystinuria, hyperlysinemia (persistent), sulfite-oxidase deficiency
Retina	Macular cherry red spot	GM_1, GM_2, gangliosidosis, mucolipidosis I, neuraminidase deficiency (sialidosis), Niemann-Pick, metachromatic leukodystrophy
	Pigment retinopathy	Albinism, cystinosis, Refsum's disease, neuronal ceroid lipofuscinosis, Hunter's, Hurler's, mitochondrial disorders
	Optic atrophy	GM_2 gangliosidosis, Krabbe's disease, Leigh syndrome, metachromatic leukodystrophy

*_MSUD_, Maple syrup urine disease; _PKU_, phenylketonuria; _MMA_, methylmalonic acidemia; _PA_, propionic acidemia; _UCED_, urea cycle enzyme deficiency.

- Blood ammonium: pulmonary hemorrhage or primary respiratory alkalosis may be first clue of hyperammonemia
- Routine urinalysis: Ketonuria in newborn is pathological until proven otherwise
- Clinitest for urine: negative test does not rule out reducing substances in galactosemia; infant must be feeding lactose- and galactose-containing formula
- Plasma Ca, Mg
- Liver function tests, including PT, PTT
- Urate: elevated in glycogen storage disease type 1 and Lesch-Nyhan disease
- Galactosemia screen (from RBCs before transfusion): galactosemia in infants often presents with *E. coli* sepsis
- Urine 2,4-DNPH: detects branched-chain ketoacids (MSUD), pyruvate, acetoacetate
- Urine nitroprusside: detects disulfides in cystinuria and homocystinuria
- Amino acid screen: detects abnormally high amino acids by chromatography
- Urine organic acids: done by gas chromatography/mass spectrometry; diagnostic in organic acidemias, in which abnormal peaks appear on chromatogram as compared to reference; history of medications should be included as drug metabolites may complicate interpretations
- Plasma *quantitative* amino acids: abnormal high and low values are important in aminoacidopathies and urea cycle defects
- CSF glycine: may be elevated in presence of normal urine and plasma screens in nonketotic hyperglycinemia
- Free fatty acid: 3-OH-butyrate ratio > 4, suspect fatty acid oxidation defects
- Inital evaluation for storage diseases:
  - Urine mucopolysaccharide and oligosaccharide screen
  - X-rays of hands, chest, spine to look for dysostosis multiplex
  - Peripheral smear for leukocyte inclusions
  - Bone marrow for storage cells

15

ACUTE ENCEPHALOPATHY (Fig. 15-2)

- Poor feeding, vomiting, lethargy, irritability, seizures, and cerebral edema

AMINOACIDOPATHY

- Abnormal metabolism/transport of amino acids
- Most common: Maple syrup urine disease (MSUD): deficiency of keto-acids dehydrogenase required for branched chain amino acids (leucine, isoleucine, valine) metabolism

ORGANIC ACIDOSIS

- Enzyme defects in catabolic pathways of amino acids
- Two classic diseases: Propionic acidosis
                        Methylmalonic acidosis
- AG > 20, metabolic acidosis, hypoglycemia, neutropenia, thrombocy-

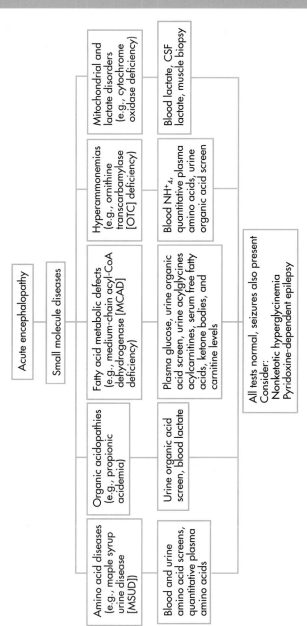

Fig. 15-2   Acute encephalopathy. (From Rudolph AM, Kamei RK, editors: *Rudolph's fundamentals of pediatrics*, ed 1, 1994, Appleton & Lange.)

topenia, ± hyperammonemia (because of inhibition of urea cycle by metabolites)

FATTY ACID OXIDATION DEFECTS

- Fasting hypoglycemia, acute hepatomegaly, ± skeletal or cardiomyopathy
- Most common: Medium-chain acyl CoA dehydrogenase deficiency (MCAD)-high FFA: 3-β-OH butyrate ratio, low carnitine, abnormal fatty acid metabolites (medium-chain dicarboxylic acids) in urine
- Treatment: avoid prolonged starvation; carnitine may be beneficial

HYPERAMMONEMIA

- Most common in urea cycle defect, however can be seen in organic acidosis and fatty acid oxidation defects
- Most common urea cycle defect: ornithine transcarbamylase (OTC) deficiency
- Treatment: limit protein intake; replenish urea cycle intermediates (e.g., arginine); provide alternate pathways of ammonium excretion (e.g., sodium benzoate)

TREATMENT OF ACUTE ENCEPHALOPATHY

1. Hydration: D10W/0.2% NaCl ± KCl at 150% maintenance to promote diuresis and excretion of water-soluble metabolites; glucose to decrease catabolic state; fluid restriction may be needed if cerebral edema is present
2. Treat shock, hypoglycemia, metabolic acidosis, electrolyte imbalances, infections, and coagulopathies by conventional methods (see Emergencies, p. 6); plasma bicarbonate < 10 mmol/L should be cautiously half corrected (see p. 109); consider dialysis for resistant metabolic acidosis
3. Treat hyperammonemia:
   - Arginine hydrochloride
   - Sodium benzoate and sodium phenylacetate (promote conversion of ammonium to water-soluble nontoxic form)
   - Hemodialysis or CVVH for severe cases
4. Treat potential vitamin-responsive enzymopathies
   - Thiamine 100 mg IV: PDH deficiency, thiamine-responsive MSUD
   - Biotin 20 mg IV: propionic acidemia, MCAD
   - Vitamin B_{12} 1 mg IV: methylmalonic acidemia
   - Pyridoxine 100-200 mg IV: intractable seizures, homocystinuria
5. Nutritional modifications: when in doubt of diagnosis, discontinue dietary or parenteral intake of protein and fat

CHRONIC ENCEPHALOPATHY (Fig. 15-3)

SMALL MOLECULE DISEASES

- Less severe variants of enzymopathies that are also associated with acute encephalopathy (see Fig. 15-2)
- Distinct group that causes only chronic encephalopathy:
- Phenylketonuria (PKU)
  - Phenylalanine → Tyrosine

Text continued on p. 278.

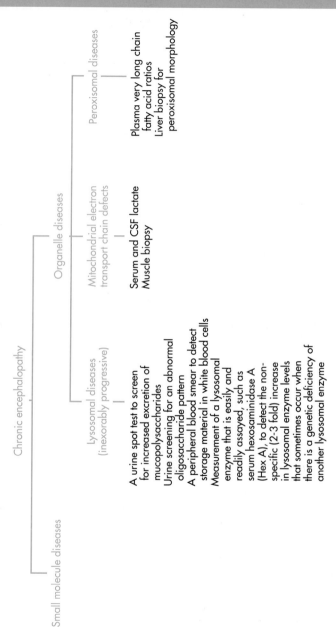

Fig. 15-3   Chronic encephalopathy. (From Rudolph AM, Kamel RK: *Rudolph's fundamentals of pediatrics, 1994, Appleton & Lange.*)

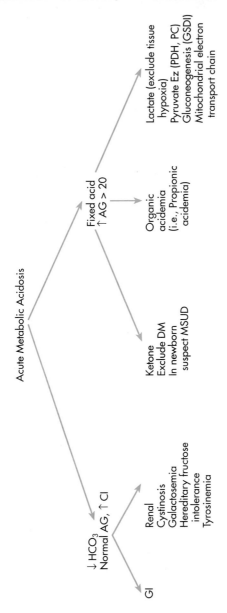

Fig. 15-4 Acute metabolic acidosis.

Acute Metabolic Acidosis

↓ HCO₃ Normal AG, ↑ Cl

GI

Renal
Cystinosis
Galactosemia
Hereditary fructose intolerance
Tyrosinemia

Fixed acid ↑ AG > 20

Ketone
Exclude DM
In newborn suspect MSUD

Organic acidemia (i.e., Propionic acidemia)

Lactate (exclude tissue hypoxia)
Pyruvate Ez (PDH, PC)
Gluconeogenesis (GSDI)
Mitochondrial electron transport chain

Table 15-2 Hepatic Disorders

Disorder	Special features	Results of investigation	Specific treatment
Galactosemia	Newborn: hepatomegaly, jaundice, hypoglycemia Older children: cirrhosis, mental retardation, recurrent hypoglycemia	Negative urine for reducing substances Confirm by RBC enzyme assay before blood transfusion Proportion presents with gram-negative sepsis	Restriction of galactose and lactose foods Despite restrictions, subtle decrease in intellectual functions
Hereditary fructose intolerance (HFI)	Symptoms only upon ingestion of fructose, sucrose, sorbitol; variable in severity Seizures, colic, vomiting, diarrhea, jaundice, hepatomegaly May cause acute liver failure or renal Fanconi syndrome	Hypoglycemia, marked metabolic acidosis, ↑ uric acid, ↓ phosphate Urine: negative Clinistix (glucose), positive Clinitest tablets (reducing substances) Chromatography of urine shows generalized aminoaciduria	Elimination of fructose, sucrose, sorbitol from diet
Tyrosinemia, type I	Presents acutely at 8-12 wk or with acute-on-chronic liver disease, ↑ bleeding, ↑ risk of hepatocellular carcinoma	↑ Plasma methionine and tyrosine, ↑ α-fetoprotein ↑ PT, ↑ PTT, abnormal LFTs ↑ Urinary succinylacetone, renal tubular defects	Diet restricted in tyrosine and phenylalanine Liver transplant
α₁-Antitrypsin deficiency	Pulmonary dysfunction, emphysema, Liver disease (cirrhosis, cholestatic jaundice, hepatomegaly, ↑ risk of hepatocellular carcinoma)	Abnormal pulmonary function tests, abnormal LFTs, serum α₁-antitrypsin, missing α₁-globulin peak on protein electrophoresis; PI typing Characteristic liver biopsy	Supportive therapy

Glycogen storage disease, type IV: brancher glycogenosis	Hepatosplenomegaly, ascites, liver failure, early cirrhosis	Abnormal LFTs, liver biopsy: electron microscopy	Supportive therapy
Glycogen storage disease, type III	Hepatomegaly, may be hypoglycemic, hypotonic; short stature	Glucagon stimulation test; Liver biopsy for debrancher enzyme assay	Supportive therapy
Glycogen storage disease, type I: von Gierke	Characteristic facies, massive hepatomegaly, hypoglycemic seizures, short stature, bleeding diathesis	Hypoglycemia, $\uparrow$ lactate, $\uparrow$ uric acid, $\uparrow$ triglycerides, $\uparrow$ urinary ketones, $\uparrow$ bleeding time (platelet dysfunction), response to glucagon	Overnight glucose, uncooked corn-starch before bed
Wilson's disease: hepatolenticular degeneration	Possible presentations: hepatitis-like illness, acute liver failure, cirrhosis, hemolytic anemia, neurologic, psychiatric, Kayser-Fleischer rings (slit lamp)	Abnormal LFTs, serum ceruloplasmin, total serum copper, $\uparrow$ urinary copper after penicillamine loading; Peripheral smear may show hemolysis; Renal tubular dysfunction, generalized aminoaciduria; Liver biopsy: copper deposition	D-penicillamine
Systemic carnitine deficiency	Recurrent attacks resembling Reye's syndrome of hypoglycemia, hyperammonemia, and hepatic encephalopathy; Skeletal myopathy; May have cardiomyopathy	Abnormal LFTs, $\uparrow$ NH_4^+, glucose, may have metabolic acidosis, $\downarrow$ carnitine in plasma, muscle (skeletal and cardiac), and liver; Decarboxylic acids in urine	Fat restriction; Glucose supplementation; L-carnitine administration

15

- Persistent hyperphenylalaninemia is neurotoxic, leading to mental retardation and seizures
- Treatment is dietary restriction of phenylalanine
- Homocystinuria: defect in cystathionine-B-synthase
  - Presents as nonprogressive encephalopathy, high myopia, lens dislocation, osteoporosis, Marfan's-like habitus

ORGANELLES
Lysosomes (Table 15-3)

- Enzyme defects that impair degradation of macromolecules (glycosaminoglycans, glycoproteins, sphingolipids) in lysosomes or disrupt transport of these molecules out to cytoplasm
- Diseases are restricted to tissues in which these macromolecules are degraded

Table 15-3　Clinical Differentiation of Organelle Disease and Small Molecule Disease

Feature	Organelle disease	Small molecule disease
Onset	Gradual	Often sudden, even catastrophic
Course	Slowly progressive	Characterized by relapses and remissions
Physical findings	Characteristic features	Nonspecific
Histopathology	Often reveals characteristic changes	Generally nonspecific changes
Response to supportive therapy	Poor	Brisk

Table 15-4　General Clinical Characteristics of Defects of Organelle Metabolism

Lysosomal	Peroxisomal	Mitochondrial
Disease limited to nervous system ± RES*	Multisystem disease	Multisystem disease
Chronic course	Severe chronic course	Acute-on-chronic course
Hepatosplenomegaly, variable	Failure to thrive	Failure to thrive
Leukodystrophy, often severe	Profound hypotonia	Cerebral dysgenesis
Cerebellar atrophy, marked	Cerebral dysgenesis	Sensorineural hearing loss
Skin lesions (angiokeratomata)	Hepatocellular dysfunction	Peripheral neuropathy
"Cherry red" macular spot	Sensorineural hearing loss	Myopathy
Behavior/psychiatric problems	Neuropathy	Extraocular ophthalmoplegia
Seizures, late	Cystic disease of kidneys	Cardiomyopathy
	Seizures, early and intractible	Retinitis pigmentosa
		Seizures variable

RES, Reticuloendothelial system.

Table 15-5 Lysosomal Storage Disorders

Disorder	Clinical features	Investigations
Mucopolysaccharidoses		
Hurler's	Coarse facies, cornea clouding, dysostosis, mental retardation, HSM*	Abnormal urine MPS. Deficiency of α-L-iduronidase tested on leukocyte or cultured fibroblast
Hunter's	Coarse facies, dysostosis, mental retardation (normal intelligence in mild form), HSM	Abnormal MPS. Deficiency of iduronate sulfatase
Glycoproteinoses		
Sialidosis	Coarse facies, mental retardation of variable severity; HSM, cherry red spot, myoclonic seizures	Abnormal urine oligosaccharide pattern, deficiency of sialidase in fibroblasts
Gangliosidoses		
GM1 gangliosidosis	Coarse facies, mental retardation, HSM, dysostosis, cherry red spot	Urine oligosaccharide consistently abnormal; deficiency of leukocyte β-galactosidase
Tay-Sachs	Normal until 5-6 mo, severe hypotonia, hyperacusis, cherry red spot, lack of visceral storage, seizures	Deficiency of hexosaminidase A in serum, leukocytes, or cultured fibroblasts

HSM, Hepatosplenomegaly.

Continued.

15

Table 15-5 Lysosomal Storage Disorders—cont'd

Disorder	Clinical features	Investigations
Sphingolipidoses		
Gaucher's (nonneuropathic form; most common of lysosomal diseases)	Neuronopathic: very rare, strabismus, trismus, opisthotonos in association with progressive spasticity and seizures Nonneuronopathic: HSM, pancytopenia, degenerative bony changes	Deficiency of glucocerebrosidase in leukocytes or fibroblasts
Niemann-Pick	Nonneuronopathic: HSM, foam cells in bone marrow Neuronopathic: as above and progressive neurologic deterioration	Some have deficiency of acid sphingomyelinase in leukocytes or fibroblasts
Leukodystrophies		
Metachromatic leukodystrophy	Onset at age 1-2 yrs of gait abnormalities, ataxia, clumsiness, weakness, behavior changes, and developmental delay, subsequent spastic quadriplegia, blindness, dementia, and seizures	Deficiency of arylsulfatase A in leukocytes or fibroblasts Delayed nerve conduction velocities (NCV), elevated CSF protein

- Almost always progressive
- Neurologic deterioration leading to dementia
- Coarse facies, retinal and peripheral nerve degeneration, hepatospleno-megaly, dysostosis multiplex
- Diagnose by lysosomal enzyme assays

Mitochondria

- Mitochondrial electron transport chain and proteins (i.e., Leigh disease: progressive dementia within first year + pyramidal tract signs, ataxia, optic neuropathy, nystagmus, respiratory irregularities)
- Mitochondrial DNA mutation: maternal inheritance or sporadic (i.e, myoclonic epilepsy with ragged red fiber [MERRF]; mitochondrial myopathy, encephalopathy, lactic acidosis, and strokelike syndrome [MELAS]; Kearns-Sayre syndrome [KSS])

Peroxisomes

- Zellweger syndrome: profound neurologic impairment, severe hypotonia and weakness, seizures, typical dysmorphic face, hepatic and renal dysfunction; majority die within 6 mo
- Diagnose by elevated very long chain fatty acids (VLCFAs), liver biopsy, enzymatic and immunologic studies of skin fibroblast and tissues

15

CHAPTER 16

NEONATOLOGY

Guy V. Widrich

ABBREVIATIONS

CAH	congenital adrenal hyperplasia
CHF	congestive heart failure
CNS	central nervous system
CPAP	continuous positive airway pressure
DIC	disseminated intravascular coagulopathy
ECMO	extracorporeal membrane oxygenation
ETT	endotracheal tube
F_iO_2	fraction of inspired oxygen
GBS	group B *Streptococcus*
GI	gastrointestinal
HIE	hypoxic ischemic encephalopathy
IDM	infant of diabetic mother
IPPV	intermittent positive pressure ventilation
IVH	intraventricular hemorrhage
LGA	large for gestational age
MAP	mean arterial pressure
NEC	necrotizing enterocolitis
NPT	nasopharyngeal tube
P_aCO_2	arterial partial pressure of carbon dioxide
P_aO_2	arterial partial pressure of oxygen
PDA	patent ductus arteriosus
PPHN	persistent pulmonary hypertension of newborn
PROM	premature rupture of membranes
PVL	periventricular leucomalacia
RDS	respiratory distress syndrome
SEH	subependymal hemorrhage
SGA	small for gestational age
UAC	umbilical artery catheter
UVC	umbilical venous catheter

Text continued on p. 290.

FLEMINGDON HEALTH CENTRE
10 GATEWAY BLVD.
DON MILLS, ONT. M3C 3A1

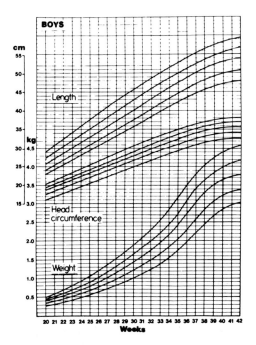

Fig. 16-1 Growth parameters: boys (means ± 1 and 2 Sds). (From Keen DV, Pearse RG: Weight, length, and head circumference curves for boys and girls of between 20 and 42 weeks gestation, *Arch Dis Child* 60:440, 1985.)

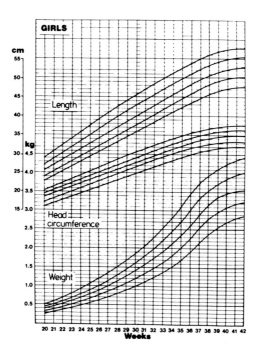

Fig. 16-2   Growth parameters:girls (means ± and Sds). (From Keen DV, Pearse RG: Weight, length, and head circumference curves for boys and girls of between 20 and 42 weeks gestation, *Arch Dis Child* 60:440, 1985.)

BOX 16-1 Parkin Assessment of Gestational Age

Soft Tissue Assessment
Skin Texture
Tested by picking up fold of abdominal skin between finger and thumb and by inspection
  0: Very thin, with gelatinous feel
  1: Thin and smooth
  2: Smooth and of medium thickness; irritation rash and superficial peeling may be present
  3: Slight thickening and stiff feeling with superficial cracking and peeling; especially evident in hands and feet
  4: Thick and parchmentlike with superficial or deep cracking

Skin Color
Estimated by inspection when baby is quiet
  0: Dark red
  1: Uniformly pink
  2: Pale pink, although color may vary in different parts of body; some parts may be very pale
  3: Pale; nowhere really pink except on ears, lips, palms, and soles

Breast Size
Measured by picking up breast tissue between finger and thumb
  0: No breast tissue palpable
  1: Breast tissue palpable on one or both sides, neither being more than 0.5 cm in diameter
  2: Breast tissue palpable on both sides, one or both being 0.5-1.0 cm in diameter
  3: Breast tissue palpable on both sides, one or both being more than 1.0 cm in diameter

Ear Firmness
Tested by palpation and folding of upper pinna
  0: Pinna feels soft and is easily folded into bizarre positions without springing back into position spontaneously
  1: Pinna feels soft along edge and is easily folded but returns in places
  2: Cartilage can be felt to edge of pinna, although it is thin in places, and pinna springs back readily after being folded
  3: Pinna firm with definite cartilage extending peripherally; springs back immediately into position after being folded

16

Score	Gestational age (in weeks)
1	27
2	30
3	33
4	34½
5	36
6	37
7	38½
8	39½
9	40
10	41
11-12	>41

From Parkin M, Hey EN, Clowes JS: Rapid assessment of gestational age at birth, *Arch Dis Child* 51:259, 1976.

GESTATIONAL AGE ASSESSMENT (Ballard)

NAME _____

HOSPITAL NO. _____

RACE _____

APGAR SCORE: 1 MINUTE _____ 5 MINUTES _____

DATE TIME OF BIRTH _____

DATE TIME OF EXAM _____

AGE WHEN EXAMINED _____

SEX _____

BIRTH WEIGHT _____

LENGTH _____

HEAD CIRC. _____

EXAMINER _____

SCORE

Neuromuscular _____

Physical _____

Total _____

NEUROMUSCULAR MATURITY

NEUROMUSCULAR MATURITY SIGN	SCORE						RECORD SCORE HERE
	0	1	2	3	4	5	
POSTURE							
SQUARE WINDOW (WRIST)	90°	60°	45°	30°	0°		
ARM RECOIL	180°		100°-180°	90°-100°	<90°		
POPLITEAL ANGLE	180°	160°	130°	110°	90°	<90°	
SCARF SIGN							
HEEL TO EAR							
					TOTAL NEUROMUSCULAR MATURITY SCORE		

PHYSICAL MATURITY

PHYSICAL MATURITY SIGN	0	1	2	3	4	5	RECORD SCORE HERE
SKIN	gelatinous, red, transparent	smooth, pink, visible veins	superficial peeling and or rash, few veins	cracking, pale area, rare veins	parchment, deep cracking, no vessels	leathery, cracked, wrinkled	
LANUGO	none	abundant	thinning	bald areas	mostly bald		
PLANTAR CREASES	no crease	faint red marks	anterior transverse crease only	creases anterior 2/3	creases cover entire sole		
BREAST	barely perceptible	flat areola, no bud	stippled areola, 1-2mm bud	raised areola, 3-4mm bud	full areola, 5-10mm bud		
EAR	pinna flat, stays folded	slightly curved pinna, soft with slow recoil	well-curved pinna, soft but ready recoil	formed & firm with instant recoil	thick cartilage, ear stiff		
GENITALS (Male)	scrotum empty, no rugae		testes descending, few rugae	testes down, good rugae	testes pendulous, deep rugae		
GENITALS (Female)	prominent clitoris & labia minora	flat areola...	majora & minora equally prominent	majora large, minora small	clitoris & minora completely covered		

TOTAL PHYSICAL MATURITY SCORE

Reference
Ballard JL, Novak KK, Driver M. A simplified score for assessment of fetal maturation of newly born infants. *J Pediatr* 95:769-774, 1979
Reprinted by permission of Dr. Ballard and *Journal of Pediatrics*

MATURITY RATING

TOTAL MATURITY SCORE	GESTATIONAL AGE (WEEKS)
5	26
10	28
15	30
20	32
25	34
30	36
35	38
40	40
45	42
50	44

GESTATIONAL AGE (weeks) _____
By dates _____
By ultrasound _____
By score _____

Fig. 16-3 **Modified Dubowitz assessment.** Sample of a form used to estimate gestational age by evaluation of various aspects of maturity. Note: Accuracy is ± 1 wk at more than 32 wk; unreliable at less than 32 wk; neurologic component in compromised infants is unreliable. (From Mead Johnson Nutritional Group, Evansville, Indiana.)

Neonate delivered
→

Transfer to radiant warmer
Dry thoroughly
Position neonate on his or her back with neck slightly extended
Assess the need for suctioning (if necessary do gently to avoid vagal stimulation)
Assessment of respiratory effort, heart rate, and color

HR >100 min
RR slow, irregular
Color: blue extremities

Gentle tactile stimulation
± gentle nasopharyngeal suction
↓
Minimal or no improvement
↓
100% O₂ by bag and mask with tight seal (IPPV)

HR <100, >50
RR slow, irregular
Color: blue

Gentle suction,
tactile stimulation,
100% O₂ by bag and mask
(IPPV) 40-60/min
↓
Minimal or no improvement

HR <50
RR, apneic
Color: blue, pale

Nasal/oropharyngeal
suction + immediate
IPPV with bag and mask or ETT;
100% O₂
IPPV 40-60/min
Peak pressures
30-40 mm Hg
initially thereafter,
decrease to minimum pressure
required to move chest

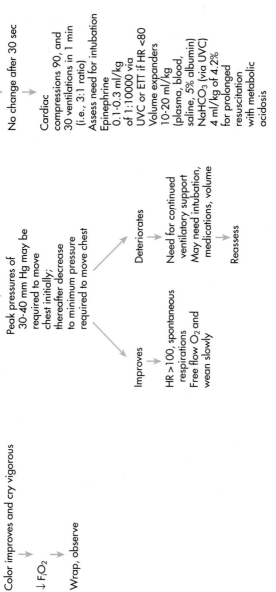

Fig. 16-4 Guide to assesment and management of neonate at delivery.

Color improves and cry vigorous

↓ F₁O₂

Wrap, observe

Peak pressures of
30-40 mm Hg may be
required to move
chest initially;
thereafter decrease
to minimum pressure
required to move chest

Improves

HR >100, spontaneous
respirations
Free flow O₂ and
wean slowly

Deteriorates

Need for continued
ventilatory support
May need intubation,
medications, volume

Reassess

No change after 30 sec

Cardiac
compressions 90, and
30 ventilations in 1 min
(i.e., 3:1 ratio)
Assess need for intubation
Epinephrine
0.1-0.3 ml/kg
of 1:10000 via
UVC or ETT if HR <80
Volume expanders
10-20 ml/kg
(plasma, blood,
saline, 5% albumin)
NaHCO₃ (via UVC)
4 ml/kg of 4.2%
for prolonged
resuscitation
with metabolic
acidosis

16

Table 16-1   APGAR Score*

Sign†	0	1	2
Heart rate	Absent	<100 beats/min	>100 beats/min
Respiratory effort	Absent	Gasping; slow, irregular	Regular, good lusty cry
Reflex irritability	No response	Grimace	Cry
Muscle tone	Limp, flaccid	Some flexion of extremities	Active, well flexed
Color	Blue, pale	Body pink; extremities blue	Completely pink

Modified from Ostheimer GW: Resuscitation of newborn infant, *Clin Perinatal* 9(1):183, 1982.

*Apgar scoring system provides mechanism for documenting newborn's condition at specific intervals after birth; it should not be used to determine need for resuscitation because resuscitative efforts, if required, should be initiated promptly after birth. APGAR score should be done at 1 and 5 min and thereafter at 5-min intervals until score of 7 is achieved.

†The sign components of the Apgar score can be remembered by mnemonic: How Ready Is This Child.

Table 16-2   Endotracheal Tube Size

Weight	Gestational age	Size
<1000 g	<28 wk	2.5 mm
1000-2000 g	28-34 wk	3.0 mm
2000-3000 g	34-38 wk	3.5 mm
>3000 g	>38 wk	3.5-4.0 mm

DELIVERY OF HIGH-RISK NEONATE (Fig. 16-4)

- Equipment in case room
  1. Laryngoscope
  2. Endotracheal tubes (sizes 2.5, 3.0, 3.5, 4.0) (Table 16-2)
  3. Magill forceps
  4. Radiant heater on
  5. Clean warm towels
  6. O_2 bagging equipment with masks (sizes 0, 1, 2)
  7. Suction *on*
  8. Meconium aspirator (Box 16-2)
  9. Umbilical catheterization tray (catheter sizes 3.5, 5.0 F)
  10. Emergency drugs.
      - Epinephrine 1:10,000
      - Na bicarbonate, 4.2% concentration (0.5 mEq/ml)
      - Dextrose (10%)
      - 5% albumin, normal saline
      - Naloxone
- Normal sequence of response to resuscitation: increased heart rate → reflex activity → color improves → apnea resolves → tone and responsiveness improve
- Threshold for intubating premature infants (<32 wk) is low

BOX 16-2 Thick ("Pea Soup") Meconium-Stained Liquor Noted During Delivery*

Mouth, pharynx, and nasal suction by obstetrician when "crowning" occurs
Radiation heater; supine; do not stimulate
Residual meconium in hypopharynx should be removed by suctioning under direct vision
Intubate (only if baby "flat" before onset of spontaneous respiration)
Suction trachea by using ETT as suction catheter, connected to wall suction by meconium aspirator
Reintubate and suction until clear
Dry thoroughly; place dry blanket under infant; do not wrap
O_2 by mask, keeping tight seal, to improve color if necessary (may need some IPPV)
Aspiration of stomach early to avoid further aspiration of swallowed meconium
Presence of meconium in premature delivery may represent *Listeria* infection

---

Modified from Merritt TA: Respiratory distress. In: Ziai M, Clarke TA, Merritt TA, eds: *Assessment of the newborn*, Boston, 1984, Little, Brown.
*Thinly stained liquor in a well baby requires gentle nasopharyngeal suction only.

- Special problems in initial management
  1. SGA infant: hypothermia, hypoglycemia, hyperviscosity syndrome- (secondary to polycythemia)
  2. LGA infant: birth trauma, asphyxia, hypoglycemia, hyperbilirubinemia

---

ASPHYXIA

16

ASSOCIATED PATHOLOGY

- CNS: HIE (Table 16-4)
- Pulmonary: PPHN, meconium aspiration
- Renal: oliguria, acute renal failure
- Cardiovascular: tricuspid regurgitation, transient myocardial ischemia, shock
- Metabolic: acidosis, hypoglycemia, hypocalcemia, hyponatremia
- GI: NEC, hepatic dysfunction
- Hematologic: thrombocytopenia, DIC

INVESTIGATIONS

- Appropriate investigations depend on individual patient and availability in each institution
- CBC, differential (to exclude sepsis, neutropenia, thrombocytopenia)
- Glucose, Ca, blood gas
- Urinalysis for hematuria
- Creatinine, electrolytes
- Liver-function tests
- PT, PTT
- ECG
- Head ultrasound (US), CT scan, MRI
- EEG
- Visual-, sensory-, auditory-evoked potentials

Table 16-3　Survival Rates for Low Birth Weight*

Birth weight (g)	Survival (%)	Intact survival (%)
500-600	36	30
600-800	67	56
800-1000	85	77
1000-1200	93	73
1200-1500	96	77

*Figures adapted from Vermont Oxford Neonatal Network, 1994. Note: Figures may vary within each institution, so one should quote own statistics when counseling parents.

Table 16-4　Sarnat and Sarnat Classification of HIE

Signs	Stage 1*	Stage 2†	Stage 3‡
Level of consciousness	Hyperalert	Lethargic	Stuperous, coma
Tone	Normal	Hypotonic	Flaccid
Posture	Normal	Flexed	Decerebrate
Reflexes	Hyperactive	Hyperactive	Absent
Pupils	Mydriasis	Miosis	Unequal, poor light reflex
Seizures	None	Common	Decerebrate
EEG	Normal	Low voltage with seizures	Burst suppression to isoelectric

*Stage 1 associated with excellent prognosis with full recovery.
†Stage 2 associated with variable outcome depending on clinical course.
‡Stage 3 associated with moderate to severe handicap or death.

NEONATAL SEIZURES

- "Jitteriness" can be differentiated from seizures by restraint or change in position: will stop jitteriness, but not seizure activity
- Causes include birth asphyxia; CNS anomalies; intracranial bleeds and infections; SGA; hyperviscosity (usually secondary to polycythemia); decreased glucose, Ca, or Mg levels (Table 16-5)

SEIZURE CONTROL

- ABCs (see pp. 2 and 14)
- Phenobarbital is first choice; apnea, hypotension may occur
- Lorazepam, diazepam
- Phenytoin
- Paraldehyde pr or IV
- Treat underlying cause

INVESTIGATIONS

- Always check glucose, Ca, Mg, electrolytes, arterial blood gases
- CBC, differential
- Septic workup (blood, CSF, urine cultures, CXR examination); workup of congenital infection as indicated (see p. 245)
- Head US, CT scan, MRI
- Neurologic function, EEG, evoked potentials

Table 16-5 Etiology of Neonatal Seizures and Approximate Time of Onset

	0-3 Days	4-7 Days	After 10 Days
Brain Injury*	+		
Complicated hypocalcemia	+		
Benign hypocalcemia		+	
Hypoglycemia	+		
Pyridoxine dependency	+	+	+
Infection (congenital, meningitis, sepsis)	+	+	+
Malformation	±	+	+
Metabolic defects†	+	+	+
Subdural injury			+
Drug withdrawal	+	+	+
IVH/SEH	+		

Modified from Weiner HL, Bresnan MJ, Levitt LP, eds: *Pediatric neurology for the house officer,* ed 2, Baltimore, 1982, Williams & Wilkins.

*Most common cause (includes asphyxia, trauma).

†Urea cycle disorders (e.g., MSUD, PKU) (see Chapter 15, Metabolic Disease).

Table 16-6 Guidelines for Fluid and Electrolye Therapy—Prediuretic Phase*

Weight	Water†	Na‡	K	Ca	Glucose§
(g)	(ml/day)		(mmol/kg/day)		(%)
<750	125-150	nil	nil	—	5
750-1000	75-125	nil	nil	—	5-10
1000-1500	60-80	nil	nil	—	10
>1500	50-60	nil	nil	—	10

From Perlman M, Kirpalani H: *Residents handbook of neonatology,* St Louis, 1992, Mosby.

*Prediuretic phase (days 1-2, urine output <1-2 ml/kg/h).

†Add 30% for radiant heater, add 10% for phototherapy, subtract 10% for heat shield and/or cellophane wrap.

‡In infants <750 g with tendency to early hypernatremia, saline may be hazardous even in arterial line.

§Change up or down may be needed, according to blood glucose concentration.

- Metabolic screen, NH_4, lactate, liver-function tests, as indicated
- Consider drug withdrawal

FLUIDS AND ELECTROLYTES (Tables 16-6 and 16-7)

- High surface-area-to-weight ratio
- Immature renal function
- Immature skin; higher losses in premature infants
- Insensible fluid losses (approximate values):
  1. <1500 g: 30-60 ml/kg/24 hr
  2. 1500-2500 g: 15-35 ml/kg/24 hr
  3. >2500 g: 10-15 ml/kg/24 hr

Table 16-7   Guidelines for Fluid and Electrolyte Therapy—
Postdiuretic Phase*

Weight	Water†	Na‡	K§	Ca	Glucose
(g)	(ml/day)		(mmol/kg/day)		(mg/kg/min)
<750	150-200	3-4	1-2	1-2	4-8
750-1000	120-160	3	1-2	1-2	4-8
1000-1500	80-150	3	1-2	1-2	4-8
>1500	70-130	2-3	1-2	1-2	4-8

From Perlman M, Kirpalani H: *Residents handbook of neonatology,* St Louis, 1992, Mosby.

*"Obligatory" diuretic phase (water and Na balance negative by definition, 1-5 days of age) and "postdiuretic" phase (water and Na balance stabilize and then should become positive after >2-4 days of age).

†Adjust water intake according to environmental conditions as indicated in Table 16-6.

‡Add Na to IV fluid when diuretic phase established (urine output >1-2 ml/kg/h for >6-8 h). Serum Na is <140 mmol/L and not rising. Much larger doses may be required in postdiuretic phase in infants <750 g in whom urine losses of Na may be excessive. This must be determined by measurement of urine Na concentration and urine output before large IV doses of sodium are given, owing to tendency of these infants to become hypernatremic from excessive IWL.

§Add K to IV fluid when diuretic phase established. Serum K is <5.5 mmol/L and not rising.

- Urine output: 50-100 ml/kg/day
- Weight is most useful parameter of fluid status monitoring
- High urinary Na losses (up to 10-12 mmol/kg/day in premature infants)
- 3% NaCl = 0.5 mmol/ml = 0.5 mEq/ml; KCI = 2 mmol/ml = 2 mEq/ml; 10% Ca gluconate = 0.2 mmol/ml = 0.4 mEq/ml

HYPONATREMIA

- Na < 130 mmol/L

Excess Na Loss

- Renal tubular immaturity, hypoxic injury
- Diuretics
- GI losses
- Salt-losing 21-hydroxylase deficiency
- "Late hyponatremia of prematurity" (>1 wk) may be caused by inadequate intake in addition to above causes

Treatment
- Calculate deficit ($Na_{desired} - Na_{actual}$) × 0.6 × wt (kg)
- Replace over 24-48 hr in addition to providing maintenance and estimate of ongoing losses
- Calculated deficit is often underestimate in infants weighing < 1500 g
- Monitor serum Na q6-12h

Water Retention

- Iatrogenic overload (excess dextrose solutions)
- SIADH
- CHF

Treatment
- Fluid restriction (½-⅔ maintenance)
- If symptomatic: 3% NaCl to correct to 125 mmol/L ± diuretics
- Monitor serum Na q6-12h

HYPERNATREMIA

- Na > 150 mmol/L

Excess H$_2$O Loss

- Dehydration from increased insensible losses (especially from radiant warmer)
- GI losses
- Osmotic diuresis (rare)

Excess Na Administration

- Normal saline
- NaHCO$_3$

Treatment (dehydration most common)

- Assume fluid deficit 10%-15% (100-150 ml/kg), and correct by replacing deficit over 24-48 hr to avoid too rapid decrease in Na
- If patient hypotensive, resuscitate with 10-15 ml/kg colloid or crystalloid, subtracting volume given from total deficit to be replaced
- If initial Na>160, use normal saline to replace deficit, use 5% dextrose and 0.45 saline (D$_5$/0.45 NS) or 3.33 dextrose and 0.33 saline (⅔-⅓) as maintenance fluid (to provide usual requirements of 3 mmol/kg/day)
- If initial Na < 160, use D5/0.45 NS for deficit; continue as above
- For infants <1.5 kg, deficits may be 20%-25% of body weight; initially use 5% dextrose with or without 0.2 saline for replacement of deficit; monitor and adjust further based on Na, weight, urine output, urine Na

HYPOKALEMIA

- Most commonly iatrogenic (e.g., inadequate intake, excessive urinary losses from diuretic therapy, or respiratory alkalosis)

HYPERKALEMIA

- K > 7 mmol/L
- Excess input (IV)
- Cellular leak (damage, necrosis, resorbed blood)
- Renal failure
- Adrenal insufficiency (CAH, hemorrhage, infarct; associated with decreased Na)

Management

- Ensure that blood sample not hemolyzed
- Obtain ECG; monitor continuously
- Serum K ≥ 8 mmol/L without ECG changes, ≥ 7 mmol/L with ECG changes

  Alkalinize with NaHCO$_3$, 1.5-2 mmol/kg/15 min + kayexalate 1 g/kg PR

  ↓ (if no effect)

  10% Ca gluconate 0.5-1 ml/kg over 2-3 min with ECG monitoring

  ↓ (if no effect)

  Glucose 1 g/kg + insulin 0.1 U/kg IV over 30 min

  ↓ (if no effect)

  Dialysis if hyperkalemia from renal failure

16

ACID-BASE STATUS

RESPIRATORY ACIDOSIS

- Corrected by ventilation, *not* $NaHCO_3$

RESPIRATORY ALKALOSIS

- Generally in ventilated infants

METABOLIC ACIDOSIS

- $HCO_3^- < 20$ mmol/L
- Sepsis (consider septic workup)
- Hypoxia
- Shock
- PDA with CHF
- HCO_3^- losses (renal tubular acidosis)
- Metabolic (amino acidemia, organic acidemia, congenital lactic acidosis)
- Excess protein load
- SEH, IVH

Management

- Treat underlying cause
- $NaHCO_3$ (4.2%) for pH < 7.2 and base excess > 10
- Base deficit: $(HCO_3\text{ desired} - HCO_3\text{ actual}) \times$ Wt (kg) $\times 0.6$
- Correct half of calculated deficit initially, usually over 1-4 hr; do not infuse in Ca-containing solutions
- 2 mmol/kg of $NaHCO_3$ increases pH by 0.1 unit

METABOLIC ALKALOSIS

- Usually secondary to excessive $NaHCO_3$ therapy
- May be seen with hypokalemia, PO_4 excess, hypochloremia, and post-exchange transfusion

HYPERGLYCEMIA

- Glucose > 10 mmol/L $\pm$ glycosuria
- Iatrogenic (TPN, dextrose solutions, steroids)
- Stress: sepsis must be excluded

Management

- Monitor urine, blood glucose, Chemstrip
- Decrease glucose infusion in stages of 2.5% Dextrose
- Monitor weight, fluid balance
- Insulin therapy rarely required

HYPOGLYCEMIA

- Full term: glucose < 2.2 mmol/L
- Preterm: glucose $< 1.65\text{-}2.5$ mmol/L
- Clinical: lethargy, apnea, cyanosis, tremor, tachypnea, seizures

- Decreased carbohydrate stores (SGA, postmature, premature, RDS, maternal hypertension)
- Endocrine: excess insulin, often LGA, IDM, erythroblastosis fetalis, Beckwith-Wiedemann syndrome, islet cell dysplasias, suppression of hypothalamopituitary adrenal axis
- Metabolic disease
- Miscellaneous mechanisms (not fully understood): shock, asphyxia, sepsis, hypothermia, polycythemia, rapid wean of IV glucose
- Critical sample: in presence of hypoglycemia take blood for glucose, insulin, cortisol, growth hormone, β-hydroxybutyrate, lactate, ammonia, acid-base status

Management

- Identify and monitor infants at risk q3-4h prefeed; every second or third feed after 48-72 hr
- Optimize oral feeds
- IV glucose if above inadequate
  1. Asymptomatic: IV glucose, 5-8 mg/kg/min (3-5 ml/kg/hr of 10% dextrose); may increase infusion as necessary
  2. Symptomatic: IV glucose bolus, 2-4 ml/kg of 10% dextrose followed by infusion of 5-8 mg/kg/min; increase infusion as necessary
  3. In presence of hyperinsulinism, requirement for glucose may be as high as 10-12 mg/kg/min
  4. If unsuccessful, consider glucagon, 0.5-1 mg/24 hr infusion; dose may be increased to 2 mg/24 hr
  5. Prednisone, diazoxide for refractory cases (consult with endocrinologist)

16

HYPOCALCEMIA

- Full term: Ca < 1.9 mmol/L
- Preterm: Ca < 1.75 mmol/L (because of lower albumin)
- Ionized Ca < 0.9 mmol/L
- Monitor Mg

Management

- Identify high-risk infants (premature, SGA, sepsis, cardiovascular compromise)
- Treat high-risk infants with maintenance Ca as continuous infusion for 48-72 hr starting at 6 hr: 0.6-1 mmol/kg/day or 25-45 mg/kg/day elemental Ca (see p. 565)
- Acute symptomatic hypocalcemia: irritability, jitteriness, cyanosis, stridor, increased reflexes, prolonged QT interval, seizures (may be multifocal or migratory with alert periods between spells)
- Dilute 10% Ca gluconate solution to 2% and give 0.05-0.1 mmol/kg infusion over 10 min with ECG monitoring (bradycardia, asystole can occur), followed by maintenance infusion as above
- Asymptomatic infants: variable, may treat when Ca < 1.8 mmol/L with oral supplementation or IV infusion as for high-risk infants
- Observe IV sites closely for extravasation
- Vitamin D PO for high-risk infants: 400-800 IU/day

NEONATAL RESPIRATORY DISTRESS (Fig. 16-5 and Tables 16-8 and 16-9)

- Goal of therapy: to maintain $PCO_2 < 50$ mm Hg; PO_2 50-70 mm Hg; and pH > 7.25
- All term neonates with respiratory distress should be treated with antibiotics (penicillin or ampicillin and aminoglycoside) until sepsis ruled out
- Criteria for ventilation:
  1. Marked hypoxia, rising PCO_2
  2. Shock with poor perfusion and hypotension, regardless of arterial blood gases
  3. Frequent apnea

SEDATION AND PARALYSISA

- Sedation can generally be accomplished with morphine in boluses, or by continuous infusion, if necessary
- Paralysis: pancuronium bromide, 0.1 mg/kg q2-4h prn
- Morphine should be used routinely when paralyzing

APNEA (Table 16-10)

- Cessation of respiration of >15-20 sec duration, with fall in heart rate to <100 beats/min or cyanosis; after 30-45 sec of apnea, pallor and hypotonia occur; apnea may be central, obstructive, or mixed

Table 16-8 Differential Diagnosis of Respiratory Distress in Newborn Period

Pulmonary disorders	
Common	Less common
Respiratory distress syndrome	Pulmonary hypoplasia
Transient tachypnea (TTN)	Upper airway obstruction
Meconium aspiration	Rib cage anomalies
Pneumonia	Space-occupying lesions (e.g., diaphragmatic hernia)
Pneumothorax	Pulmonary hemorrhage
	Immature lung syndrome

Extrapulmonary disorders		
Vascular	Metabolic	Neuromuscular
Persistent pulmonary hypertension of newborn	Acidosis	Cerebral hypertension
Congenital heart disease	Hypoglycemia	Cerebral hemorrhage
Hypovolemia-anemia	Hypothermia	Muscle or NMJ disorders
Polycythemia		Spinal cord problems
		Phrenic nerve palsy
		Drugs (morphine, phenobarbital)

Modified from Klaus MH, Fanaroff AA, eds: *Care of the high risk neonate*, Philadelphia, 1986, W.B. Saunders.

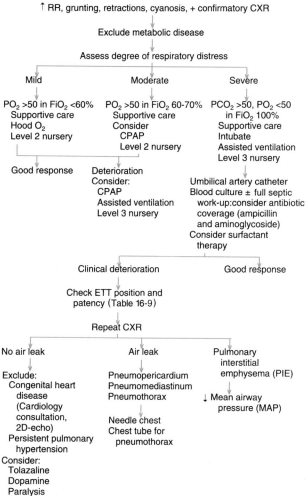

Fig. 16-5 Initial management of respiratory distress syndrome. (Adapted from Berman S, ed: *Pediatric decision making*, Toronto, 1985, B.C. Decker.)

Table 16-9   Management of Nonresponse to IPPV

Cause of nonresponse	Diagnostic features	Action
ETT not in correct location	Observe chest movement Auscultate for asymmetric air entry CXR to confirm	Reposition if ETT in right main stem bronchus Reintubate and reassess
Tension pneumothorax	Displaced apex beat ± hemodynamic compromise Decreased or unequal air entry CXR or transilluminate to confirm	Urgent drain with butterfly needle until stable; then insert chest tube
Massive meconium aspiration	History of fetal distress and "pea-soup" liquor staining Characteristic CXR ↑ Risk of PFC ↑ Risk of pneumothorax	Suction trachea and oropharynx using ETT Intubate and ventilate, if indicated
Diaphragmatic hernia	Scaphoid abdomen noted at birth ± respiratory distress Bowel sounds heard over chest CXR diagnostic ↑ Risk of PPHN	Pass N/G tube and connect to low-gomco Intubate IPPV and transfer to tertiary center Sedate and paralyze
Hypoplastic lungs	History of oligohydramnios ± PROM ± Potter's facies Characteristic CXR	Urgent intubation Ventilatory support Require high peak pressures
Sepsis neonatorum ± congenital pneumonia	History of PROM, GBS, or maternal fever CXR suspicious, but may look like RDS Cultures may be positive	Antibiotics Ventilatory support ± Volume expanders ± Inotropes

Table 16-10   Management of Apnea

Immediate Resuscitation
Surface stimulation
Gentle nasopharyngeal suction
Ventilation with inflating bag and mask
Intubation and IPPV

	Cause	Action
1. Infection	Neonatal sepsis	Full septic workup, including LP
	Meningitis	
	Necrotizing enterocolitis (NEC)	Antibiotics
2. Thermal instability	Hypo/hyperthermia	Assess body and isolette temperature
3. Metabolic disorders	Hypoglycemia	Dextrostix ± blood glucose
	Hypocalcemia	Serum Ca, ECG
	Hypo/hypernatremia	Electrolytes, BUN; fluid balance, weight
	Hyperammonemia	Serum NH_4, amino acids, organic acids, liver function tests
4. CNS problems	Asphyxia	Observation
	Intracranial hemorrhage	EEG, head US
	Cerebral malformation	Head US ± CT scan
	Seizures	Consider anticonvulsants
5. Decreased O_2 delivery	Hypoxemia	Check ETT
	Worsening RDS ± complication	CXR
	Anemia/shock	CBC, electrolytes, BUN, ABG
	Left to right shunt (PDA)	ECG, 2D-ECHO
	Pneumothorax	Needle + chest tube
6. Upper airway obstruction	Choanal atresia	Attempt passage of N/G tube
	Macroglossia	Oropharyngeal airway
	Reflux	CXR for aspiration
7. Drugs	Maternal prenatal or postnatal exposure	Drug/toxic screen, depending on history and clinical findings

16

Continuing Management to Prevent Recurrences; Monitoring
Continuous $TCPO_2$ monitoring; adjust F_IO_2 accordingly
Minimize handling of small infants
± "Rocking mattress" stimulation
Consider altering feeding pattern (i.e., slow continuous orogastric or IV)
Drug therapy:
1. Caffeine citrate; lower incidence of side effects with caffeine vs. theophylline
2. Aminophylline or theophylline are alternatives
Recurrent attacks: Consider short-term assisted ventilation:
1. NPT or nasal prong CPAP
2. ETT CPAP
3. IPPV; often need only slow rate (i.e., ~6-10/min)

Modified from Forfar JL, Arneil GC: *Textbook of paediatrics,* ed 2, New York, 1978, Churchill Livingstone.

- Do not attribute apnea automatically to prematurity, especially in infants of gestational age >30 wk
- Always exclude underlying cause

PATENT DUCTUS ARTERIOSUS (PDA)

- Common association with RDS in premature infants; 80% of infants <1000 g, 20% of all premature infants
- Clinical signs: characteristic harsh systolic murmur continuing into diastole, active precordium, bounding pulses, wide pulse pressure, worsening respiratory status, CHF (Box 16-3)
- Signs may be absent ("silent ductus")
- When available, 2D-ECHO to confirm diagnosis
- Decision to treat depends on clinical significance of duct; includes increasing ventilatory and F_iO_2 requirements, apnea and bradycardia events, CHF, and poor growth

Management

- Fluid restriction: ⅔ maintenance
- Indomethacin: 0.2 mg/kg for three doses, at 12-hr intervals or 0.1 mg/kg for five doses at 24-hr intervals; second course can be repeated 48 hr later in absence of side effects
- Adverse effects of indomethacin: platelet dysfunction, decreased renal artery flow leading to decreased GFR and urine output, fluid retention ± hyponatremia, increased creatinine, bowel perforation (rare)
- 80% success rate after first dose with 25% reopening; 18% reclose without further therapy

---

BOX 16-3 Cardiac Failure in the Neonatal Period

1. Birth
   Arrhythmias
   Anemias
   A-V fistula
   Perinatal asphyxia
2. Day 1
   As in *A* plus:
   Hypoplastic left heart syndrome
   Metabolic abnormalities
   Tricuspid atresia/Ebstein's
   Critical pulmonary stenosis
3. Weeks 1-2
   As in *B* plus:
   Arrhythmias
   Coarctation
   TGA with VSD
   TAPVR (obstructed)
   Myocarditis
   Endocardial fibroelastosis
   Pompe's disease
   PDA in premature infant
4. Weeks 2-4
   As in *C* plus:
   TAPVR (unobstructed)
   Truncus arteriosus
   A-V canal

---

*For management, see p. 65; for abbreviations, see p. 54.

- Contraindications to indomethacin:
  1. Increased creatinine (>100-120 μmol/L)
  2. Increased urea (>7 mmol/L)
  3. Oliguria < 0.5-1 ml/kg/hr
  4. Necrotizing enterocolitis
  5. Thrombocytopenia < 80,000
  6. Hyperbilirubinemia
  7. IVH
- Surgical approach: ligation or division

PERSISTENT PULMONARY HYPERTENSION OF NEWBORN (PPHN)

- Right-to-left shunt occurs through foramen ovale and/or PDA; associated with pulmonary arteriolar spasm or thickening (primary)
- May be 1 or 2 degrees
- Most are term or postterm infants
- Secondary causes include
  1. Transient tachypnea of newborn
  2. Meconium aspiration syndrome
  3. Hyaline membrane disease (respiratory distress syndrome)
  4. Group B streptococcal pneumonia
  5. Pulmonary hypoplasia ± diaphragmatic hernia
  6. Severe asphyxia
  7. Polycythemia
- Clinical: marked cyanosis, acidosis, and RV heave

16

INVESTIGATIONS

- Hyperoxic challenge (see p. 66)
- CXR: oligemic lung fields or consistent with underlying disease; cardiomegaly; may look normal
- ECG: RV strain
- $\text{O}_2 \text{ Index} = \dfrac{\text{MAP F}_i\text{O}_2 \times 100}{\text{P}_a\text{O}_2}$
  If >40, consider ECMO; MAP = mean airway pressure

TREATMENT

- Sedation ± paralysis usually required
- Ventilate to achieve P_aO_2 60-80 mm Hg and P_aCO_2 35-45 mm Hg and increase pH to 7.45-7.5 with judicious use of alkali infusion; causes pulmonary arteriolar vasodilatation and decreases pulmonary vascular resistance
- Inotropes: dopamine, dobutamine to increase systemic resistance and decrease right-to-left shunting
- Tolazoline: 1-2 mg/kg IV bolus then 0.5-2 mg/kg/hr; patients should be on continuous inotrope infusion to counteract fall in systemic BP; may need colloid/crystalloid support
- Nitric oxide: continuous inhaled gas 40-80 ppm NO

JAUNDICE

<24 HR OF AGE

- Hemolytic (Rh or ABO incompatibility) anemia until proven otherwise
- Sepsis or congenital infection should be considered

24-72 HR OF AGE

- Mostly "physiologic;" premature infants have later onset (day 6 or 7) and longer duration (up to day 14) of physiologic jaundice
- Hemolytic anemia (unrelated to major blood group incompatibility): G6PD deficiency, pyruvate kinase deficiency, spherocytosis, Duffy or Kell incompatibility
- Polycythemia (SGA, late clamping of cord, maternal-fetal and fetofetal transfusions)
- Sepsis or congenital infection
- Bruising, hemorrhage, or swallowed blood

>72-96 HR OF AGE

- "Physiologic" ± breast milk jaundice most common
- Infection: sepsis (including UTI) or hepatitis (congenital infection)
- GI obstruction (increased enterohepatic circulation)

>1 WK OF AGE (PROLONGED NEONATAL JAUNDICE)

- Hypothyroidism (may not have typical features)
- Galactosemia
- Breast milk (benign)
- Prolonged physiologic (e.g., preterm)
- Crigler-Najjar syndrome, Gilbert's disease
- Obstructive jaundice (e.g., "neonatal hepatitis," biliary atresia, inspissated bile syndrome, choledochal cyst, α-1-antitrypsin deficiency)

INVESTIGATIONS (Box 16-4)
Jaundice Occurring <1 Wk of Age

- Family history of jaundice, maternal history, blood group and Rh status, previous pregnancies, transfusions, Rhogam
- Physical exam: hepatosplenomegaly, enclosed hemorrhage
- Laboratory: infant's blood group, direct Coombs' test (negative test does

---

BOX 16-4 Nonphysiologic Jaundice (Jaundice Requiring Investigation or Treatment)

Clinically apparent jaundice in first 24 hr of life
Increase in total serum bilirubin concentration of >85 mmol/L per day
Direct serum bilirubin concentration higher than 34 mmol/L
Visible jaundice lasting >1 wk in term infants or 2 wk in premature infants

---

Modified from Foetus and Newborn Committee, Canadian Paediatric Society: Use of phototherapy for neonatal hyperbilirubinemia, *Can Med Assoc J* 134:1237, 1986.

not rule out hemolytic anemia), total bilirubin or microbilirubin, CBC, hematocrit ± reticulocyte count, blood smear
- Septic workup as indicated

Prolonged Jaundice (>1 Wk of Age)

- Above features and investigations plus thyroid-function tests, galactosemia screen (including urine for nonglucose-reducing substances), total and direct bilirubin, liver-function tests

PHOTOTHERAPY (Table 16-11)

- Should be first line of therapy, depending on rate of rise and independent of etiology
- More effective when combined with oral feeds
- More effective in controlling bilirubin in high-risk situations if initiated at low levels than in abruptly reducing established high levels
- Blue light most effective, but affects ongoing assessment of infant by altering observer perception
- "Double" phototherapy indicated when bilirubin levels approach within 35 mmol/L of exchange level (but may be initiated earlier)

Table 16-11 Management of Hyperbilirubinemia in Healthy Neonates

Age (hrs)	Consider phototherapy/repeat bilirubin (μmol/L)	Phototherapy (μmol/L)	Exchange transfusion if phototherapy fails (μmol/L)*	Exchange transfusion (μmol/L)
Birth weight > 2.5 kg†				
≤24	≥171	≥257	≥342	≥342
25-48	≥222	≥308	≥428	≥513
49-72	≥257	≥342	≥428	≥513
>72	≥291	≥376	≥428	≥513
Birth weight 1.5-2.5 kg†				
<36	130	150-240		290
36-72	180	200-250		290
72-120	210	250-280		305
>120	235	270-300		320
Birth weight 1.0-1.5 kg†				
<36	105	125-200		240
36-72	150	170-220		240
72-120	175	210-230		250
>120	185	225-250		265
Birth weight < 1.0 kg†				
<36	90	110-170		200
36-72	125	145-180		200
72-120	150	180-200		215
>120	165	190-210		225

Based on the Provisional Committee on Quality Improvement, American Academy of Pediatrics.
*Failure of phototherapy is defined as failure of bilirubin level to stabilize or decline by at least 17 to 34 μmol/L within 4 to 6 hr in infants exposed to intensive phototherapy; guidelines based on healthy neonates; neonates with hyperbilirubinemia in first 24 hr of life may not have physiologic jaundice and should be investigated for another cause.
†Guidelines for premature neonates are those used at Hospital for Sick Children, Toronto, Canada.

16

- Insensible fluid loss may increase by up to 35%, necessitating increased fluid intake, especially in very low–birth weight (VLBW) infants
- Serum bilirubin levels should be followed every 6 hr or more often, depending on level and cause
- Delaying initiation of phototherapy until bilirubin levels are >200 mmol/L by 24 hr after birth may significantly reduce number of infants receiving phototherapy for ABO incompatibility without increasing need for exchange transfusions, assuming no other high-risk factors present (e.g., preterm)
- Exclude treatable causes of jaundice (e.g., sepsis, metabolic); many initially respond to phototherapy, thus delaying primary treatment
- Phototherapy treatment can be used prophylactically in high-risk infants (e.g., markedly bruised premature infants) and as adjunct to, but not replacement for, exchange transfusion (controversial)
- Contraindicated in presence of conjugated hyperbilirubinemia ("bronzed" baby)
- Complications and adverse effects include hypernatremic dehydration, hyperthermia, masking of potentially serious underlying cause (e.g., sepsis), possible retinal damage if eyes uncovered, transient rashes, loose stools
- Watch for "delayed" anemia in hemolytic disease of newborn; often overlooked during initial management of hyperbilirubinemia

EXCHANGE TRANSFUSION (Table 16-12)

- Indications in hemolytic disease of newborn:
  1. Cord hemoglobin < 120 g/L or cord bilirubin > 85 mmol/L
  2. Postnatal rate of rise of unconjugated bilirubin > 17 mmol/L/hr in Rh incompatibility
  3. Serum unconjugated bilirubin > 340 mmol/L in first 48-72 hr of life (controversial)

Table 16-12   Exchange Transfusion Guidelines

	Serum Bilirubin Concentration (μmol/L)					
	Birth Weight Groups (g)					
	<1000	1000-1249	1250-1499	1500-1999	2000-2500	>2500
A*	171	222	256	291	308	342
B†	171	171	222	256	291	308

*A, Healthy.

†B, At risk of any of following factors:

Apgar < 7	Hypoalbuminemia
Hypoxia + acidosis	Hypoglycemia
Hypothermia	Sepsis
Clinical deterioration of any cause	

Levels for these various interventions should be individualized, if additional risk factors are present (see rationales and correction factors in text). Authorities differ on question of whether these criteria should refer to "indirect" bilirubin or total bilirubin. "Indirect" bilirubin should be used in patients with high "direct" bilirubin concentrations (i.e., >17 mmol/L [>1 mg/dl]).

4. Rapid progression of anemia despite satisfactory control of jaundice
5. Hydrops fetalis may require immediate exchange transfusion with packed cells to correct anemia
- Postexchange (30-60 min); anticipate "rebound" rise in bilirubin because of redistribution (of bilirubin)
- Much controversy exists about safe or critical levels of unconjugated bilirubin; threshold for intervention in "sick," low–birth weight (LBW) or VLBW infant should be low
- Complications:
  1. Embolization of air bubbles or small thrombi
  2. Hypocalcemia, hypoglycemia, acidosis, hyperkalemia
  3. Hypothermia, hyperthermia
  4. Sepsis
  5. Volume overload, cardiac arrhythmias

NUTRITION (Table 16-13)

TPN

- See p. 364; principles for starting and maintaining TPN are similar to those in older children; for lower glucose needs or intolerance, 5% or 7.5% glucose solutions (P 7.5) are available; monitoring and complications are similar to those in older children

RETINOPATHY OF PREMATURITY (ROP)

STAGING OF ROP*

- Stage I: demarcation line; a thin line separates anterior avascular retina from posterior vascularized retina
- Stage II: ridge; line of stage I has developed height, width, and volume, extending out of plane of retina; small isolated tufts of neovascularization may be seen posterior to ridge
- Stage III: ridge with fibrovascular proliferation; to ridge of stage II is added extraretinal fibrovascular proliferation
- Stage IV: partial retinal detachment; partial retinal detachments are typically exudative or traction
- Stage V: total retinal detachment; usually funnel-shaped detachment
- "Plus" disease describes abnormal tortuosity and dilation of retinal vessels of posterior pole; represents very active phase of acute disease; it signifies poor prognosis
- Cicatricial disease represents changes in peripheral and posterior retina associated with regression of more severe forms of ROP

WHOM TO SCREEN FOR ROP

- All infants born weighing <1300 g or <30-wk gestation, irrespective of oxygen use
- Infants of <1800 g birth weight or <35-wk gestation, if they received supplemental oxygen

*Based on Committee for International Classification of Retinopathy of Prematurity.

Table 16-13 Approximate Daily Nutritional Requirements of Term and Preterm Infants

	Term	Preterm*
Energy (kcal/kg)	100	110-165
Protein (g/kg)	2.2	2.9-4.0
Carbohydrate (g/kg)	10	8-16
Fat (g/kg)	3.3	4.0-9.0
Na (mmol/kg)	2-3	3-5
Cl (mmol/kg)	1-2	2.1-3.3
K (mmol/kg)	1-2	2.0-5.0
Ca (mmol/kg)	1.0-1.1	2.2-4.5
P (mmol/kg)	0.7	2.1-3.8
Vitamin A (μg/kg)	200-400	120-195
Vitamin D (IU/day)	400	400-1000
Vitamin E (mg/100 kcal)	2.0-2.5	0.6
Vitamin K	0.5-1.0 mg at birth	

From Perlman M, Kirpalani H: *Residents handbook of neonatology,* St Louis, 1992, Mosby.
*Requirements should be computed according to BW until BW is regained, after which actual weight is used; "requirements" are based on *enteral* nutrition.

WHEN TO SCREEN FOR ROP

- Initial examination should take place 5 to 7 wk after birth, but not before 32 wk after conceptual age
- Infants <35 wk receiving supplemental oxygen should be screened before discharge from hospital

INDICATIONS FOR ULTRASOUND INVESTIGATION OF HEAD (Box 16-5)

- In babies with high index of suspicion of intracranial pathology, neurologic symptoms, or acute unexplained blood loss
- In babies at risk for IVH
  1. All infants of BW < 1.25 kg, in first week, then repeat at 4 wk of age
  2. Infants of BW > 1.25 kg at high risk, in first wk, then repeat at 4 wk of age
- Suspected hydrocephalus
- Following episodes of severe hypoxia or shock at later ages, within 3-5 days, then repeat 4 wk later
- US screening used mainly to diagnose grades 3 and 4 IVH and PVL for prognostic purposes and to diagnose posthemorrhagic hydrocephalus in those at risk
- Monitoring by serial cranial US should be done weekly to exclude posthemorrhagic hydrocephalus in all cases of SEH-IVH until ventricular size stabilizes

BOX 16-5 Staging of IVH

Grade 1	Subependymal hemorrhage (SEH) only
Grade 2	Intraventricular hemorrhage (IVH): small (filling $< \frac{1}{2}$ of lateral ventricle $\pm$ slight dilation) $\pm$ SEH
Grade 3	IVH: large (filling $> \frac{1}{2}$ of lateral ventricle with ventricular dilation)
Grade 4	IVH + intraparenchymal hemorrhage

INFECTION (Fig. 16-6)

- High-risk infants include <37-wk gestational age, prolonged membrane rupture (>24 hr), maternal fever, instrumental vaginal delivery, indwelling catheters, maternal UTI, use of broad-spectrum antibiotics
- Wide spectrum of clinical presentation; must consider in any infant with following:
  1. Respiratory distress
  2. Apnea
  3. Increasing O_2 and ventilation requirements
  4. Feed intolerance
  5. Abdominal distension or ileus
  6. Temperature instability
  7. Seizures, lethargy
  8. Metabolic: hyperglycemia, hypoglycemia, acidosis, hyperbilirubinemia
  9. Obvious focus: skin, bones, joints, omphalitis
- Recommendations for babies born to HBsAg-positive mothers (see p. 218)

INVESTIGATIONS

- "Surface" and ETT cultures may be of little value
- Blood cultures
- Urinalysis, microscopy, urine culture: suprapubic aspiration is preferred method, see p. 500; catheter sample acceptable
- CSF Gram stain, protein, glucose; culture (LP not performed if cardiorespiratory instability)
- CXR (nonspecific for infection)
- Urine, CSF for antigen detection (latex agglutination); may be useful in infant in whom antibiotics already initiated

ANTIBIOTIC THERAPY

- Common organisms include group B *streptococci,* coliforms, *Listeria,* and coagulase-negative *staphylococci* (in infants >7 days who have had intravenous catheters)
- Consider *S. aureus* in skin, bone, and joint disease; *Shigella* or *Salmonella* in gastroenteritis
- Superinfection with *Candida* must be considered in all infants with pro-

Flow Chart for Infants Born with Antenatal Risk Factors for GBS Indicating Chemoprophylaxis
For use only for Babies *Without Clinical Signs of Sepsis*

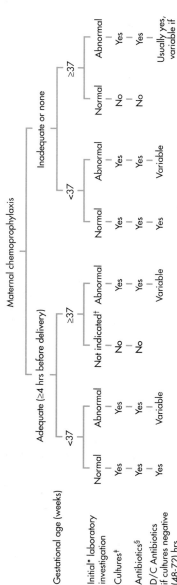

Based on CPS Statement, *Can J Paediat* 1(8):247-252, 1994.

Note: All babies born with clinical signs of sepsis should be investigated, and treated with antibiotics, regardless of maternal GBS colonization or chemoprophylaxis.

*Laboratory investigation (not routinely required such as complete blood count with differential, erythrocyte sedimentation rate, or C-reactive protein) may assist clinical decisions regarding risk of GBS sepsis.

†Investigation, culture, and treatment of the neonate not necessarily indicated for all high-risk GBS situations; may be indicated in the presence of maternal chorioamnionitis, regardless of maternal chemoprophylaxis.

‡When obtained, should include a blood culture. Other cultures, including CSF, are at the discretion of the attending physician.

§Antibiotics should always include ampicillin. With positive cultures, the baby should receive a full course of therapy. With negative cultures, a variable length of therapy may occur based on the physician's assessment of the likelihood of infection, which may include laboratory abnormalities and potential influence of prior treatment of the mother.

Fig. 16-6 Flowchart for asymptomatic infants born with antenatal risk factors for GBS, indicating chemoprophylaxis.

longed or recurrent illness, indwelling shunt or intravenous catheter, or congenital heart disease (bacterial endocarditis)
- *Ureaplasma urealyticum* increasingly implicated in respiratory infection
- Initial coverage depends on clinical presentation:
    1. Ampicillin + aminoglycoside

        or

    2. Ampicillin + cefotaxime

        ±

    3. Cloxacillin if *Staphylococcus* is consideration
- Vancomycin used in prolonged or recurrent illness, especially if indwelling shunt or catheter
- *Pseudomonas* requires coverage with ceftazidime or ticarcillin
- NEC (see p. 479)
- For *Candida* sepsis, treat with amphotericin B

DRUG WITHDRAWAL

- Opiates, cocaine, alcohol most common; usually incomplete history; must have high index of suspicion for multiple drug use
- CNS: high-pitched cry, sleeplessness, hyperactive Moro's reflex, tremors, increased muscle tone, myoclonus, seizures, areas of skin excoriation secondary to excess activity
- GI: excessive sucking, poor feeding, regurgitation and vomiting, loose and watery stools, prolonged postnatal weight loss
- Autonomic: fever, tachypnea, apnea, nasal stuffiness, mottling, fever, sneezing, yawning
- Time of onset: usually within 72 hr after birth; may appear up to age 2 wk; will vary depending on drug, timing of use before delivery, labor, presence of other illness
- Duration ranges from 6 days-8 wk; may last up to several mo
- Neonatal abstinence scoring sheets used to monitor symptoms and response to pharmacotherapy; scores are dynamic (every 2-4 hr), based on CNS, GI, vasomotor, respiratory, and metabolic disturbances

TREATMENT

- Phenobarbital (loading dose followed by titrated maintenance dose based on abstinence scores and/or clinical picture); usually 20 mg/kg load followed by 6-12 mg/kg/day
- Paregoric 0.8-2 ml/kg/day, titrated as above; morphine as alternative
- Treatment generally 3-5 days, then gradually taper
- Must follow for long-term effects of prenatal and perinatal drug exposure, general increase in caloric requirements, risk of HIV infection, neurodevelopmental delay, child abuse

USEFUL HINTS

- Morphine infusion: ½ infant's weight (kg) in mg added to 50 ml D5W

$$1 \text{ cc/hr} = 10 \text{ μg/kg/hr}$$

16

- Dopamine infusion: 15 × infant's weight (kg) in mg added to 50 ml D5W

$$1 \text{ cc/hr} = 5 \text{ } \mu\text{g/kg/min}$$

- Dobutamine infusion: same as for dopamine
- Prostaglandin E_1 infusion: 500 μg added to 80 ml D5W; run infusion at infant's weight (kg) per hour (i.e. 0.1 μg/kg/min)
- D12.5W: mix 94 ml D10W + 6 ml D50W
- D15W: mix 90 ml D10W + 13 ml D50W
- Bicarbonate infusion: to alkalinize infant infuse, 0.5-1 mEq/kg/hr; measure blood gas frequently and monitor closely
- 10% calcium gluconate = 0.2 mmol/ml
- 3% sodium chloride = 0.5 mmol/ml

D5W = 5% dextrose water; D10W = 10% dextrose water;
D12.5W = 12.5% dextrose water; D15W = 15% dextrose water;
D50W = 50% dextrose water

CHAPTER 17

NEPHROLOGY

ASHER SCHACHTER

CLINICAL EVALUATION OF RENAL FUNCTION

HISTORY

- Thorough, with focus on:
  1. Manifestations of genito-renal dysfunction:
     - Hematuria, dysuria, polydipsia, polyuria, nocturia, urinary stream
     - Anorexia, fatigue, headache, seizures
     - Dyspnea, chest pain, abdominal pain, nausea/vomiting
     - Bone pain/deformities, numbness/paresthesiae, edema
  2. Associated symptoms:
     - Fevers, recent infections, deafness, bloody diarrhea
     - Collagen-vascular diseases (mouth sores, eye symptoms, rashes, joint pain)
  3. Medications/toxins: aminoglycosides, amphotericin, cisplatin, NSAIDs
     - Radiocontrast agents
  4. Perinatal: polyhydramnios, oligohydramnios, single umbilical artery, umbilical catheter
     - Perinatal asphyxia, congenital infection (e.g., syphilis)
  5. Family history (FHx): hypertension, renal failure, renal cystic disease, hematuria, deafness

PHYSICAL EXAM

- Thorough, with focus on:
  - Growth (especially height), pallor, hydration, dysmorphism (facial, auricular)
  - BP, pulses, fundi, cardiac exam, signs of pulmonary edema, jugular venous pressure
  - Abdo masses/renomegaly, bladder, costovertebral angle tenderness, bruits, genitalia
  - Rashes, edema, deep-tendon reflexes, bony deformities, arthritis

LABS

- Urinalysis; renal function as indicated by history and physical exam

USEFUL CALCULATIONS
Bladder volume

- (ml) = [age (yr) + 2] × 30

Glomerular Filtration Rate (GFR)

- Expressed as ml/min/1.73 m^2
- Normal values:

- Birth: (full-term) 20
- 1 wk 45
- 3-5 wk 60
- 6 wk-6 mo 75
- 6 mo-2 yr 75-120
- 2-15 yr males 98-155
  females 95-122
- Adults males 91-120
  females 77-113
- Schwartz formula: GFR based on plasma creatinine and length or height

$$GFR = K \times L \div serum\ Cr$$

where L = length in cm; Cr in $\mu mol/L$; K = 30 (prem), 40 (term), 48 (children <12 yr, female adult), 62 (male adult)
- Creatinine clearance: volume of plasma completely cleared of Cr/unit time (see p. 543)
  - Requires plasma Cr measurement and timed urine collection
  - Assess completeness of urine collection based on $\mu mol/kg/d$ Cr
  Normal: neonates: 70-90 $\mu mol/kg/day$
  1 mo-1 yr: 105-130
  girls/prepubertal boys: 135-175
  adult males: 170-220

$$Cl_{Cr}\ (ml/min/1.73\ m^2)$$

$$= \frac{U_{Cr}\ (\mu mol/L) \times volume\ urine\ (ml) \times 1.73}{P_{Cr}\ (\mu mol/L) \times 1440\ min/day\ (if\ 24\ hr\ urine) \times BSA\ (m^2)}$$

$$BSA = body\ surface\ area = \sqrt{\frac{Ht\ (cm) \times Wt\ (kg)}{3600}}$$

(see also p. 543)

Tubular Functions

- Fractional excretion of X: $FEx = \dfrac{(Ux/Px)}{(U_{Cr}/P_{Cr})} \times 100$ (equation can be used for Na, P, etc.)
- Tubular reabsorption of phosphate = $(100 - FE_P)$
  - Normal > 85% (TR_P < 85% seen in Fanconi syndrome)
- Protein (PTN) excretion:
  - Total PTN (g/hr) = total PTN in urine (g/L) $\times$ urine vol (L) $\div$ 24 hr
  - Total PTN $(mg/m^2/hr) = \dfrac{total\ PTN\ (g/hr) \times 1000\ (mg/g)}{body\ surface\ area\ (m^2)}$
  > 4 $mg/m^2/hr$ = significant proteinuria; >40 $mg/m^2/hr$ = nephrotic range
  - Spot urine PTN:Cr ratio = (g/L protein divided by $\mu mol/L$ Cr) $\times$ 8800
  normal is < 0.2, nephrotic > 3.5
  (e.g., ratio of 0.2 reflects protein excretion of 0.2 g/24 hr/1.73 m^2)
- Calcium excretion: normal < 0.1 mmol/kg/day
  - Spot urine Ca:Cr ($\mu mol : \mu mol$); normal < 0.56-0.7

- Transtubular Potassium Gradient (TTKG)
  - Used to assess integrity of renal K excretory mechanisms

    $\dfrac{(U/P)_K}{(U/P)_{osm}}$ when (U/P) osm > 1 and urine Na > 25 mmol/L

  - < 4 = low aldosterone; > 6 = aldosterone present

RENAL IMAGING

- US: renal size/position, architecture, cortical-medullary differentiation, lower tract
- VCUG: bladder contour, VUR (see p. 487), urethral anatomy
- DMSA: binds to cortical tubular cells → parenchyma: scars, infarcts, masses
- DTPA: filtered and not reasorbed → renal perfusion/extraction/excretion, differential GFR
- MAG3: cleared by tubular secretion → useful in neonates (immature GFR)

RENAL BIOPSY
Indications

- Diagnosis of renal disease of unclear etiology
- To provide information that may help guide choice of therapy of renal disease, including suspected renal allograft rejection

Prebiopsy

- Check/treat coagulopathy, thrombocytopenia, hypertension, UTI/pyelonephritis
- Ensure two kidneys are present (except in transplant recipient)

Postbiopsy

- Pressure over site, bedrest, encourage fluids (IV/PO)
- Monitor BP, urine output, gross hematuria, abdominal pain
- Microhematuria occurs in 100% postbiopsy
- CBC 4-6 hr after biopsy and following morning

Complications

- Perirenal hematoma, renal AV fistula
- Infection
- Trauma to nearby structures: GI, liver, lumbar arteries; pancreatic pseudocyst

---

HYPERTENSION (HTN)

- For management of hypertensive emergencies, see p. 23

DEFINITION

- BP > 95th percentile for age on at least three separate measurements with appropriately sized cuff (Tables 17-1 and 17-2)
- Age < 10 yr: likely secondary etiology

Text continued on p. 320.

Table 17-1 Blood Pressure Levels for 90th and 95th Percentile of Blood Pressure for Girls 1 to 17 Yrs of Age by Percentiles of Height

Age (yr)	% ile	Systolic BP (mm Hg) by percentile of height							Diastolic BP (DBP5) (mm Hg) by percentile of height						
		5%	10%	25%	50%	75%	90%	95%	5%	10%	25%	50%	75%	90%	95%
1	90th	98	98	99	101	102	103	104	52	52	53	53	54	55	55
	95th	101	102	103	104	106	107	108	56	56	57	58	58	59	60
2	90th	99	99	101	102	103	104	105	57	57	58	58	59	60	60
	95th	103	103	104	106	107	108	109	61	61	62	62	63	64	64
3	90th	100	101	102	103	104	105	106	61	61	61	62	63	64	64
	95th	104	104	106	107	108	109	110	65	65	66	66	67	68	68
4	90th	101	102	103	104	106	107	108	64	64	65	65	66	67	67
	95th	105	106	107	108	109	111	111	68	68	69	69	70	71	71
5	90th	103	103	105	106	107	108	109	66	67	67	68	69	69	70
	95th	107	107	108	110	111	112	113	71	71	71	72	73	74	74
6	90th	104	105	106	107	109	110	111	69	69	69	70	71	72	72
	95th	108	109	110	111	113	114	114	73	73	74	74	75	76	76
7	90th	106	107	108	109	110	112	112	71	71	71	72	73	74	74
	95th	110	111	112	113	114	115	116	75	75	75	76	77	78	78
8	90th	108	109	110	111	112	114	114	72	72	73	74	74	75	76
	95th	112	113	114	115	116	117	118	76	77	77	78	79	79	80

Age	%ile														
9	90th	110	111	112	113	114	116	116	74	74	74	75	76	77	77
	95th	114	115	116	117	118	119	120	78	78	79	79	80	81	81
10	90th	112	113	114	115	116	118	118	75	75	76	77	77	78	78
	95th	116	117	118	119	120	122	122	79	79	80	81	81	82	82
11	90th	114	115	116	117	119	120	120	76	77	77	78	79	79	80
	95th	118	119	120	121	122	124	124	81	81	81	82	83	83	84
12	90th	116	117	118	119	121	122	123	78	78	78	79	80	81	81
	95th	120	121	122	123	125	126	126	82	82	82	83	84	85	85
13	90th	118	119	120	121	123	124	124	79	79	79	80	81	82	82
	95th	122	123	124	125	126	128	128	83	83	83	84	85	86	86
14	90th	120	121	122	123	124	126	126	80	80	80	81	82	83	83
	95th	124	125	126	127	128	130	130	84	84	85	85	86	87	87
15	90th	121	122	123	124	126	127	128	80	81	81	82	83	83	84
	95th	125	126	127	128	130	131	131	85	85	85	86	87	88	88
16	90th	122	123	124	125	127	128	129	81	81	81	82	83	84	84
	95th	126	127	128	129	130	132	132	85	85	86	87	87	88	88
17	90th	123	123	124	126	127	128	129	81	81	82	83	83	84	85
	95th	127	127	128	130	131	132	133	85	86	87	88	88	88	89

17

From Rosner B, Prineas RJ, Loggie JMH, Daniel SR: Blood pressure nomograms for children and adolescents by height, sex, and age in the United States, *J Pediatr* 123(6):874, 1993.

Table 17-2   Blood pressure levels for 90th and 95th percentiles of blood pressure for boys 1 to 17 years of age by percentiles of height

Age	% ile	Systolic BP (mm Hg) by percentile of height							Diastolic BP (DBP5) (mm Hg) by percentile of height						
		5%	10%	25%	50%	75%	90%	95%	5%	10%	25%	50%	75%	90%	95%
1	90th	94	95	97	99	101	102	103	49	49	50	51	52	53	54
	95th	98	99	101	103	105	106	107	54	54	55	56	57	58	58
2	90th	98	99	101	103	104	106	107	54	54	55	56	57	58	58
	95th	102	103	105	107	108	110	110	58	59	60	61	62	63	63
3	90th	101	102	103	105	107	109	109	59	59	60	61	62	63	63
	95th	105	106	107	109	111	112	113	63	63	64	65	66	67	68
4	90th	103	104	105	107	109	110	111	63	63	64	65	66	67	67
	95th	107	108	109	111	113	114	115	67	68	68	69	70	71	72
5	90th	104	105	107	109	111	112	113	66	67	68	69	69	70	71
	95th	108	109	111	113	114	116	117	71	71	72	73	74	75	76
6	90th	105	106	108	110	112	113	114	70	70	71	72	73	74	74
	95th	109	110	112	114	116	117	118	74	75	75	76	77	78	79
7	90th	106	107	109	111	113	114	115	72	73	73	74	75	76	77
	95th	110	111	113	115	117	118	119	77	77	78	79	80	81	81
8	90th	108	109	110	112	114	116	116	74	75	75	76	77	78	79
	95th	112	113	114	116	118	119	120	79	79	80	81	82	83	83

Age	Percentile	Systolic							Diastolic						
9	90th	109	110	112	114	116	117	118	76	76	77	78	79	80	80
	95th	113	114	116	118	119	121	122	80	81	81	82	83	84	85
10	90th	111	112	113	115	117	119	119	77	77	78	79	80	81	81
	95th	115	116	117	119	121	123	123	81	82	83	83	84	85	86
11	90th	113	114	115	117	119	121	121	77	78	79	80	81	81	82
	95th	117	118	119	121	123	125	125	82	82	83	84	85	86	87
12	90th	115	116	118	120	121	123	124	78	78	79	80	81	82	83
	95th	119	120	122	124	125	127	128	83	83	84	85	86	87	87
13	90th	118	119	120	122	124	125	126	78	79	80	81	81	82	83
	95th	121	122	124	126	128	129	130	83	83	84	85	86	87	88
14	90th	120	121	123	125	127	128	129	79	79	80	81	82	83	83
	95th	124	125	127	129	131	132	133	83	84	85	86	87	87	88
15	90th	123	124	126	128	130	131	132	80	80	81	82	83	84	84
	95th	127	128	130	132	133	135	136	84	85	86	86	87	88	89
16	90th	126	127	129	131	132	134	134	81	82	82	83	84	85	86
	95th	130	131	133	134	136	138	138	86	86	87	88	89	90	90
17	90th	128	129	131	133	135	136	137	83	84	85	86	87	87	88
	95th	132	133	135	137	139	140	141	88	88	89	90	91	92	93

17

From Rosner B, Prineas RJ, Loggie JMH, Daniel SR: Blood pressure nomograms for children and adolescents by height, sex, and age in the United States, *J Pediatr* 123(6):874, 1993.

- Age > 10 yr with strong family history of HTN: likely primary/essential HTN

ETIOLOGY

- Primary/essential: suspected when FHx positive for HTN and absence of secondary causes
- Secondary
  - Renal: chronic glomerulonephritis, chronic pyelonephritis, obstructive uropathy
  - Cystic renal disease, hemolytic uremic syndrome
  - Renal vascular: renal artery stenosis, fibromuscular dysplasia, vasculitis
  - CVS: coarctation of aorta
  - Neuro/endocrine: CNS mass, pheochromocytoma, neuroblastoma, Conn's syndrome
  - Medications: corticosteroids, oral contraceptives, nasal decongestants, cocaine

SYMPTOMS/SIGNS

- Headache, epistaxis, Bell's palsy, encephalopathy, seizures, cortical blindness
- Congestive heart failure, failure to thrive, abdominal pain
- Manifestations of underlying disease (if present)

INVESTIGATIONS

- Nature/extent is dictated by history, physical exam; confirmation of HTN
- Complete urinalysis, urine culture
- Baseline renal function, electrolytes, blood gases
- Renal US; end-organs: echocardiogram for LV mass, fundoscopy
- Consider: angiogram, renal vein renin sampling; endocrine studies, including VMA, catecholamines, 17-OH progesterone

MANAGEMENT

- Treat underlying cause, if present
- Nonpharmacologic: no-added-salt diet, aerobic exercise, no smoking
- Pharmacologic: (Box 17-1)
  1. Use medication aimed at underlying mechanism for HTN (e.g., diuretics for fluid overload, ACE inhibitor for renin-mediated HTN)
  2. If not well controlled, maximize dosage or add other first-line drug

PROTEINURIA (Box 17-2)

DEFINITION

- >4 mg/m^2/hr; nephrotic > 40 mg/m^2/hr

INVESTIGATIONS

- History, physical exam, urinalysis
- Split 24-hr urine protein and Cr (rule out [R/O] orthostatic proteinuria; recumbent/overnight urine sample is collected separately from daytime/upright sample)

BOX 17-1 Antihypertensive Agents

Calcium channel blockers: act on vascular smooth muscles
  Nifedipine: no effect on cardiac conduction; short (SA)/prolonged (PA)/long-acting (XL)
  Verapamil: depresses cardiac pacemaker, inhibits cyclosporin metabolism
  Amlodipine: once-daily dosage, tasteless, odorless, dissolvable
ACE-Inhibitors: captopril, enalapril; block angiotensin I → angiotensin II
  Side effects: rash, cough, angioedema, proteinuria, marrow depression, hyperkalemia
  ↓ GFR and ARF in sick neonates with HTN
  Contraindications: solitary kidney with renal artery stenosis (RAS), bilateral RAS
β-Blockers ↓ HR, ↓ cardiac output, ↓ renin release; may cause nightmares, impotence,
  hyperlipidemia, decreased school performance
  Selective β$_1$-Blockers
    Metoprolol: fatigue, dizziness, headache ± bronchospasm
    Atenolol
  Nonselective β-Blockers
    Propranolol: contraindications include asthma, diabetes, CHF, Raynaud's
    Nadolol: once-daily dosage; same contraindications as propranolol
α$_1$-blockers: Prazosin: blocks vasoconstriction; effective in renal failure
Combined α and β blocker: Labetalol (↓ peripheral resistance, ↓ HR); postural hypotension
Diuretics
  Thiazide: effective for primary HTN; not effective when GFR < 50% of normal; side
    effects: hypokalemia, hypercalcemia, hyperuricemia, hyperlipidemia
  Furosemide: useful in renal failure; side effects include hypokalemia, hyponatremia,
    ototoxic (high-dose IV)
  K-sparing: spironolactone (with thiazide = Aldactazide), triamterene, amiloride
Centrally acting alpha stimulators
  Stimulate the brainstem α2-receptors → peripheral adrenergic drive; sudden with-
    drawal → rebound HTN
  Clonidine: agitation, insomnia, diaphoresis
  α-Methyldopa: side effects include sedation, nasal congestion, GI
Vasodilators: hydralazine, nitroprusside, minoxidil
  Direct action on vascular smooth muscle; reflex ↑ HR, Na and water retention →
    therefore combine with diuretics, β-blockers

17

- If active urine sediment, edema, HTN, or systemic disorder is present,
  then do renal function, blood gas, electrolytes, C$_3$, total protein, albumin, cholesterol, and CBC and consider ANA, ASOT, HBV and HCV
  serology, HIV, VDRL, abdominal US, renal biopsy

NEPHROTIC SYNDROME (NS)

DEFINITION

- Proteinuria > 40 mg/m^2/hr, hypoalbuminemia, edema, hypercholester-
  olemia
- See Box 17-3

Other Possible Manifestations

- U/A: oval fat bodies, maltese crosses as observed under polarized light
- Ascites, pleural effusion

Differential Diagnosis of Proteinuria

I. Orthostatic
II. Transient: Fever, exercise, cold exposure, stress, epinephrine infusion
III. Glomerular
  Congenital: Congenital nephrosis (Finnish), diffuse mesangial sclerosis, CMV, syphilis
  Acquired:
  • Primary: minimal change, FSGS, membranous, MPGN
  • Secondary:
    • Infection: PSGN/PIGN, shunt GN, SBE, HBV, HCV, HIV, malaria, syphilis
    • Multisystem: SLE, HUS, HSP, sickle cell, PAN, Wegener, Goodpasture, Wilson
    • Drugs: penicillamine, NSAIDs, captopril, gold, mercury, lithium, heroin
    • Neoplasia: leukemia, lymphoma, carcinoma
    • Renal/vascular: renal vein thrombosis, renal artery stenosis, HTN
IV. Tubular (light-chain Ig, β2-microglobulin, lysozyme, albumin)
  Congenital/genetic
  • Syndromes: Fanconi, Lowe's, Laurence-Moon-Biedl
  • Cystic/dysplastic renal disease
  • Metabolic: RTA, cystinosis, oxalosis
  Acquired: Interstitial nephritis, pyelonephritis, ATN, transplant rejection, hypokalemic nephropathy, reflux nephropathy, drugs (aminoglycosides, analgesics, cyclosporine, *cis*-platinum)
V. Overload
  Hemoglobin (intravascular hemolysis), myoglobin (rhabdomyolysis) lysozyme (monocytic and myelocytic leukemias), light chains (plasma cell dyscrasias)

Differential Diagnosis of Nephrotic Syndrome (NS)

Primary NS
Minimal change (MCNS): 75% of cases of NS
Chronic GN: FSGS, membranous, MPGN, mesangial proliferative GN/Berger (IgA)
Congenital NS (Finnish type), diffuse mesangial sclerosis
Secondary NS
Vasculitis: SLE, HSP
Infection: HBV, HIV, VZV, malaria, congenital/secondary syphilis, FMF, bacterial endocarditis, ventriculoatrial shunt
Metabolic: diabetes mellitus
Medications: gold, penicillamine, NSAIDs, captopril, heroin, mercury
Hereditary: Alport's, sickle cell
Neoplasia: lymphomas

• Hypercoagulability $\rightarrow$ renal vein thrombosis (loss of antithrombin III, protein S, protein C, plasminogen)
• Infections (loss of factor B $\rightarrow$ $\downarrow$ opsonization $\rightarrow$ *E. coli, Pneumococcus*): cellulitis, peritonitis, bacteremia

MANAGEMENT
Nonpharmacologic

• No-added-salt diet; fluid restriction usually not necessary
• Avoid albumin infusions (risk of rebound pulmonary edema, HTN)

- Thiazide diuretic (if uncomfortable from edema)
- Avoid aggressive diuresis (risk of hypercoagulability)

Pharmacologic

1. Prednisone (generally 2 mg/kg/day × 4-8 wk)
   - 95% of minimal change nephrotic syndrome (MCNS) responds to prednisone within 8 wk
   - Remission: no PTN on urine dipstick for 4-7 consecutive days
   - Relapse: dipstick PTN 2+ or more for at least 3-5 consecutive days
   - Frequent relapse: 2 relapses in 6 mo or 4 relapses in any 12-mo period; 25% is MCNS; 75% is FSGS or mesangial proliferative
   - Steroid-dependent: relapse while on steroids or within 2 wk of stopping steroids
   - Treat relapses with prednisone
   - Third relapse: induce remission with prednisone then use cytotoxic therapy × 8 wks
2. Cyclophosphamide: maximum cumulative dose 165 mg/kg, gonadal toxicity, carcinogenesis, hemorrhagic cystitis
3. Chlorambucil: total cumulative dose 8.4-11 mg/kg; leukopenia, azoospermia
4. Other medications
   - Levamisole: anthelminthic, effects on T cell
   - Cyclosporine: often induces remission, but relapse may occur after drug withdrawal

HEMATURIA (Box 17-4)

DEFINITION

- >3-5 RBC/HPF in spun urine

INVESTIGATIONS

- History, physical exam, urinalysis
- Urine RBC morphology; U/A on first-degree relatives (Alport's, familial hematuria)
- Significant associated proteinuria suggests glomerular disease
- Urine culture
- Consider
  - Renal function, electrolytes, Ca, P, total PTN, albumin, cholesterol
  - C_3, ANA, ASOT, ANCA
  - 24-hr urine for protein, Cr, and Ca
  - Throat culture, TB skin test
  - Abdominal US, VCUG, renal biopsy, cystoscopy, audiogram

NEPHRITIC SYNDROME

DEFINITION

- Gross hematuria, hypertension, edema, azotemia

BOX 17-4   Differential Diagnosis of Hematuria

Upper Tract
Glomerular: (brown-, tea-, or cola-colored)
Benign, sporadic, familial, exercise, fever
Acute GN: PSGN, HSP, HUS, SLE, MPGN, RPGN
Alport's, IgA, Goodpasture's, SLE
Tubulointerstitial
Cystic disease: PCKD, medullary cystic disease
Nephrocalcinosis/hypercalciuria, RTA, cystinosis, oxalosis, nephrolithiasis
Transplant rejection
Medication toxicity: aminoglycoside, cyclosporine, cisplatin, analgesics
Medication hypersensitivity: penicillins, sulfa drugs, NSAIDs, diuretics
Toxins: radiocontrast, heavy metals, radiation
Infection (bacterial, viral, TB), reflux nephropathy, obstructive uropathy
Tumors: Wilms, leukemia, lymphoma
Vascular
Renal vein thrombosis, renal artery thrombosis
AVM (arteriovenous malformation)
Lower Tract (red/pink colored)
UTI, cystitis/cyclophosphamide, urethritis, prostatitis
Calculi, trauma, foreign body
Obstructive hydronephrosis
Bleeding Diathesis
Hemophilia, thrombocytopenia, anticoagulants

ETIOLOGY (GLOMERULONEPHRITIS)
Congenital/Inherited

- Alport's

Acquired

- Primary: IgA (Berger's) nephropathy, rapidly progressive glomerulonephritis (RPGN)
- Secondary:
  - Infection: poststreptococcal [PSGN/postinfectious GN (APIGN)] endocarditis, shunt nephritis, HBV, HIV
  - Multisystem disease: HSP, SLE, HUS, other vasculitides, sickle cell
  - Drugs: NSAIDs, penicillamine, captopril, gold salts
  - Neoplasia: carcinoma, leukemia, lymphoma

CLASSIFICATION BASED ON C_3 LEVEL

	Only renal ds	Systemic ds
↓ C_3	APIGN, PSGN	SLE, SBE
	MPGN type 1	shunt nephritis

- All others have normal C_3

ALPORT'S SYNDROME

- X-linked dominant inheritance; also AR, AD inheritance; more severe in males
- FHx of deafness, renal failure

- Persistent microhematuria; proteinuria; HTN, renal failure
- Bilateral sensorineural hearing deficit; anterior lenticonus
- May have platelet dysfunction
- Pathology: split/laminated glomerular basement membrane (GBM) on electron microscopy (EM); lack of Goodpasture's antigen on immunofluorescence
- Rx: supportive, dialysis/transplantation

IgA NEPHROPATHY
Primary (Berger's nephropathy)

- More common in males
- Macrohematuria within 72 hr of onset of URI, exercise
- Mild/moderate proteinuria (variable)
- Pathology: mesangial matrix/cellular proliferation; IgA on immunofluorescence
- Hematuria usually lasts up to 1 wk; no specific treatment

Secondary Causes

- Infection: CMV, HBV, mycosis fungoides, dermatitis herpetiformis
- Collagen-vascular diseases: JRA, ankylosing spondylitis
- Vasculitis: HSP, SLE
- GI/liver disease: cirrhosis, celiac disease

POSTSTREPTOCOCCAL GLOMERULONEPHRITIS (PSGN)

- Immune reaction induced by nephritogenic strains of *streptococci*
- Nephritis onset 1-2 wk poststrep pharyngitis or otitis media; 3 wk postimpetigo
- May develop hypertensive encephalopathy, oliguria as part of nephritic syndrome
- Low C_3; positive ASOT, antihyaluronidase, antistreptozyme, anti-DNase B (see p. 553)
- May have positive throat culture
- Treatment (supportive): antihypertensives, diuretics, fluid restriction $\pm$ dialysis; penicillin or erythromycin if culture positive for strep

HENOCH-SCHÖNLEIN PURPURA

- Immune-mediated small-vessel vasculitis
- Ages 5-15 yr; late winter-early summer; majority have history of preceding URI
- Palpable purpura on lower limbs and buttocks (100% of cases), edema (scalp, scrotal)
- Arthralgia/arthritis: knees, ankles, feet (70%)
- GI (45%): abdo pain, vomiting, diarrhea, hematochezia, melena, ileus, intussusception
- Renal (20%-30%): 10%-40% of these cases have residual renal dysfunction
- ⅔ of cases with renal manifestations have hematuria or hematuria and proteinuria
- ⅓ of cases have acute nephritis, nephrosis, or nephritis/nephrosis
- Normal C_3, high serum IgA

17

Treatment

- Supportive, analgesics, monitor for complications
- Monitor mild renal cases for persistent hematuria/proteinuria, HTN, azotemia
- Severe renal disease: antihypertensives, fluid/electrolyte management, dialysis

Prognosis

- Nephritic or nephritic/nephrotic at presentation: 44% have persistent renal dysfunction
- Hematuria ± proteinuria at presentation: up to 18% can have persistent renal dysfunction
- Poor prognosis: HTN, ARF, crescentic GN

HEMOLYTIC UREMIC SYNDROME (HUS)

- Common cause of acute renal failure in children <5 yr of age; April-September
- Triad of microangiopathic hemolytic anemia, thrombocytopenia, uremia
- *E. coli* 0157:H7 verotoxin is most common cause of epidemic form
- Other associations: *Salmonella, Shigella, Yersinia, Campylobacter*
  Pneumococcal infection
  HIV, DPT/MMR vaccines
  Cyclosporine, renal transplantation, chemotherapy, Kawasaki
- Pathology: verotoxin binds to GB3 receptor → endothelial damage → microthrombi
- Clinical course: Bloody diarrhea → resolves → HUS
- May have CNS involvement → seizures; R/O bleed if thrombocytopenic
- May have GI/pancreatic involvement
- Normal C_3, negative Coombs' (direct and indirect)

Treatment

- ARF: antihypertensives, appropriate fluid and electrolyte therapy, dialysis
- Blood transfusions only if hemodynamically unstable; no platelet transfusions

Prognosis

- Guarded if anuria >2 wk, dialysis >1 wk; multiorgan involvement (CNS, GI/pancreas); older children/adolescents, nonendemic/familial forms

ACUTE RENAL FAILURE

DEFINITION

- Sudden reduction in renal function resulting in azotemia and disturbed metabolic, fluid, and electrolyte homeostasis

DIFFERENTIAL DIAGNOSIS

- Prerenal: shock, hypovolemia, dehydration, hemorrhage, burns, third-space losses
- Renal: ATN—ischemia (prolonged prerenal failure), nephrotoxins; HUS, glomerulonephritis, renal vascular diseases, interstitial nephritis; rhabdomyolysis, tumor lysis syndrome
- Postrenal: posterior urethral valves (PUV)/other structural lower-tract abnormalities; clots, tumors, stones

CLINICAL MANIFESTATIONS

- Intrinsic renal failure may be oliguric or nonoliguric
- Symptoms/signs of underlying cause and volume overload, HTN, metabolic dysfunction

DIAGNOSIS

- History, physical exam, urinalysis

Test	Prerenal azotemia	Intrinsic ARF	Postrenal
Urine SG	>1.02	<0.015	—
Urine osmolality	>500	<300	300-400
Urine/plasma osm	>1.3	<1.3	—
Urine/plasma Cr	>40	<20	<20
Urine Na (mEq/L)	<20	>40	>40
FE_{Na}	<1%	>2%	>3%

MANAGEMENT

- Treat underlying cause; volume challenge if prerenal
- Antihypertensives if needed
- Treat: hyperkalemia (see p. 24); hypocalcemia, hyperphosphatemia: Calcium carbonate 100-300 mg/kg/day
- Fluids: insensibles (400 ml/m^2/day) with D10W, no potassium and losses with solution appropriate to type of loss
- Dialysis: HTN, volume overload, hyperkalemia, intractable acidosis
- Monitor vitals/BP, weight, urine output, input/output, renal function, serum electrolytes
- Aggressive nutritional therapy: high-carbohydrate, low-protein diet

17

CHRONIC RENAL FAILURE

DEFINITION

- Irreversible chronic loss of renal function
- Mild renal failure: GFR 50%-80%
- Moderate renal failure: GFR 25%-50%
- Severe renal failure: GFR 10%-25%
- End-stage renal disease (ESRD): GFR < 10%

ETIOLOGY

- Congenital: renal hypoplasia/dysplasia, cystic renal diseases
- Anatomic: obstruction/reflux (i.e., VUR, PUV)

- Hereditary: Alport's syndrome (XL-D), juvenile nephronophthisis (AR), polycystic kidney disease
- Metabolic: cystinosis, oxalosis
- Vasculitis: HUS, SLE, PAN, HSP
- Primary glomerulonephritis

CLINICAL MANIFESTATIONS
Uremia

- Syndrome that is result of CRF
- Anorexia, fatigue, nausea/vomiting, hiccups, peptic ulcer, pancreatitis, seizures, coma, pericarditis
- Edema, hyponatremia, hyperkalemia, hypocalcemia

Failure to Thrive (FTT)

- Multifactorial
- Energy malnutrition, acidosis, anemia, HTN, renal osteodystrophy, delayed bone age

NEURO

- Hypertensive encephalopathy, seizures, peripheral neuropathy

CVS

- HTN, pericarditis, uremic cardiomyopathy

MSK

- Renal osteodystrophy (ROD): $\downarrow$ 1,25(OH)$_2$-D3 $\rightarrow$ rickets, hyperparathyroidism
- Rickets: osteomalacia, widened metaphyses, valgus/bowing, epiphyseal slipping
- Hyperparathyroidism: osteitis fibrosa cystica, subperiosteal resorption, osteosclerosis
- $\uparrow$ALP, $\uparrow$PTH, $\uparrow$P, $\downarrow$Ca; serum vitamin D rarely helpful

HAEM

- Normochromic normocytic anemia, prolonged bleeding time

Metabolic

- Acidosis, hyponatremia, hypernatremia, hyperkalemia; $\uparrow$ triglycerides, $\uparrow$ VLDL

Imaging

- Small kidneys on renal US

MANAGEMENT
Nutrition

- Low P, low K, no-added-salt diet (NAS)
- Protein: lower limit of recommended daily allowance (RDA); high biologic value (dairy, meat)
- PM 60/40 formula (whey:casein 60:40): low protein, low Na, low phosphate

- Oliguric/anuric: dialyze off extra fluid to allow for adequate caloric intake
- Vitamins: Diavite 1 tablet daily

Fluids

- Insensibles + urine output → maximum fixed daily intake if in steady state

Electrolytes

- Na 1—2 mEq/kg/day, low K diet (avoid citrus fruits, bananas, chocolate)
- See p. 24 for management of hyperkalemia

Prevention of Renal Osteodystrophy

1. GFR < 75%
   - Phosphate restriction (dairy, meats, soft drinks, snack foods)
   - Calcium supplements: 100-300 mg/kg/day
   - Calcium carbonate: when with meals → acts as phosphate binder
   - TUMS, calcium
2. GFR < 50%
   - Vitamin D: alfacalcidol, rocaltrol

Acidosis

- Dialysis, $NaHCO_3$, citrate

Anemia

- Fe supplements; recombinant erythropoietin (EPO) 100 U/kg 2-3 ×/wk

Hypertension

- Medical therapy (see p. 315), fluid restriction

Short Stature

- Recombinant growth hormone may be indicated

Dialysis

- See following discussion

DIALYSIS

HEMODIALYSIS (HD)

- Difficult vascular access in neonates/infants; requires anticoagulation
- Circuit volume must not exceed 10% of patient's blood volume (8 ml/kg)
- Not first choice if hemodynamically unstable or bleeding diathesis
- Main problems: clotting, hypotension, infections, dialysis disequilibrium

PERITONEAL DIALYSIS (PD)

- Can be done at home; various schedules possible to function around school, play
- Easier access than HD; no anticoagulation needed

- Requires well-motivated patient/family
- Not recommended if previous abdo surgery, ostomies, VP shunts, Wilms' tumor (seeding)
- Main problems: exit site/tunnel infection, peritonitis, catheter leak/obstruction
  1. Exit site infection: red, tender → treat early with PO cloxacillin or cefazolin; cleansing
  2. Tunnel infection: if tender along subcutaneous path, use IV antibiotics; may need to replace catheter at another site
  3. Peritonitis: fever, nausea, abdominal pain, cloudy dialysate, dialysate WBC > 100/mm^3; *S. epidermidis, S. aureus,* gram-negative organisms; 10% are culture negative
     - Intraperitoneal (IP) heparin 500 units/L dialysate until clear effluent
     - Intraperitoneal (IP) Cefazolin 500 mg/L load → 250 mg/L maintenance and tobramycin 1.7 mg/kg load → 4-6 mg/L maintenance
  4. Obstruction
     - Fibrin clots (inflow and outflow obstruction): urokinase 5000 U IP × 1-2 hr
     - Wrap of omentum (outflow obstruction): saline irrigation or replace catheter
  5. Leakage: catheter used too soon after insertion
     - Decrease dwell volume → gradually increase as tolerated

URINARY TRACT INFECTION (UTI)

DEFINITION

- More than two clean voided urine specimens with ≥10^5 colonies/ml of single organism or ≥10^3 colonies/ml in catheter specimen or any concentration in suprapubic specimen

BACTERIOLOGY

- *Escherichia coli* in 85% of females, *Proteus* species in males; also, *Streptococcus faecalis, Klebsiella, Pseudomonas, Staphylococcus epidermidis*

DIFFERENTIAL DIAGNOSIS

- Pyuria: bacterial UTI, fever, dehydration, mycoplasma, appendicitis

INVESTIGATIONS

- Diagnostic tests (e.g., WBC dipstick, nitrite dipsticks)
- Urine for microscopy (cell count, bacteria, casts)
- Urine culture and sensitivity
- In systemic illness, CBC, blood culture, renal-function tests

MANAGEMENT

- Encourage fluids → promotes urine flow
- Antibiotics: trimethoprim-sulphamethoxazole (TMP-SMX), amoxicillin or pivampicillin, or nitrofurantoin orally for uncomplicated cases × 7-10

days; ampicillin plus aminoglycoside parenterally initially for systemic illness, then change to PO once afebrile

FOLLOW-UP
Cultures

- Repeat cultures at 48 hr (should be sterile), then 3 days after cessation of therapy
- Monthly cultures × 3 (if anatomy normal), then only if symptomatic or febrile

Radiologic Evaluation

- US: first UTI under 6 yr of age
- VCUG in all boys and in girls <6 yr with first UTI; done 1-2 wk after UTI treated (see p. 487)
- DMSA: if VCUG is abnormal, history of pyelonephritis (assess renal shape, scarring)

Chemoprophylaxis

- TMP-SMX, amoxicillin, pivampicillin indicated for all grades of reflux and/or >3 UTIs/yr
- For children <2 mo, TMP-SMX is relatively contraindicated because of sulfa component and potential for hyperbilirubinemia; may use trimethoprim alone, 2 mg/kg/day (single or divided doses) or amoxicillin/pivampicillin; for children >2 mo: TMP-SMX and nitrofurantoin are best choices
- Amoxicillin and pivampicillin are inadequate for prophylaxis; cephalexin may be used

Reflux

- See p. 487

RENAL TUBULAR ACIDOSIS (RTA)

- Suspect in child with FTT and/or normal anion gap metabolic acidosis (Fig. 17-1)
- Urine net charge: positive (Na + K > Cl) → ammonium not present in urine (cannot trap H^+); negative (Na + K < Cl) → ammonium present in urine
- Urine-blood PCO_2: indicator of terminal nephron's ability to trap protons; in RTA; U-B $PCO_2 \leq 10$-15 mm Hg, when urine pH ≥ 7.5

Type 1 RTA (Distal)

- Distal H^+ trapping defect
- Large DDx: tubulointerstitial disease, nephrocalcinosis, hereditary fructose intolerance (HFI); amphotericin B, lithium

Type 2 RTA (Proximal)

- Proximal HCO_3 reabsorption defect
- Large DDx: carbonic anhydrase inhibition; cystinosis, tyrosinemia, galactosemia, HFI, glycogen storage disease; Lowe's syndrome, Wilson's dis-

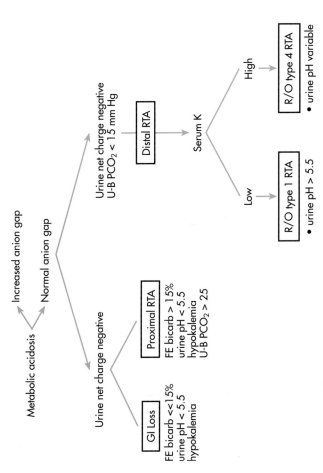

Fig. 17-1   Renal Tabular Acidosis

ease; early renal transplant rejection, medullary cystic disease, nephrotic syndrome; gentamicin, lead, mercury

Type 4 RTA (distal, hyperkalemic)

- Obstructive uropathy, Addison's disease, congenital adrenal hyperplasia, pseudohypoaldosteronism

TREATMENT OF RTA
Types 1 and 2

- Alkali therapy in form of K and Na salts (e.g.: $NaHCO_3$, dicitrate)
- K supplementation

Type 4

- Relieve obstruction, if present
- Treat hyperkalemia; aldosterone replacement, if deficient

UROLITHIASIS

CLINICAL FEATURES

- Colic (abdomen, flank, groin), dysuria, fever
- Gross or microscopic hematuria; urinary passage of stone, gravel, or sludge; anuria
- Family history of urolithiasis

DIFFERENTIAL DIAGNOSIS
Calcium

- Calcium is constituent of 90% of calculi
- Calcium phosphate (precipitates in alkaline urine)
- Calcium oxalate (precipitates in acid urine)
- Hypercalciuria
  - Hypercalcemic: hyperparathyroidism, hyperthyroidism, hypervitaminosis D
  - Normocalcemic: familial, sporadic, distal RTA, loop diuretics, acetazolamide
  - Hyperoxaluria: primary hyperoxaluria, inflammatory bowel disease, hyperglycinuria

Magnesium Ammonium Phosphate (struvite)

- Precipitates in alkaline urine
- UTI from urea-splitting organism *(Proteus)*
- Urinary tract foreign body and urinary stasis

Uric Acid

- Precipitates in acid urine
- Leukemia/lymphoma, gout, Lesch-Nyhan, type I glycogen storage disease

Cystine

- Precipitates in acid urine
- Cystinuria

17

DIAGNOSIS

- High index of suspicion
- Compositional analysis of passed stone or sediment from strained urine
- Plain radiograph: calcium and struvite stones are radiopaque; uric acid stones are radiolucent
- US: assess urinary-tract anatomy, obstruction, nephrocalcinosis
- Blood: gas, electrolytes, Cr, Ca, P, ALP, uric acid
- Urine: urinalysis, pH (anaerobic), culture, spot urine Ca:Cr, cyanide-nitroprusside (cystine); 24-hour urine: Cr, Ca, oxalate, uric acid

TREATMENT

- Minimum daily fluid intake of 2400 ml/m^2
- Thiazide diuretics: reduce urinary calcium excretion
- Alkali therapy for uric acid and cystine stones
- Specific therapy for underlying cause (e.g., allopurinol for gout)
- Treat UTI if present
- Surgical correction for anatomic abnormalities causing predisposition to stones or infections
- Extracorporeal shock-wave lithotripsy (ESWL) for large stones, refractory cases

CHAPTER 18

NEUROLOGY/NEUROSURGERY

Sʜᴀʀᴏɴ Mɪᴇʟᴋᴇ Dᴇʟʟ

DEFINITIONS

MUSCLE TONE

- Resistance of muscle to passive range of movement (velocity dependent)

HYPERTONIA
Spasticity

- Different extents of hypertonia in different muscle groups
- Clasp-knife phenomenon (greatest tone at initiation of passive movement)
- Caused by UMN lesion involving pyramidal tract

Rigidity

- Hypertonia independent of direction of movement
- Lead-pipe and cogwheel rigidity are descriptive terms
- Caused by extrapyramidal dysfunction (basal ganglia)

CEREBRAL PALSY

- Nonprogressive disorder of posture and movement
- Prenatal, perinatal, and postnatal causes; most cases idiopathic

CLINICAL CLASSIFICATION

- Spastic
  - Hemiplegia (one-sided spasticity, UL > LL)
  - Diplegia (spasticity mostly LL)
  - Quadriplegia (spasticity LL > UL)
  - Monoplegia and triplegia rare
- Dyskinetic
  - Athetosis
  - Other
- Ataxic
- Mixed

ASSOCIATIONS

- Seizures, developmental delay
- Visual, hearing, and speech problems
- Orthopedic problems: joint contractures, dislocated hips, scoliosis
- Gastroesophageal reflux and aspiration
- Drooling and dental problems
- Feeding problems
- Mesenteric artery syndrome

EARLY SIGNS

- Delayed milestones, abnormalities in muscle tone, and primitive reflexes (Box 18-1)
- Must rule out progressive disorder of CNS

MANAGEMENT

- Multidisciplinary approach: pediatrics, orthopedics, neurology, ophthalmology, dentistry, occupational and physical therapy, speech and audiology, dietician
- Referral to pediatric rehabilitation center
- Assistive devices: splints, walkers, wheelchairs, lifts
- Drugs for spasticity (questionable efficacy): dantrolene sodium, benzodiazepines, baclofen
- Surgery: soft tissue releases for lengthening of heel cords, hamstrings, posterior tibial tendons; rhizotomy

HYPOTONIA: FLOPPY BABY

- Differentiate *hypotonia* from muscle *weakness*

ETIOLOGY BY ANATOMIC LOCALIZATION
Central

- Neonatal asphyxia and/or intracranial hemorrhage (evolve to spasticity)
- Chromosomal disorders (trisomy 21, Prader-Willi)
- CNS malformations
- Dysmorphic syndromes
- Metabolic/endocrine causes
- Benign congenital hypotonia (diagnosis of exclusion)

BOX 18-1   Primitive and Protective Reflexes*

Primitive Reflexes (present at birth, disappear between 3 and 5 mo)
Local
   Head: rooting, righting response
   Upper limbs: palmar grasp
   Lower limbs: plantar grasp, placing, stepping
General
   Asymmetric tonic neck reflex (ATNR)
   Moro's response
Secondary Reflexes (appear between 4 and 10 mo and persist)
Rolling
Balancing
Protective: parachute, lateral propping

---

*Abnormalities include absent or asymmetric reflexes and persistent or obligatory primitive reflexes.

Anterior Horn Cell

- Spinal muscular atrophy

Peripheral Nerve

- Guillain-Barré syndrome (congenital or neonatal form), hereditary neuropathies, metabolic, toxins, trauma

Neuromuscular Junction

- Myasthenia gravis, botulism, organophosphates

Muscle

- Muscular dystrophies, congenital myopathies, myotonic dystrophy, myositis, metabolic myopathies

Other

- Elastin disorders (Ehlers-Danlos)

DIAGNOSTIC APPROACH

History

- Onset and progression, detailed birth history, family history, history of seizures (suggests central cause)

Physical Exam (Table 18-1)

- Dysmorphic features (suggests central cause)
- Shake mother's hand (myotonia)

Investigations

- Consider head ultrasound (US), CT, MRI, LP if central cause likely
- Muscle enzymes, especially CPK
- Chromosomes for dysmorphic features
- DNA analysis for dystrophies
- EMG, nerve conduction studies
- Tensilon test for myasthenia gravis
- ±Muscle/nerve biopsy
- ±Metabolic workup, if indicated

18

BOX 18-2 Deep Tendon Reflexes

Deep Tendon Reflex	**Segmental Level**
Jaw jerk	Pons → trigeminal nerve
Biceps	C5-C6
Triceps	C7-C8
Brachioradialis	C5-C6
Knee	L3-L4
Ankle	S1-S2

Table 18-1 Neurologic Signs by Anatomic Localization in the Floppy Baby

	Central	Anterior horn cell	Peripheral nerve	Neuromuscular junction	Muscle
Muscle power	Normal or decreased	Decreased	Decreased	Fluctuating weakness	Decreased
Muscle bulk	Normal or decreased	Proximal atrophy	Distal atrophy	Normal	Decreased
Fasciculation	Absent	Present	Variable	Absent	Absent
Tendon reflexes	Increased	Decreased to absent	Decreased	Normal to decreased	Decreased
Primitive reflexes	Persistent/reappear	Absent	Absent	Absent	Absent
Plantar response	Extensor	Flexor to nonreactive	Flexor to nonreactive	Flexor	Flexor to nonreactive
Sensation	Normal	Normal	Loss	Normal	Normal

GUILLAIN-BARRÉ SYNDROME

- Airway protection and ventilation: monitor respiratory parameters (e.g., forced vital capacity [FVC]) with respiratory therapist on daily or twice-daily basis during acute phase
- Intubation (airway protection) and ventilation necessary if
  1. Bulbar involvement (dysphagia, dysarthria, hoarseness, weak cough) with inability to protect airway
  2. Worsening respiratory parameters
  3. Cardiovascular instability
- Monitor for
  1. Cardiac arrhythmias, BP instability
  2. Bowel and bladder hypofunction
  3. Deep-vein thrombosis
- Specific management (in consultation with neurologist)
  1. Gammaglobulin infusion
  2. Plasmapheresis

SEIZURES

HISTORY

- Precipitating factors
  - Fever, illness
- Description of seizure (Box 18-3, Fig 18-1)
  - Aura
  - Duration
  - Simple

18

BOX 18-3   Classification of Seizures*

I. Partial seizures
   A. Simple
      1. With motor signs (Jacksonian seizures, focal motor seizures)
      2. With somatosensory or special signs (sensory seizures)
      3. With autonomic symptoms or signs (abdominal epilepsy or epileptic equivalent)
      4. With psychic symptoms
   B. Complex partial seizures
   C. Partial seizures with secondary generalization
I. Generalized seizures
   A. Absence seizures
      1. Typical (petit mal)
      2. Atypical (petit mal variant, complex petit mal)
   B. Myoclonic seizures (minor motor seizures)
   C. Clonic seizures (minor motor seizures)
   D. Tonic seizures (minor motor seizures)
   E. Atonic seizures (akinetic seizures or drop attacks)
   F. Tonic-clonic seizures (grand mal, major motor seizures)

---

*ILAE Classification (old terminology).

- Partial (focal) versus generalized
- Motor signs (tonic, clonic, atonic, myoclonic movements) and progression
- Autonomic, somatosensory, or psychic signs
- Associated cyanosis, vocalizations, incontinence
- Postictal state
  - Drowsiness or stupor, headache, transient paralysis
- Seizure pattern (if previous seizures)
  - Frequency, time of day, precipitating factors, alterations in types
  - Associated symptoms, drugs, development, family history

PHYSICAL EXAM

- Growth parameters, dysmorphism, skin lesions (use Wood's lamp), neurologic signs, fundi
- Hyperventilation for 3 to 4 min: precipitates absence seizure

DIFFERENTIAL DIAGNOSIS

- Syncope, breath holding, gastroesophageal reflux, migraine, tics, benign paroxysmal vertigo, sleep disorders, daydreaming, pseudoseizures, psychiatric (rage attacks)

INVESTIGATIONS

- Bloodwork
  - Glucose, electrolytes, calcium, magnesium ± anticonvulsant levels

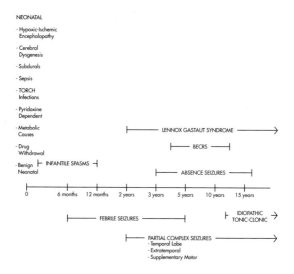

Fig. 18-1 **Types of seizures in children.** *BECRS,* Benign epilepsy of childhood with rolandic spikes; *GTC,* Generalized tonic-clonic seizures.

- Routine EEG
  - May have normal interictal EEG; increased yield with sleep deprivation, photic stimulation
- Video EEG recording
  - For complex cases, possible surgery, query pseudoseizures
- Neuroimaging
  - CT ± MRI
  - ± CSF for suspected infection, demyelinating disorder, metabolic disorder
  - ± Metabolic workup

MANAGEMENT

- See p. 14 for treatment of status epilepticus

Parental Education

- First aid for seizures: remove from danger and place in recovery position; do not put fingers or other object in mouth
- Helmet for young children
- Supervision for swimming, bicycle riding

Anticonvulsant Therapy

- Only 50% of children with first afebrile seizure will go on to have recurrent seizures; therefore therapy usually not necessary with first seizure
- Select drug appropriate for seizure type (Table 18-2)
- Need monitoring with serum levels or CBC, LFTs; frequency determined by seizure control (Table 18-3)
- Try to use monotherapy, if possible
- Be aware of many drug interactions between anticonvulsants and with antibiotics (especially erythromycin) and other drugs

18

Table 18-2   Long-Term Seizure Management

Seizure type	First choice	Alternates
Generalized tonic-clonic	Carbamazepine or valproate	Phenobarbital*
		Phenytoin
		Primidone
Partial	Carbamazepine	Phenobarbital
		Valproate
		Phenytoin
		Primidone
		Vigabatrin†
		Gabapentin†
		Lamotrigine†
Absence	Ethosuximide	Valproate
		Clonazepam
Myoclonic	Valproate	Nitrazepam
		Clonazepam
Infantile spasms	ACTH or vigabatrin	Nitrazepam

*First choice for seizures in children < 2 yr old.
†Can also be considered for generalized tonic-clonic seizures.

Table 18-3   Selected Anticonvulsant Drugs*

Drug	Monitoring	Major side effects
Carbamazepine (Tegretol)	Levels† CBC LFT‡	Diplopia, dizziness, drowsiness, rash, leukopenia, hepatocellular damage, renal toxicity
Clonazepam (Rivoitril)		Tolerance, drowsiness, irritability, weight gain, ataxia, dysarthria
Ethosuximide (Zarontin)	Levels	GI upset, rash, reversible leukopenia, abdominal pain, and irritability
Gabapentin (Neurontin)		Somnolence, dizziness, ataxia, nystagmus
Lamotrigine (Lamictal)		Diplopia, dizziness, somnolence, headache, fatigue, GI upset, rash
Phenobarbital	Levels	Drowsiness, hyperactivity, impaired cognition, rash, Stevens-Johnson syndrome
Phenytoin (Dilantin)	Levels	Gingival hyperplasia, hirsutism, nystagmus, ataxia, confusion, lupus, lymphadenopathy, Stevens-Johnson syndrome, decreased serum folate, rickets
Valproate (Epival/Depakene)	Levels CBC LFT	GI upset, weight gain, hepatocellular damage, thrombocytopenia, hyperammonemia, pancreatitis, behavioral changes
Vigabatrin (Sabril)		Sedation, insomnia, GI upset, ataxia, agitation, and hyperactivity

*See formulary for drug dosages.

†See p. 624 for therapeutic drug monitoring levels and sampling guidelines.

‡*LFT*, Liver function tests.

Surgery

- For selected intractable seizure disorders with focality
- Anterior temporal lobectomy, amygdalohippocampectomy, hemispherectomy, corpus collosotomy

WEANING ANTICONVULSANTS

- Trial when seizure-free for minimum 2 yr
- Chance of recurrence: < 25% if no risk factors; usually recur in the first 6 mo after discontinuing therapy
- Risk factors for recurrence include fixed neurologic deficit, focal seizures, and long duration of epilepsy before control
- Wean over 3-6 mo

FEBRILE SEIZURES

- Occur in 4% of children under 5 years of age, often with family history of febrile seizures
- Frequently associated with roseola, otitis, upper respiratory tract infection, gastroenteritis, pneumonia
- High index of suspicion for meningitis is needed in children < 1 yr old or with recurring or prolonged seizures in previous 24 hr

- Hospitalization not necessary if seizure is "typical," cause of fever is identified and treated, and follow-up is arranged

TYPICAL FEATURES

- Previously normal development and neurologic exam
- Generalized seizure
- Duration of seizure < 15 min
- Only one seizure in 24-hr period
- Normal neurologic exam after seizure

PARENTAL EDUCATION

- Febrile seizures are common and benign
- ⅔ of children will have only one seizure
- Recurrent febrile seizures are more likely if there is positive family history of febrile seizures or if first febrile seizure occurs at < 1 yr of age
- Subsequent nonfebrile seizures are more likely if seizure has atypical features or if there is positive family history of epilepsy in parents or siblings
- Prophylactic anticonvulsants are usually unnecessary; in recurrent, prolonged febrile seizures, consider use of rectal lorazepam
- Acetaminophen should be given with fevers, but may not prevent febrile seizure
- Parents should know first aid for seizures and call ambulance if seizure lasts more than 5-10 min or child is turning blue; if seizure is short and typical, they can visit their doctor to establish cause of fever and treatment

ACUTE ATAXIA

HISTORY

- Recent headache, vomiting, fever, stiff neck, viral illness (e.g., varicella), head trauma
- Presence of vertigo, focal neurologic findings, seizures
- Drug or toxin exposure (e.g., phenytoin, alcohol)
- Recurrent acute ataxia (e.g., with migraine, metabolic disorders, or benign paroxysmal vertigo)
- Family history (migraine, familial ataxia, metabolic disorders)

EXAMINATION

- Raised ICP
- Skin rash
- Meningitis
- Nystagmus, opsoclonus (conjugate jerking of eyes in random directions)
- ENT exam for otitis media, mastoiditis
- Differentiate ataxia from weakness or abnormal tone

INVESTIGATIONS

- Depend on history and physical exam
- Urgent CT scan (or MRI) if signs of ↑ ICP
- Lumbar puncture (if no elevation of ICP)

18

- Electrolytes, glucose, CBC, NH_4, LFTs, plasma amino acids, urine organic acids
- Urine catecholamines (neuroblastoma)
- Toxic screen (blood, urine) if there is specific history
- Vitamins B_{12} and E if history of malabsorption
- Titers for varicella, mumps, coxsackievirus, echo, influenza A and B, mycoplasma (see p. 555)
- EEG
- May need further metabolic investigations

STROKE

HISTORY

- Past history of strokes, migraine, seizures
- Family history of cardiac, cerebrovascular disease or deep venous thrombosis
- Underlying medical problems such as cardiac disease, bleeding diathesis, leukemia, febrile illness, dehydration
- Medications likely to affect coagulation (e.g., aspirin or intravenous drug abuse)
- Recent trauma, including intraoral trauma

EXAMINATION

- Evidence of increased ICP (see p. 13)
- Meningismus
- Cranial bruits
- Focal neurologic findings
- Cardiovascular exam: cardiac murmur, heart rhythm, blood pressure
- Evidence of bleeding diathesis
- Sepsis: scalp or facial lesions, mastoiditis, retropharyngeal abscess, fever
- Presence of neurocutaneous disorder or hemangioma suggestive of arteriovenous malformation

INVESTIGATIONS

- CBC, ESR, PT, PTT, sickle cell prep (when appropriate), glucose, gas, electrolytes
- Emergency or urgent CT scan or MRI as indicated (include C-spine if there are features of vertebrobasilar stroke)
- LP if CT negative: may reveal evidence of subarachnoid bleed
- MRV if considering sinus venous thrombosis
- MRA and/or cerebral angiography as indicated
- Other as indicated
  1. ECG and 2-D echocardiogram
  2. Coagulopathy workup: protein S, protein C, antithrombin III, fibrinogen, lipid profile, anticardiolipin antibody, ANA, anti-DNA, rheumatoid factor
  3. Metabolic workup: serum and CSF lactate and amino acids (MELAS), urine nitroprusside test (homocystinuria), urine organic acids (organic acidopathies)
  4. EEG if history and physical consistent with postictal event

MANAGEMENT

- Monitor for raised ICP, which may be maximal a few days after onset of stroke
- Correct underlying etiology where possible
- Anticoagulation may be required in specific situations after initial investigations done

HEADACHE

TYPES OF HEADACHE
Tension-Type Headache

- Continuous pain throughout day
- Often feels like tight band around the head (sharp or pressure sensation)
- Does not usually interfere with sleep
- Often associated with ongoing anxiety or depression

Headache Because of Raised ICP

- Recent onset (usually wks)
- Increasing severity of headache
- Lethargy, drowsiness
- Morning vomiting
- May have increasing unsteadiness of gait
- May be recent history of significant head trauma

Migraine

- Migraine with aura (classic)
- Migraine without aura (common)
- Complicated (hemiplegia, ophthalmoplegia, basilar signs, or acute confusional state)
- Cluster (associated with conjunctival injection, tearing, nasal discharge)
- Presence of at least three of following:
  - Intermittent throbbing headache
  - Complete relief with sleep
  - Aura
  - Unilateral pain
  - Nausea, vomiting, or abdominal discomfort
  - Family history of migraine

EXAMINATION

- Fundi for papilledema
- Cranial nerve abnormalities, especially of cranial nerve VI with diplopia on lateral gaze
- Hypertension
- Enlarging head circumference, cranial bruit
- Evidence of sinusitis, otitis media, mastoiditis
- Presence of ataxia, weakness, or spasticity, especially in lower limbs
- Skin stigmata of neurocutaneous syndrome (Table 18-4) or nonaccidental injury

18

Table 18-4 Neurocutaneous Syndromes

	NF	TS	SW	AT	IP
Inheritance	AD (50%)	AD (30%)	Sporadic	AR	XLD
Skin findings	CAL Freckling (axilla and groin) Neurofibromas	Ash leaf spots Shagreen patch Adenoma sebaceum CAL Periungal fibroma	Port wine in V1 Other cutaneous vascular malformations	Telangiectases (conjunctival and cutaneous) CAL	Bullae as neonates Splashes or whorls of hyperpigmentation
Other findings	Lisch nodules Sz DD Osseous lesions	Infantile spasms DD & MR Calcified tubers in brain Retinal lesions	Sz Glaucoma Hemihypertrophy Intracranial AVM MR	Ataxia Immunodeficiency	Sz DD & MR Strabismus Female
Tumors	Plexiform neuroma Optic glioma Acoustic neuroma (NF II) Astrocytoma Meningioma Leukemia Pheochromocytoma Neuroblastoma Wilms' Tumor	Optic glioma Astrocytoma Cardiac rhabdomyoma Renal hamartoma Lung angiomyolipoma	Intracranial calcifications	Leukemia Lymphoma Solid tumors	

AD, Autosomal dominant; *AR,* autosomal recessive; *XLD,* x-linked dominant; *NF,* neurofibromatosis; *TS,* tuberous sclerosis; *SW,* Sturge Weber syndrome; *AT,* ataxia telangiectasia; *IP,* incontinentia pigmenti; *CAL,* café-au-lait spots; *DD,* developmental delay; *MR,* mental retardation; *Sz,* seizure disorder; *AVM,* arteriovenous malformation.

INVESTIGATIONS

- If abnormal neurologic exam or history suggestive of increased ICP, obtain CT scan or MRI
- If CT scan or MRI abnormal, consult neurosurgeon; if normal and symptoms/signs of ↑ ICP; lumbar puncture, including measurement of opening pressure, CSF for cytology, culture, microscopy, virology, latex agglutination
- If normal neurologic examination with no history consistent with increased ICP, no investigations required, but follow-up essential

SPECIFIC MANAGEMENT FOR MIGRAINE

- Acute management: acetaminophen, dark, quiet environment; may use dimenhydrinate (PO or PR) if severe vomiting; chlorpromazine or meperidine if migraine severe or prolonged (in emergency department only)
- History of complicated migraine: use acetominophen in prodromal stage
- Migraine with aura in adolescents only: use sublingual ergotamine in prodromal stage (contraindicated in complicated migraine)
- Prophylaxis (individualized) approach: behavioral techniques are initial approach; if these fail and there is recurrent, severe headache with significant school absence, warrants neurology referral ± prophylactic medications

MYELOMENINGOCELE

INITIAL EVALUATON AND MANAGEMENT

- Initial stabilization (ABC)
- Keep NPO for possible surgery; establish maintenance IV of D5/0.2% saline
- Determine size of lesion, distal motor paralysis of legs and sphincters, associated neurogenic foot deformities, knee and hip contractures, evidence of hydrocephalus, associated congenital anomalies
- Transport for neurosurgic management: keep infant prone with moistened sterile saline dressings applied to open defect (must be kept wet at all times and changed as necessary)
- Initial diagnostic assessment includes head US or CT to look for hydrocephalus

TREATMENT

- Operative repair ± ventriculoperitoneal shunt
- Multidisciplinary team, including pediatrician, neurosurgeon, urologist, orthopedic surgeon, physiotherapist
- Assess important neurologic levels re: future function; prognosis is difficult; independent ambulation more likely with lower lesion
- Urologic: even very distal lesions (S2) will have some degree of neurogenic bladder; usually require clean intermittent catheterization and prophylactic antibiotics (see p. 488)
- Orthopedic: legs extended with lesions as low as L3; scoliosis increases with more proximal lesions; universal above L2
- Need counseling about recurrence and risks and folic acid supplementation with future pregnancies

18

BLOCKED CSF SHUNT

HISTORY

- Progressive history of increasing lethargy, vomiting, and headache
- May be associated with abdominal pain or fever
- Most useful indication of shunt malfunction is prior similar history with proven malfunction
- Consider shunt infection

INVESTIGATIONS

- Determine shunt patency by depressing subcutaneous pump, usually located in occipital scalp regions; should depress easily and refill within 5-15 sec
- CT scan or MRI to compare ventricular size with that found on previous CT scans; if ventricular size unchanged but symptoms persist, consider radionuclide shunt scan
- X-ray of skull, chest, abdomen ("shunt series") to rule out shunt-tube disconnection
- If symptoms intermittent or associated with abdominal pain and fever, sample CSF through subcutaneous reservoir for culture

ACUTE SPINAL CORD LESION

- Neurosurgic emergency
- Back pain
- Deteriorating gait with weakness in lower extremities
- Alteration in bladder (increased or decreased urination) or bowel (constipation) function

PHYSICAL EXAMINATION

- Altered pinprick sensation in lower extremities, including perianal area; if there is altered sensation, determine sensory level by moving from area of reduced sensation to normal areas; in young child, observe facial expression in response to stimuli; helpful dermatomes (Fig. 18-2):
  1. Nipples T4-5
  2. Umbilicus T10
  3. Dorsal aspect of big toe L5
  4. Perianal area S4, S5, coccygeal
- Hypotonia and depressed reflexes followed by hyperreflexia
- In older child, examine position and vibration sense in lower extremities, after establishing that reliable responses given with upper-limb testing
- Bladder may be enlarged and palpable
- Palpate spine for tenderness or fluctuant mass over spine
- Spinal bruits

INVESTIGATIONS

- Urgent MRI (myelogram if MRI not available)
- Of MRI normal, may still have transverse myelitis or cord infarction

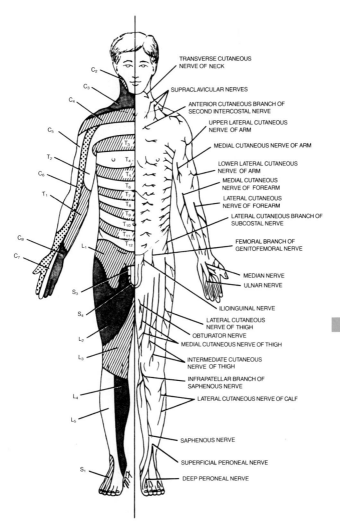

Fig. 18-2 A, Dermatomes and distribution of cutanious nerves on anterior aspect of body. (From Snell R, Smith M: *Clinical anatomy for emergency medicine,* St Louis, 1993, Mosby.)

Continued.

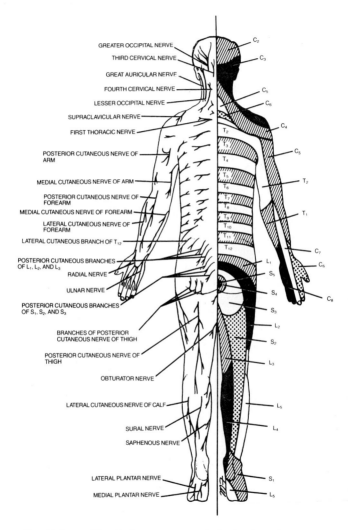

Fig. 18-2, cont'd.   B, Dermatomes and distribution of cutaneous nerves on posterior of body.

CHAPTER 19

NUTRITION

HANSA BHARGAVA AND FRANCY PILLO-BLOCKA

BREAST FEEDING

- Proper positioning: baby horizontal and anteriorly against mother (cradle hold) or to improve visibility, baby tucked under mother's arm along her side with hand supporting neck at level of breast (football hold); mouth at level of nipple; thumb on top of breast; fingers underneath well away from nipple
- Proper latching: stimulate wide-open mouth by running nipple along lower lip; use arm holding baby's head to bring him or her quickly onto breast; use index finger to pull baby's chin down and flange lower lip out to improve latch if soreness occurs
- Complications such as sore nipples or insufficient milk supply may sometimes be corrected with proper positioning or use of lactation aid if necessary; oral candidiasis may be contributing factor in sore nipples or poor latching
- Lactation device (improvised): #5 Fr. 36" feeding tube inverted into bottle through enlarged hole in bottle nipple; run tube along breast before latch, or insert at side of mouth once latched; baby nurses from breast and supplements via tube simultaneously; tube should not pass end of mother's nipple; supplement in bottle should be positioned at baby's head level or slightly above; manufactured supplemental nurser system available; follow-up with health professional recommended if supplement devices used
- Breast milk jaundice: do not discontinue breast feeding
- Breast abscess or mastitis: treat with antibiotics (cover *S. aureus*) and continue to breast feed unless incision and drainage required
- If gaining weight poorly consider dehydration and failure to thrive; treat with proper instruction on how to breast feed and lactation device (can fortify expressed breast milk to increase strength)
- Most newborn infants breast feed 6-9 times over 24 hr; stools every 3 hr

CONTRAINDICATIONS TO BREAST FEEDING

- Mothers receiving chemotherapy or radioactive compounds for diagnosis or treatment
- Excessive maternal alcohol intake
- Maternal drug abuse
- Maternal HIV or active tuberculosis
- Maternal CMV, hepatitis, and mastitis treated with antibiotics are *not* contraindications

BOTTLE FEEDING

FORMULA SELECTION (Table 19-1)

- First choice: iron-fortified cow's milk-based formula; preterm formula for prems < 1800 g
- Lactose intolerance: lactose-free cow's milk-based formula or soy-based formula
- Allergy to cow's-milk protein:
  1. Moderate-severe allergic reaction and high-risk infants (strong family history): protein hydrolysate formula (Nutramigen)
  2. Mild or questionable allergic reaction: trial of soy-based formula (∼ 50% cross-sensitivity) or partially hydrolyzed protein formula (Good Start)
- Protein and/or fat malabsorption: elemental formula (Pregestimil)
- Milk (cow; goat)
  - Do not give before 9-12 mo; no skim, 1% or 2% before 1 yr of age
  - Should be pasteurized

VITAMIN SUPPLEMENTATION

- Breast-fed
  Vitamin D (10 μg/day)
  Iron if exclusively breast-fed past 6 mo
  Fluoride (Table 19-2)
- Formula-fed
  None required if iron-fortified version used and adequate fluoride in water supply (see Table 19-2)
- Goat's milk
  Possibly folate, vitamins A and D (supplementation voluntary by manufacturer)

INTRODUCTION OF SOLIDS

- Introduce one new food every 2-3 days; single flavors first; introduce more slowly if higher risk of allergies (Table 19-3)
- Avoid raw vegetables, grapes, hot dogs, nuts, small candies, raisins, raw peas, popcorn, and beans in children < 4 yr because of choking and aspiration risks
- Peanut butter should not be given alone (sticky bolus can compromise airway)
- Discourage bedtime bottle in crib to avoid nursing caries (see "Common Feeding Problems")

SELF-FEEDING

- Child should self-bottle-feed at age 6 mo
- Child should feed by cup at 7-9 mo
- Child should feed by spoon at 7-12 mo

Text continued on p. 360.

Table 19-1 Composition of Milks and Formulas per 100ml Normal Dilutions

	Milks	
	Human (mature)	Cow's (whole)
Calories	75	64
Protein (g)	1.1	3.2
Source	Lactalbumin, casein	Casein, whey
Whey:casein	70:30	18:82
Fat (g)	4.5	3.6
Source	Human butterfat	Butterfat
CHO (g)	7.1	4.8
Source	Lactose	Lactose
No (mmol)	0.7	2.2
K (mmol)	1.3	4.0
Cl (mmol)	1.1	2.7
Ca (mmol)	0.9	3.1
P (mmol)	0.5	3.0
Fe (mg)	0.05	0.04
Vit. A (RE)	61	32
Vit. C (mg)	5.2	0.8
Vit. D (μg)	0	0.9
Osmolality (mOsm/kg/H_2O)	290	315
Indications for use	Desired feeding for preterm and term infants	Not recommended for infants < 9-12 mo old
Manufacturer	—	—

19

Note: 68 kcal/dl = 2800 kJ/L = 20 kcal/oz; 80 kcal/dl = 3300 kJ/L = 24 kcal/oz; 90 kcal/dl = 3800 kJ/L = 27 kcal/oz; 100 kcal/dL = 4200 kJ/L = 30 kcal/oz.

Continued.

Table 19-1   Composition of Milks and Formulas per 100ml Normal
Dilutions—cont'd

	Cow's-milk-based formula		
	Enfalac with Fe	Similac with Fe	Good Start
Calories	67	68	67
Protein (g)	1.5	1.5	1.6
Source	Demineralized whey, skim milk	Skim milk	Partially hydrolysed demineralized whey
Whey:casein	60:40	18:82	100:0
Fat (g)	3.8	3.7	3.5
Source	Palm, soy, coconut, sunflower oils	Safflower or sunflower, coconut, soy oils	Palm, soy, coconut, safflower oil
CHO (g)	6.9	7.2	7.3
Source	Lactose	Lactose	Lactose, maltodextrins
No (mmol)	0.8	0.8	0.7
K (mmol)	1.8	1.8	1.7
Cl (mmol)	1.2	1.2	1.1
Ca (mmol)	1.3	1.2	1.1
P (mmol)	1.1	1.2	0.8
Fe (mg)	0.7	1.2	1.0
Vit. A (RE)	63	60	60
Vit. C (mg)	5.5	5.5	5.5
Vit. D (μg)	1.0	1.0	1.0
Osmolality (mOsm/ kg/H_2O)	300	290	265
Indications for use	For term and preterm infants when breast feeding not chosen		Risk of cow's-milk protein allergy; delayed gastric emptying
Manufacturer	Mead Johnson	Ross	Carnation

	Soy-based			Premature	
Enfalac lactose free	Isomil	Enfalac Soy	Prosobee	Similac special care 20	24
67	6.8	67	67	68	81
1.5	1.7	2.0	2.0	1.8	2.2
Skim milk	Soy protein isolates	Soy protein isolates	Soy protein isolates	Skim milk, demineralized whey	
18:82	—	—	—	60:40	
3.7	3.7	3.6	3.6	3.7	4.4
Palm, soy, coconut, sunflower oil	Soy and coconut oils	Palm, soy, coconut, sunflower oils	Palm, soy, coconut, sunflower oils	MCT (50%), soy, coconut oils	
7.0	7.0	6.7	6.8	7.2	8.6
Corn syrup solids	Corn syrup solids, sucrose (50%), modified corn starch	Corn syrup solids, sucrose (40%)	Corn syrup solids	Maltodextrins, lactose	
0.8	1.3	1.1	1.1	1.3	1.5
1.9	1.9	2.0	2.0	2.1	2.6
1.3	1.2	1.4	1.4	1.5	1.8
1.4	1.8	1.7	1.6	2.8	3.3
1.4	1.6	1.6	1.6	1.9	2.3
1.2	1.2	1.2	1.2	0.25	0.3
63	61	63	63	78	94
5.5	5.5	5.5	5.5	25	30
1.0	1.0	1.0	1.0	1.05	1.25
165	240	255	160	250	235
Lactose intolerance		Lactose intolerance; risk of cow's-milk protein allergy; galactosemia		Preterm infants who weigh < 2000g	
Mead Johnson	Ross	Mead Johnson	Mead Johnson	Ross	

19

Continued.

Table 19-1 Composition of Milks and Formulas per 100ml Normal Dilutions—cont'd

	Premature	Therapeutic		
	Fortified human milk*	Nutramigen	Alimentum	Pre-gestimil
Calories	74	67	68	67
Protein (g)	1.6	1.9	1.9	1.9
Source	Lactalbumin, casein, whey, skim milk	Hydrolysed casein	Hydrolysed casein	Hydrolysed casein
Whey:casein	65:35	0:100	0:100	0:100
Fat (g)	4.2	2.6	3.8	2.7
Source	Human butterfat, MCT (25%) soy and coconut oils	Corn, soy oils	MCT (50%) safflower, soy oils	Corn, MCT (40%), soy oils
CHO (g)	7.9	9.1	6.9	9.1
Source	Lactose, corn syrup solids	Corn syrup solids, modified corn starch	Sucrose, modified tapioca starch	Corn syrup solids, modified corn starch
No (mmol)	1.2	1.4	1.3	1.4
K (mmol)	2.1	1.9	2.1	1.9
Cl (mmol)	1.6	1.6	1.5	1.6
Ca (mmol)	2.5	1.6	1.8	1.6
P (mmol)	1.6	1.4	1.6	1.4
Fe (mg)	0.17	1.2	1.2	1.3
Vit. A (RE)	116	51	61	63
Vit. C (mg)	17	5.5	6.0	5.5
Vit. D (μg)	1.5	0.9	1.0	1.05
Osmolality (mOsm/kg/H_2O)	295	320	370	350
Indications for use	Human milk fortifier for low–birth weight infants	Allergy to intact protein	Protein +/or fat malabsorption	
Manufacturer	Ross	Mead Johnson	Ross	Mead Johnson

*Fortified human milk=human milk, mature: Similac Natural Care (1:1).

	Therapeutic		Dehydration	Enteral formulas	
				Tube feeds	
Portagen	Similac PM 60/40	S44	Lytren	Pediasure	Isocal
68	68	68	10	100	100
2.4	1.5	1.7	0	3.0	4.2
Na caseinates	Whey, Na caseinates	Demineralized-whey, whey	—	Na caseinates, whey	Na + Ca caseinates, soy protein isolates
0:100	60:40	100:0	0	5.0	3.3
3.2	3.8	2.2	—	Safflower, soy oils MCT (20%)	Canola oil, MCT (40%)
MCT (86%), corn oil	Corn, coconut, soy oils	Coconut, safflower or sunflower, soy oils			
7.7	6.9	9.7	2.0	11.0	13.3
Corn syrup solids, sucrose	Lactose	Lactose	Dextrose	Maltodextrins, sucrose	Maltodextrins, sucrose
1.5	0.7	0.05	5.0	1.6	3.8
2.2	1.5	0.8	2.5	3.3	3.8
1.6	1.1	0.06	4.5	2.8	3.8
1.6	1.0	0.4	0	2.4	2.1
1.5	0.6	0.6	0	2.6	2.7
1.3	0.15	1.27	0	1.4	1.5
68	61	0	0	78	75
2.6	6.1	0	0	10	25
0.46	1.0	0	0	0.9	0.9
220	280	360	220	310	305
Fat malabsorption	Hyperphosphatemia	Idiopathic hypercalcemia-formula is incomplete	Achieve and maintain hydration in acute diarrhea	Children 1-10 yr old; can use orally	Children older than 10 yr
Mead Johnson	Ross	Wyeth	Mead Johnson	Ross	Mead Johnson

19

Continued.

Table 19-1   Composition of Milks and Formulas per 100ml Normal
Dilutions—cont'd

| | Enteral formulas | | | |
| | Tube feeds | Oral supplements | | Malabsorption |
	Jevity	Ensure	Ensure Plus	Vital HN
Calories	106	106	150	100
Protein (g)	4.4	3.7	5.7	4.2
Source	Na + Ca caseinates	Na + Ca caseinates, soy protein isolates	Na + Ca caseinates, soy protein isolates	Partially hydrolyzed whey, meat + soy, amino acids
Whey: casein	3.6	3.7	5.4	1.1
Fat (g)	Sunflower or safflower canola oils MCT (50%)	Corn oil	Corn oil	Safflower oil, MCT (45%)
Source				
CHO (g)	14.1	14.5	19.9	18.6
Source	Maltodextrins, corn syrup solids, soy polysaccharides	Corn syrup solids, maltodextrins, sucrose	Corn syrup solids, maltodextrins, sucrose	Hydrolysed corn starch, sucrose
No (mmol)	3.2	3.3	4.6	2.5
K (mmol)	3.2	3.1	4.9	3.6
Cl (mmol)	3.2	3.3	4.6	2.9
Ca (mmol)	2.3	1.4	1.6	1.7
P (mmol)	2.4	1.8	2.0	2.2
Fe (mg)	1.4	1.0	1.3	1.2
Vit. A (RE)	114	79	65	100
Vit. C (mg)	23	16	21	20
Vit. D (µg)	0.8	0.5	0.4	0.7
Osmolality (mOsm/kg/H_2O)	310	450	690	460
Indications for use	14 g dietary fiber/liter	Oral nutrition supplement; may tube-feed		Semielemental; impaired GI function; tube-feed
Manufacturer	Ross	Ross	Ross	Ross

| | Modules | | | | |
| Malabsorption | Protein | Fat | | | CHO |
Pepta-men	Promod /100 g	Corn oil /100ml	MCT /100ml	Microlipid /100ml	Caloreen /100 g
100	424	813	770	450	384
4.0	76	0	0	0	0
Hydrolyzed whey	Whey	—	—	—	—
	9.1 Butterfat	92 Corn oil	93 Fractionated coconut oil	50 Safflower oil	0 —
3.9 MCT (70%) sunflower oil	10.2 Lactose	0 —	0 —	0 —	96 Hydrolyzed corn starch
12.7 Maltodextrins, corn starch					
2.2	9.9	0	0	0	<2.2
3.2	25.2	0	0	0	<0.2
2.8	0	0	0	0	tr
2.0	16.7	0	0	0	tr
2.3	16.1	0	0	0	tr
1.2	0	0	0	0	0
120	0	0	0	0	0
14	0	0	0	0	0
0.7	0	0	0	0	0
270	N/A	N/A	N/A	70	N/A
Impaired GI function; delayed gastric emptying	Protein supplement	Caloric supplement	Caloric supplement for fat malabsorption	Caloric supplement as 50% fat emulsion	Caloric supplement
Clintec	Ross		Mead Johnson	Wyeth	Clintec

19

Clinical Dietitians, The Hospital for Sick Children, Toronto, 1995.

Table 19-2   Dosage Schedule for Dietary Fluoride Supplements (mg/day)

	Fluoride conc of principle drinking water source (ppm)		
Age	< 0.3 ppm	0.3-0.6 ppm	> 0.6ppm
6 mo-3 yr	0.25 mg	0	0
> 3-6 yr	0.5 mg	0.25 mg	0
> 6-16 yr	1.0 mg	0.5 mg	0

From Canadian Paediatric Society Statement: *The use of fluoride in infants and children*, Ottawa, 1995, CPS.

Table 19-3   Timing of Introduction of Various Food Groups

Age	Food	Comments
0-4 mo	Breast milk, formula	Will meet nutritive needs exclusively until 6 mo of age
4-6 mo	Iron-enriched cereal	Introduce rice cereal first
4-7 mo	Puréed vegetables	Yellow-orange vegetables first, green last (more bulk)
		Do not give high nitrate or nitrite-containing vegetables (beets, spinach, turnips) before 12 mo of age
6-9 mo	Puréed fruits and juices	Avoid "desserts" and fruit mixtures
6-9 mo	Puréed meats, fish, and poultry; egg yolk	Do not give egg white until 12 mo of age (risk of allergy)
9-12 mo	Finger foods, peeled fruit, cooked vegetables, cheese	Should be without added sugar, fat, salt, or seasonings
		Introduce varied food textures and encourage chewing, coordination, and independence

VEGETARIAN DIET

- With careful planning can meet all requirements
- Risk for deficiencies increases if variety of foods is very restrictive (i.e., macrobiotic, Rastafarian)
- Nutrients most at risk: iron; calcium; vitamins D, riboflavin, and B_{12}; zinc

COMMON FEEDING PROBLEMS

NURSING CARIES

- Common causes: bottles at bedtime; pacifiers dipped in sugar, syrup, honey; bottle feeding past 12 mo; omit bedtime bottles or give plain water
- Can occur even before teeth erupt; severe decay warranting extraction can interfere with speech articulation and chewing

CONSTIPATION

- Infrequent passage of hard stool

Differential Diagnosis

- Dietary (usually from inadequate intake of fluids or carbohydrates); behavioral
- Hirschsprung's
- Incarcerated hernia
- Obstruction (e.g., volvulus postsurgical adhesions)
- Ileus (electrolyte imbalance, hypothyroidism)
- Meconium ileus (cystic fibrosis)
- Renal tubular acidosis
- Dehydration
- Neuromuscular (myotonic dystrophy, myelomeningocele, spinal cord tumors)
- May be perpetuated by painful defecation and formation of painful anal fissures

Management

- Rule out other causes (as listed above)
- Establish bowel routine
- Conservative
  - < 6m
    - Ensure adequate fluid intake
    - Add 10-20 g sucrose or dextrose per liter of fluid feeding
  - > 6m
    - As above plus give small amounts of prune juice
    - Increase cereal, fruit, vegetable content (fiber)
- Medical
  - < 2 yr: lactulose once a day
  - > 2 yr: mineral oil (but first may need to clean out rectum with Fleet enemas and/or Golytely)

LOW-FAT DIETS

- Restricting dietary fat not recommended until postpubertal growth complete (may jeopardize growth and development)
- No consistent evidence that fat-reduced, cholesterol-lowering diet in infancy decreases risk of atherosclerosis in adulthood

LACTOSE INTOLERANCE

- Diagnosis: hydrogen breath test in children > 3 yr
- Infants: lactose-free cow's milk-based formula or soy formula
- > 9-12 mo: vitamin D-fortified soy milk or cow's milk treated with β-galactosidase (LactAid)
- Primary: may tolerate small amounts of lactose-containing foods
- Secondary: try reintroducing small amounts of lactose at regular intervals (e.g.; in cases of transient lactase deficiency secondary to gastroenteritis)

19

FOOD ALLERGIES

- Prevalence 1%-8%; highest frequency in first yr of life
- Risk largely related to genetic predisposition and age of introduction
- Most common: milk, egg, peanut, soy, nuts, and wheat
- Rare to have allergy to more than two or three foods
- Sensitivity disappears within a few yr except to peanuts, nuts, fish, and seafood; these allergies are most severe and tend to be lifelong
- See also p. 44

EXCESSIVE CONSUMPTION OF JUICE AND/OR MILK

- Can decrease appetite for solid foods
- Energy and nutrient intakes (fat, protein, iron) can be inadequate, causing poor weight gain, chronic diarrhea, failure to thrive, nutrient deficiencies (including iron deficiency anemia)

FAILURE TO THRIVE

DEFINITION

- Weight < 3rd percentile or a fall in weight and/or height over two major percentile lines

CATEGORIES

1. Inadequate intake, persistent regurgitation or vomiting
2. Inadequate absorption and assimilation
3. Failure of utilization
4. Increased metabolism

DIFFERENTIAL DIAGNOSIS
Inorganic (includes decreased intake)

- Psychosocial factors
- Emotional deprivation
- Rumination
- Anorexia nervosa
- Diagnose by careful history and observation (hospitalization may be required)

Organic

- Inadequate intake (any reason)
- Inadequate absorption:
  GI malabsorption (multiple causes)
  Cystic fibrosis
  Parasites
  Liver disease
  Inflammatory bowel disease
- Failure of utilization or increased metabolism
  Endocrine: hyperthyroidism
  Chronic heart failure
  Chronic renal failure, renal tubular disorder
  Chronic inflammation: rheumatoid arthritis

Immunodeficiency: congenital or acquired
Malignancies: kidney, adrenal, brain, leukemias
• Other
Congenital syndromes (e.g., FAS, FPS, TORCH, Down, Williams, Noonan's)
Cerebral palsy

INVESTIGATIONS

• Careful history (including detailed diet history) and physical exam will be suggestive in > 90% of organic FTT
• Dietary history and socioeconomic status
• CBC, ESR, electrolytes, urea, creatinine, venous gas, Ca, PO_4, Mg, thyroid function tests, glucose, protein, albumin, Zn, PT, PTT
• Specific vitamin levels, if indicated by history and physical findings
• Urine for pH, culture, specific gravity, metabolic screen, reducing substances
• Stool for microscopy (fat, white cells), occult blood; consider ova and parasites; reducing substances; cultures, including *Giardia*
• Three-five day stool collection for fecal fat
• Sweat chloride
• Search for sites of chronic infection
• Anthropometry: weight, height, percentage ideal body weight, head circumference, skinfold thickness, midarm muscle circumference
• Radiologic investigations may include bone age, skull x-ray, CXR, abdominal and head US
• Depending on clinical situation: immunoglobulins, chromosomes, liver function tests, HIV test

TREATMENT

• Trial of high-calorie formula or diet may be sufficient to achieve desirable weight gain
• May require hospital admission
• Rehydrate (if necessary) with oral electrolyte rehydration or maintenance solution; rarely needed
• Treat infection, parasites

DIET

• Calories: 150-170 kcal/kg/day (↑ gradually and stop at level where catch-up weight gain is achieved)
• Protein and other nutrient needs can be met if concentrated formula is used
• May require supplemental tube feeding

COMPLICATIONS

• Diarrhea, infections, bleeding, hypothermia, hypoglycemia

ENTERAL NUTRITION

• No more than 4-8 hr supply of enteral feeds should be hung at one time to prevent bacterial contamination

- Symptoms of intolerance include abdominal distension, cramping, nausea, vomiting, diarrhea; check for lactose intolerance, hyperosmolar feeds, too rapid rate of infusion or too large a volume, cold feeds, medications associated with diarrhea (bacterial contamination)
- Discontinue tube feeding when oral intake improves to ⅔-¾ of estimated caloric and protein requirements

ROUTE

- NG if tube feeds needed for < 6-8 wk
- G-tube: long-term feeding
- NJ, GJ: use if higher risk of aspiration, GER

METHOD

- Bolus via syringe or gravity over a few min
- Intermittent: gravity from over 30-45 min; not suitable for jejunal feeds
- Continuous: pump administered; better tolerance for GER, risk of aspiration, jejunal feeds

TUBES

- Nasoenteric: 5- to 6-French for small infants; 6- to 8-French for older children and adolescents
- Silicone or polyurethane: flexible; guidewire for insertion, replace q 2-4 wk
- Polyvinylchloride: stiffer; replace q 4-7 days because of risk of intestinal perforation
- Enterostomy: 12- to 18-French; available as rubber catheter with mushroom tip (replace q 1.5 yr), silicone catheter with balloon tip (replace q 6-8 mo) or silicone catheter with external "button" device

CHOICE OF FORMULAS

- < 1 yr of age: expressed breast milk or commercial infant formula if breast milk unavailable
- > 1 - 10 yr of age: Pediasure
- For impaired pancreaticobiliary function, small-bowel obstruction, or direct delivery into small intestine use "elemental" formula (e.g., Pregestimil, Tolerex, Vital, Peptamen)

INCREASING ENERGY CONTENT OF FORMULAS
(Table 19-4)

- Concentrate formula in stepwise fashion to 1 kcal/ml (max 4 g protein/kg); increased intestinal osmolality and renal solute load
- Add fat (corn oil, Microlipid, MCT oil) or carbohydrate modules (Caloreen and Polycose)
- Protein supplements rarely indicated

TOTAL PARENTERAL NUTRITION

- TPN is indicated when patient's nutrient needs are not or cannot be met by enteral route
- To calculate TPN dosage, three requirements must be kept in mind:
  1. Amino acid/protein requirement

Table 19-4 Energy Content of Formula

Kilojoules*/liter	Kilocalories/100 ml	Kilocalories/ounce
2800	68	20
3300	80	24
3800	90	27
4200	100	30
4600	110	33

*1 kilojoule = 4.2 kilocalories.

2. Caloric requirement
3. Total daily fluid intake
- Aim is to give optimal energy/caloric requirements without superceding total fluid intake per day or total protein/lipid intake

APPROACH TO ORDERING TPN
Step One

1. Look up caloric requirements for specific age group in Table 19-5; this is eventual aim for caloric intake
2. Calculate total daily fluid intake for patient, keeping in mind fluid restriction if necessary (e.g., cardiac patients) (see p. 100)

Step Two

1. Look up protein requirement for the patient in Table 19-5
2. Choose specific TPN formula for patient, depending on age (e.g., "P" solutions are for preterm infants; "I" solutions are for infants and children) (Table 19-6)
3. Calculate amount of TPN solution needed to get protein requirement; start with 1 g/kg/day of protein for young children and infants and work up on protein content to recommended intake on daily basis
4. Calculate amount of calories in above results to find out how much of energy requirement is being met

Example: 1-yr-old boy weighing 10 kg
- Caloric requirement is ~ 100 kcal/kg/day = 100 × 10 = 1000 kcal (see Table 19-5)
- Total daily maintenance fluid requirement approximately 100 cc/kg/day = 1000 cc, therefore this is amount of IV fluids not to be superseded
- Protein requirement (Table 19-5) = 1.21 g/kg/day, but start with 1 g/kg/day; therefore it is 10 g of protein
- For age, use I-10, which contains 30g/1000 cc; by simple calculation, child will require ~ 333 cc of I-10 to get his protein requirement (10 g)
- This amount of solution will give child 0.333 × 495 kcal/1000 cc = 165 kcal (see Table 19-6); therefore he will not meet his caloric requirement by this solution alone; however, we also add lipids (10% or 20%) to meet essential fatty-acid requirements, as well as calorie requirements

Text continued p 370.

19

Table 19-5   Summary Examples of Recommended Nutrient Intakes for Canadians*†‡

Age	Sex	Energy (kcal/kg/day)	Protein (g/kg/day)	Fat-soluble vitamins			Water-soluble vitamins			Minerals					
				Vitamin A (RE/day)	Vitamin D (µg/day)	Vitamin E (mg/day)	Vitamin C (mg/day)	Folate (µg/day)	Vitamin B_{12} (µg/day)	Calcium (mg/day)	Phosphorus (mg/day)	Magnesium (mg/day)	Iron (mg/day)	Iodine (µg/day)	Zinc (mg/day)
Mo															
0-2	Both	120-100	2.15	400	10	3	20	50	0.3	250	150	20	0.3	30	2
3-5	Both	100-95	1.46	400	10	3	20	50	0.3	250	150	20	0.3	30	2
6-8	Both	95-97	.41	400	10	3	20	50	0.3	400	200	32	7	40	3
9-11	Both	97-99	1.37	400	10	3	20	50	0.3	400	200	32	7	40	3
Yr															
1	Both	101	1.21	400	10	3	20	65	0.3	500	300	40	6	55	4
2-3	Both	94	1.16	400	5	4	20	80	0.4	550	350	50	6	65	4
4-6	Both	100	1.06	500	5	5	25	90	0.5	600	400	65	8	85	5
7-9	M	88	1.03	700	2.5	7	25	125	0.8	700	500	100	8	110	7
	F	76	1.03	700	2.5	6	25	125	0.8	700	500	100	8	95	7
10-12	M	73	1.01	800	2.5	8	25	170	1.0	900	700	130	8	125	9
	F	61	1.01	800	5	7	25	180	1.0	1100	800	135	8	110	9

Age	Sex														
13-15	M	57	0.98	900	5	9	30	150	1.5	1100	900	185	10	160	12
	F	46	0.95	800	5	7	30	145	1.5	1000	850	180	13	160	9
16-18	M	51	0.93	1000	5	10	40	185	1.9	900	1000	230	10	160	12
	F	40	0.88	800	2.5	7	30	160	1.9	700	850	200	12	160	9
19-24	M	42	0.86	1000	2.5	10	40	210	2.0	800	1000	240	9	160	12
	F	36	0.86	800	2.5	7	30	175	2.0	700	850	200	13	160	9
Pregnancy (additional) (kcal/day) (g/day)															
First trimester		100	5	100	2.5	2	0	300	1.0	500	200	15	0	25	6
Second trimester		300	15	100	2.5	2	10	300	1.0	500	200	45	5	25	6
Third trimester		300	24	100	2.5	2	10	300	1.0	500	200	45	10	25	6
Lactation (additional)		500	22	400	2.5	3	25	100	0.5	500	200	65	50	6	

*Recommended Nutrient Intakes Health and Welfare, Canada, 1990.

†With exception of energy, all recommended intakes are designed to cover individual variations in essentially all of healthy population subsisting on variety of common foods available in Canada.

‡Figures for energy are estimates of average requirements for expected patterns of activity; for nutrients not shown, following amounts recommended: Thiamin, 0.4 mg/1000 kcal; riboflavin, 0.5 mg/1000 kcal; niacin, 7.2 NE/1000 kcal; vitamin B_6, 15 μg, as pyridoxine, per gram of protein.

19

Table 19-6 Composition of VAMIN-N Based Standard Solutions (per L)

| | Premature infants* | | | | Infants, children, and adolescents | | | Fluid-restricted patients |
	P-5	P-7.5	P-10	PI-10	I-10	1-20†	C-30
Protein (g)	15.0	15.0	20.0	20.0	30.0	30.0	50
Glucose (g)	50.0	75.0	100.0	100.0	100.0	200.0	300.0
Energy (kcal)‡	248.0	340.0	455.0	455.0	495.0	870.0	1320.0
Na (mmol)	20.0	20.0	14.3	30.0	30.0	30.0	30.0
K (mmol)	20.0	20.0	18.9	30.0	30.0	30.0	30.0
Cl (mmol)	21.1	21.1	15.7	31.3	32.1	32.1	32.1
Ca (mmol)	9.0	9.0	9.0	9.0	9.0	9.0	9.0
P (mmol)	9.0	9.0	9.0	9.0	9.0	9.0	9.0
Mg (mmol)	3.0	3.0	4.0	4.0	4.0	4.0	4.0

Zn (μmol)	46.0	46.0	46.0	46.0	46.0	46.0	46.0
Cu (μmol)	6.3	6.3	6.3	6.3	6.3	6.3	6.3
Mn (μmol)	1.8	1.8	1.8	1.8	1.8	5.0	5.0
I (μmol)	0.47	0.47	0.47	0.47	0.47	0.47	0.47
Cr (μmol)	0.076	0.076	0.076	0.076	0.076	0.076	0.076
Se (μmol)	0.25	0.25	0.25	0.25	0.25	0.25	0.25
Fe (μmol)§	—	—	—	—	18.0	18.0	18.0

Modified from guidelines for total parenteral nutrition, Toronto, 1986, Hospital for Sick Children.

Fat emulsion, 10%: 1100 kcal/L, 100 g fat/L, 47 g linoleic acid/L (1.1 kcal/ml).

Fat emulsion, 20%: 2200 kcal/L (2.2 kcal/ml).

*"P" solutions standard for premature infants who are not fluid restricted, "I" solutions are for premature infants who are fluid restricted and for children and infants.

†I-20 is intended for central venous line therapy only.

‡Energy unit: 1 kcal = 4.2 kJ; energy content includes potential energy from protein as well as that from glucose.

§Iron can be included in "P" solutions in neonates who have been receiving TPN for 1 mo or more and should therefore be ordered.

19

Step Three

1. For lipid component, start with 1 g lipid/kg/day; can be increased slowly by 1 g/kg/day up to 4 g/kg/day as long as serum intralipid levels (which should be measured regularly) stay below 1 g/L

Example: For the 10-kg boy, give him 10 kg × 1 g/kg/day = 10 g/day

- 10% lipid solution contains 10 g lipid/100 cc; therefore 100 cc of 10% lipid per day will give him his lipid requirement
- 10% lipid solution contains 110 kcal/100cc; therefore we will also be providing 110 kcal/day
- 20% lipid solution contains 220 kcal/100 cc (used in fluid restriction)

Step Four

1. Calculate resulting fluid intake and caloric intake from TPN administration

In example of 10-kg boy, use

I-10:	333 cc, giving him	165 kcal and 10 g protein	
10% lipid:	+100 cc, giving him	+110 kcal and 10 g lipid	
	433 cc	275 kcal	

- Therefore child needs 567 cc (1000-433) of fluids, which may be provided with saline or dextrose solutions
- Child needs 725 kcal (1000-275), which we need to work up to by increasing lipids and I-10 on daily basis

Points to Remember when using TPN

1. Appropriate monitoring required (see following discussion)
2. While weaning off TPN, decrease rate in stepwise fashion over 1-2 hr to avoid hypoglycemia
3. Certain IV drugs not compatible with TPN; check with pharmacy
4. Special solutions (e.g. additional protein, carbohydrate, minerals, lytes) are available and generally can be mixed, depending on clinical situation

COMPLICATIONS OF TPN
Short-term

1. Glucose intolerance
   - Glycosuria: infants especially may have this with normal serum glucose levels
   - Hyperglycemia: may occur especially with major surgery, trauma, steroids, or sepsis
   - ↑ monitoring of blood + urine; rule out sepsis
   - Consider IV rate and concentration of glucose in TPN solution
2. Hypoglycemia: especially in term, LGA
   - Slowly ↑ rate or concentration over 4-5 days
3. Electrolyte imbalance
4. Infection of line, bacteremia
5. Thrombophlebitis

Long-term

1. Cholestasis (see p. 199)
   - Patients on long-term TPN are at risk

- Initiation of enteral nutrition while weaning/cycling parenteral nutrition may reverse
2. Venous thrombosis: patients on longer-term TPN are at risk

LIPIDS

- Relative contraindications (because of excess of unmetabolized lipid in serum)
  1. Neonatal indirect hyperbilirubinemia (free fatty acids compete for binding on albumin)
  2. Thrombocytopenia (may interfere with platelet function)
  3. Respiratory distress (may interfere with gas exchange)
  4. Sepsis (may develop lipid intolerance): withhold lipid for 24 hr

ELECTROLYTES, VITAMINS, AND MINERALS

- Requirements vary with age and disease
- Ca, P, Mg, Zn, Cu, Mn, Cr, I, and Se must be present in TPN; for special TPN, new orders must be filled out
- Iron must be included except in premature infants < 1 mo
- Multivitamins must be supplemented

MONITORING

- Fluid balance daily
- Daily urine glucose: glycosuria may occur with normal serum glucose especially in neonates; decrease glucose concentration if this occurs
- CBC, urea, PO_4, Ca, Mg, albumin, bilirubin, LFTs, and creatinine (baseline and weekly determinations)
- Electrolytes, glucose (baseline and twice weekly)
- Lipid levels twice weekly and with sepsis and solution change; generally keep < 1 g/L.
- Growth parameters

INDICATIONS FOR CENTRAL VENOUS LINE

- Unable to meet requirements through peripheral TPN
- TPN > 2 wk (variable)
- Venous access difficulty
- Osmolality of solution (> 12.5% glucose solution)

19

OBESITY

- Definition: > 120% of ideal weight for height
- Majority are primary; secondary causes include endocrine, some genetic syndromes (Prader-Willi, Laurence-Moon-Biedl); most endocrine abnormalities are *secondary* to obesity
- History: caloric intake, activity, medications (e.g., steroids), psychosocial

INVESTIGATIONS (all are optional):

1. Thyroid function tests
2. Fasting blood glucose, HbA1c
3. ± Lipid profile

4. ± Pituitary function (GH, FSH, LH), adrenal tests (cortisol, 17-OH progesterone)
5. ± Chromosomes

MANAGEMENT

- Dietary mainstay: involve dietitian, family
- Encourage increased physical activity
- Follow blood pressure, skin (intertrigo), pubertal development, hips (risk of slipped capital femoral epiphysis), menstrual function, blood lipids, glucose tolerance
- Treat underlying cause if secondary; still requires above monitoring

CHAPTER 20

ONCOLOGY

MARYAM FOULADI

TUMOR LYSIS SYNDROME

- Occurs because of breakdown of malignant cells and release of intracellular contents, leading to:
  - Hyperkalemia
  - Hyperuricemia (from release and metabolism of nucleic acids)
  - Hyperphosphatemia (and secondary hypocalcemia)
- Most commonly in
  - Burkitt's lymphoma
  - T cell leukemia, lymphoma
- May occur in acute lymphoblastic leukemia (ALL)
- Not common in acute nonlymphoblastic leukemia (ANLL), other solid tumors (neuroblastoma may be exception)
- Occurs before therapy, particularly at initiation of therapy

MANIFESTATIONS

- Renal failure: from deposition of urate and phosphate in tubules
- Cardiac arrhythmias: from hyperkalemia, hypocalcemia
- Seizures, tetany: from hypocalcemia
- Metabolic acidosis: from massive cell lysis

MANAGEMENT

- Hydrate:
  1. ⅔-⅓ or D5/0.2 NS at 3-4 L/m^2/day (no added K)
  2. If urine output < 60% of input in 4 hr, give IV furosemide 0.5-1 mg/kg; if no response, IV mannitol 0.5-1 g/kg
- Alkalinize: With 50-100 mEq of NaHCO$_3$/L to keep urine pH between 7-7.5 with specific gravity < 1.010; at pH > 7.5, CaPO$_4$ and hypoxanthine crystals precipitate; therefore adjust NaHCO$_3$ to maintain pH in narrow range of 7-7.5
- Allopurinol: 400 mg/m^2/day divided tid PO or if vomiting, IV (inhibits xanthine oxidase, enzyme that forms uric acid from nucleic acid breakdown)
- Monitor
  1. CBC, lytes, Ca, PO$_4$, urea, creatinine, urate q6h
  2. Urine specific gravity, pH, output qvoid
  3. Accurate ins and outs
- If hyperkalemia: see p. 24
- Consider dialysis if K+ > 6, creatinine > 10 × normal, uric acid > 600 μmol/L and rising despite treatment, phosphate > 3.2 mmol/L, symptomatic hypocalcemia, volume overload, oliguria
- If hypocalcemia:
  1. ECG, cardiac monitor

373

2. Monitor for tetany, seizures
3. Correct hyperphosphatemia with Amphogel 30 mg/kg/day tid
4. No added Ca unless tetany, seizures, ECG abnormality, or critically low ionized calcium; when Ca × PO_4 product is above six, may get metastatic calcification and renal failure

FEVER AND NEUTROPENIA

DEFINITION

- Fever defined as temperature > 38° C orally in presence of absolute neutrophil count (ANC) < 500 (0.5×10^9/L); ANC is sum of mature and band forms of polymorphonuclear leukocytes (PMNs)
- High risk of morbidity and mortality

APPROACH

- Thorough history and physical exam with special attention to
  - Oral mucosa, perioral areas
  - Skin and indwelling catheters
  - Lungs
  - Perirectal areas
- Even subtle signs of inflammation are potential sites of infection

MANAGEMENT

- ABCs if any cardiorespiratory instability (see p. 2)
- CBC and differential

ANC > 500

- Blood culture from central and peripheral site
- Treat with appropriate antibiotics if any infectious source identified from history and physical exam

ANC < 500

- Admit to hospital
- Vital signs q1h until stable and then q4h or as indicated
- Discontinue all antineoplastics and cotrimoxazole prophylaxis
- IV fluids at 1.5 × maintenance via CVL or PIV (use CVL as soon as possible)
- Cultures
  - Blood from peripheral site and all indwelling venous lines
  - Urine
  - Any apparent site of infection
- Electrolytes, urea, creatinine, urinalysis
- CXR if clinically warranted
- Administer antibiotics stat (see following discussion)
- Blood products as required (after antibiotics)

Antibiotic Management

- Broad spectrum coverage: piperacillin 200 mg/kg/day IV divided q6h (max 24 g/day, 6 g/dose) and gentamycin 7.5 mg/kg/day IV divided q8h (max 100 mg/dose before serum monitoring)

- Patients with piperacillin allergy (small incidence of cross reactivity between penicillins and cephalosporins; therefore in patient with significant penicillin allergy such as anaphylaxis, consider consulting infectious disease specialist for alternate antibiotic management or desensitization): ceftazidime 150 mg/kg/day IV divided q8h (max 2 g/dose) and vancomycin 60 mg/kg/day IV divided q6h (max 1 g/dose)
- Patients with double lumen CVLs should have their antibiotic therapy alternated between lumens until CVL cultures are known to be negative
- If blood cultures (peripheral or central) are positive, then repeat cultures should be drawn; antibiotics specifically directed toward identified organism should be added to broad-spectrum coverage; broad spectrum coverage should not be replaced by specific antibiotics alone in neutropenic patient
- Antibiotic therapeutic drug level monitoring if appropriate (see p. 624), especially if receiving concurrent nephrotoxic drugs (e.g., amphotericin, acyclovir); follow renal function
- Patients who deteriorate clinically (e.g., are hemodynamically unstable or show signs of sepsis, see p. 6) should be switched to ceftazidime and vancomycin
- Persistent fever or recurrence of fever without other signs of clinical deterioration is not reason to change initial broad-spectrum therapy
- Consider addition of amphotericin after 5-7 days of persistent fever, and initiate fungal workup

Duration of Antibiotics

- Afebrile, ANC > 500, cultures negative at 48 hr: discontinue antibiotics
- Afebrile, ANC < 500, cultures negative at 48 hr: consider oral antibiotics (see following discussion)
- Afebrile, ANC < 500, cultures negative, IV antibiotic duration > 7 days: consider discontinuing antibiotics
- Afebrile, ANC > 500, cultures positive: consider discontinuing broad-spectrum antibiotics; continue specific therapy

Oral Antibiotic Therapy

- After minimum of 48 hr of IV antibiotic therapy, it may be reasonable to consider oral antibiotics and discharge for patients who meet following criteria:
  - Blood cultures (CVL and peripheral) negative
  - Afebrile for minimum of 24 hr
  - Fever must not have persisted beyond 96 hr
  - Other known infections must be caused by organism known to be sensitive to oral antibiotics used, or infection must be viral in origin (presumed or proven)
  - Clinically well and not in need of inpatient care
  - Able to ingest and absorb oral antibiotics
  - ANC at discharge is <500
- Those who are *not* suitable to start or continue oral therapy include:
  - Fever > 38° C oral (or equivalent) within 24 hr of discharge
  - On induction therapy for malignancy known to significantly involve bone marrow

20

- Known or suspected noncompliance
- Known allergy to recommended oral antibiotics
- Clinical sepsis at presentation
- Recommended oral therapy: cefixime 8 mg/kg/day once daily (max 400 mg/day) and cloxacillin 100 mg/kg/day divided qid (max 4 g/day; capsules only)
- Alternatives for cloxacillin:
  - Flucloxacillin 50 mg/kg/day divided qid (max 2 g/day; if liquid meds needed)
  - Clindamycin 30 mg/kg/day divided qid (max 2 g/day)
  - Erythromycin 40 mg/kg/day divided qid (max 2 g/day)
- Patients should be discharged home on two antibiotics, not one
- Families must have strict follow-up with treatment team
- Recurrence of fever should be approached as new fever in neutropenic host; requires immediate evaluation

SUPERIOR VENA CAVA/MEDIASTINAL SYNDROME

- Compression of vena cava $\pm$ trachea

ETIOLOGY

- Anterior mediastinal mass: NHL, Hodgkin's, germ cell tumor, Ewing's of rib, thymoma
- Infections, histoplasmosis, granuloma
- Vascular thrombosis from cardiac surgery or catheterization

SYMPTOMS

- Chest pain, cough, dyspnea, orthopnea, wheezing, hoarseness, headache, and stupor

SIGNS

- Pulsus paradoxus; swelling and plethora of face, neck, upper extremities; engorged collateral veins; engorged fundal veins; seizures

INVESTIGATIONS

- CXR (for mediastinal mass)
- CBC with diff and smear (leukemia, lymphoma)
- α-fetoprotein; β-HCG (germ cell tumor)
- Assess anesthetic risk: CT of chest without sedation with anesthesia personnel present to evaluate level and degree of airway compression $\pm$ echocardiogram for evaluation of compression
- If possible, tissue diagnosis with least invasive method

TREATMENT

- Elevate head of bed at least 45 degrees
- No sedation or stress, as may precipitate respiratory arrest
- Inform anesthesia about possibility of urgent intubation
- Do not attempt intubation yourself if not emergent as intubation beyond block may be needed or not possible
- IV access in lower limbs only

- Tissue diagnosis: involved nodes, pleural/pericardial tap; if high anesthetic risk, use fine-needle aspiration biopsy under local anesthesia
- If impending respiratory arrest or critical airway compression, treat empirically with prednisone 40 mg/m^2/day + allopurinol + hydration and defer biopsy for up to 48 hr

SPINAL CORD COMPRESSION

ETIOLOGY

- May occur with lymphoma, neuroblastoma, leukemia, and sarcoma of related tissues, drop metastases from medulloblastoma

CLINICAL

- Back pain, localized tenderness, neurologic deficit, urinary retention

INVESTIGATIONS

- Spine x-ray (may be normal)
- Urgent MRI with gadolinium (contrast)
- Urgent lumbar myelography if no MRI available

TREATMENT

- Emergency use: dexamethasone 1-2 mg/kg/day divided q6h (if neurologic dysfunction)
- Urgent neurosurgic consult
- If epidural mass and tumor type not identifiable from another investigation: surgery for decompression and identification
- If lymphoma/leukemia: chemotherapy
- If cause is neuroblastoma, emergency use of chemotherapy and intensive observation may be satisfactory
- For sarcoma: need decompression

LEUKEMIA

20

- Most common childhood malignancy (⅓ of childhood cancer)
- Peak age 2-5 yr; whites > blacks
- Acute: 95%
  ALL: 80% T cell (20%)
      B cell (5%)
      NonB/NonT (75%)
  ANLL: 15%
- Chronic: 5%; adult CML > juvenile CML

APPROACH

- Hematologic: CBC with diff, platelet count, reticulocyte count, PT/PTT
- Biochemical: electrolytes, urea, creatinine, uric acid, Ca, PO$_4$, LFTs, albumin, Igs, complement
- Infectious: varicella zoster antibodies (CMV, HSV, hepatitis)
- Urinalysis
- CXR (for mediastinal mass)

- Bone marrow aspirate: morphology (ALL versus ANLL and subtypes based on FAB classification, L1-L3 for ALL, M0-7 for ANLL), cytochemistry, flow cytometry, and cytogenetics
- For ALL, assign risk category; high risk as follows:
  - Age < 2 yr, > 10 yr
  - WBC > 20×10^9/L
  - L2, L3 morphology
  - Lymphoma syndrome (one criterion from each of clinical and lab groups)
    - Clinical criteria
      1. Lymphadenopathy > 3 cm, node groups > 5 cm
      2. Mediastinal mass
      3. Massive hepatomegaly or splenomegaly (down to umbilicus)
    - Lab criteria
      1. Hb < 100 g/L
      2. WBC > 20×10^9/L

TREATMENT
On Admission

- Prevent and treat tumor lysis: hydrate, alkalinize, allopurinol (see p. 373)
- Treat if febrile and neutropenic (see p. 374)
- Induction therapy 4 wk
- Consolidation
- Delayed reinduction and consolidation for high risk
- Maintenance therapy: total duration for 3 yr

PROGNOSIS

- Low risk: 90% long-term cure rate
- High risk: 70% long-term cure rate

ACUTE NONLYMPHOBLASTIC LEUKEMIA

TREATMENT

- Chemotherapy and CNS prophylaxis
- Bone marrow transplant: allogenic or autologous

PROGNOSIS

- 5 yr disease-free survival: 50% (high risk, 40%; low risk, 70%)

LYMPHOMA

- Third most common pediatric malignancy, 1.68/100,000/yr
- Non-Hodgkin's lymphoma (0.93) common in younger children
- Hodgkin's lymphoma (0.75) common in older children

NON-HODGKIN'S LYMPHOMA
Classification

- Lymphoblastic (30%-35%; 90% T cell, 10% B cell): adolescent with anterior mediastinal mass, cervical or axillary adenopathy, pleural effusion; rapid progression; bone marrow involvement

- Small noncleaved cell (40%-50%); Burkitt's, non-Burkitt's, B cell; abdominal intussusception in older child; fastest growing malignancy; renal failure and tumor lysis common presentation
- Large cell (15%-20%, immunoblastic B > T; anaplastic usually T): usually abdomen; mediastinal and other unusual sites possible; cytokine syndrome with fever and inflammatory features

Staging

I. Single tumor excluding mediastinum and abdomen
II. Several nodal and/or extranodal sites on one side of diaphragm
III. Tumor on both sides of diaphragm; all primary intrathoracic; extensive abdominal, epidural
IV. Confirmed involvement of BM or CNS

Approach

- Baseline: CBC, liver and renal function, urate, PO_4, Ca, LDH
- Staging: CXR, chest and abdominal CT, gallium scan, bone marrow, and CSF exam
- Tissue diagnosis: biopsy

Treatment

- Manage superior mediastinal syndrome (p. 376), tumor lysis (p. 373)
- Chemotherapy; radiation not used in primary treatment

Prognosis

- Stages I, II: 90% cure
- Stages III, IV: 60%-90% cure

HODGKIN'S LYMPHOMA

- Bimodal distribution: peak 15-34 yr and over 50 yr; rare <5 yr
- Three-seven times higher risk in family members

Signs and Symptoms

- Painless lymphadenopathy (90%)
- B symptoms: weight loss > 10%, fever > 38° C, night sweats
- Pruritis; pain with alcohol ingestion
- Baseline: CBC, LFTs, renal function, uric acid, ALK PO_4(bone, liver); ESR (active disease)
- Staging: CXR, chest/abdo/pelvis CT; gallium scan; BM aspirate + biopsy
- Tissue diagnosis: biopsy

Staging

I. Single node; organ (disease free survival [DFS] at 5yr > 90%)
II. Several nodes or extranodal sites on one side of diaphragm (DFS > 90%)
III. Tumor on both sides of diaphragm (DFS = 80%)
IV. Dissemination of extralymphatic involvement (DFS = 80%)

Treatment

- IA (high right neck): radiation
- IA (other)-IIIB: chemotherapy (MOPP/ABV), extended-field low-dose radiation (1500 cGy)
- IV: chemotherapy and radiation to bulk disease

APPROACH TO ABDOMINAL MASSES

- Two most common malignancies are Wilms' and neuroblastoma

Approach to Initial Diagnosis

- History and physical exam
- Abdominal ultrasound (US), CT scan of abdomen to delineate structure of origin (difficult to differentiate neuroblastoma from Wilms' on imaging)
- CBC (polycythemia in Wilms', anemia if bleeding into tumor)
- Electrolytes, urea, creatinine
- PT, PTT (acquired von Willebrand disease with Wilms')
- Urinalysis (hematuria in Wilms')
- VMA/HVA spot and 24-hr urine

NEUROBLASTOMA

- Most common tumor of infancy (8%-10% of cancers); peak age 2 yr

SIGNS AND SYMPTOMS
General

- Unwell child, failure to thrive, fever

Tumor Mass

- Signs and symptoms based on location

Metastases

- Bone pain, periorbital bruising ("raccoon eyes"), skin nodules ("blueberry muffin"), liver

Paraneoplastic

- Opsoclonus-myoclonus, intractable watery diarrhea (VIP), hypertension, sweating

STAGING WORK-UP

- Spot and 24-hr VMA/HVA on urine
- CT of primary tumor, abdomen, chest
- Bilateral BM aspirates + biopsies
- MIBG/bone scan
- Serum ferritin (if high, poor prognosticator)

TISSUE DIAGNOSIS

- Tissue biopsy for histologic classification and biologic predictors of outcome

TREATMENT

- Surgery, if localized
- Chemotherapy, radiation, surgery if nonlocalized
- Minimal treatment for stage IVS
- High-dose chemotherapy and autologous bone marrow transplant

PROGNOSIS (5-yr disease-free survival)

	I + II	III	IV	IVS
<1 year	90%	80%	60%	70%-90%
>1 year	90%	60%	20%	60%

Good Prognostic Factors

- Age <1 yr; paraspinal site; opsoclonus; female; stage I, II, or IVS disease; low serum ferritin; VMA/HVA ratio > 1; aneuploid; no N-myc amplification; favorable histology

WILMS' TUMOR

- Most common primary renal tumor of childhood (6% of all cancers)
- Peak 3-4 yr
- Associated with congenital anomalies (15%): aniridia, hemihypertrophy, Beckwith-Wiedemann syndrome; GU abnormalities, hamartomas

SIGNS AND SYMPTOMS

- Generally child asymptomatic
- Abdominal mass ± hypertension, hematuria
- Bleeding diathesis (acquired von Willebrand disease), polycythemia
- Wilms', aniridia, GU abnormalities, mental retardation (WAGR syndrome)
- Drash syndrome (pseudohermaphroditism, glomerulopathy, and Wilms')
- Associated congenital anomalies

INVESTIGATIONS

- CBC (polycythemia), urinalysis (hematuria), LFTs (metastases), urea, Cr
- Assessment of coagulation (PT, PTT, fibrinogen)
- Abdominal US/CT: function of opposite kidney, lymph node, liver, blood vessel involvement
- Chest CT for metastases

STAGING

- I. Limited to kidney; intact capsule
- II. Regional extension, total excision
- III. Residual tumor in abdomen
- IV. Hematogenous metastases (lung, liver, bone, brain)
- V. Bilateral renal involvement

Table 20-1 Cancer Chemotherapy

Drug*	Action	Metabolism	Excretion	Toxicity
Antimetabolites				
Methotrexate	Folic acid antagonist; inhibits dihydrofolate reductase	Hepatic	Renal, 50%-90% excreted unchanged; biliary	Myelosuppression (nadir 7-10 days), mucositis, stomatitis, dermatitis, hepatitis; renal and CNS† with high-dose administration; prevent with leucovorin, monitor levels
6-Mercaptopurine	Purine analog	Hepatic; allopurinol inhibits metabolism	Renal	Myelosuppression; hepatic necrosis; mucositis; allopurinol increases toxicity
Cytosine arabinoside (Ara-C)	Pyrimidine analog; inhibits DNA polymerase	Hepatic	Renal	Myelosuppression, conjunctivitis, mucositis, CNS† dysfunction
Alkylating Agents				
Cyclophosphamide (Cytoxan)	Alkylates guanine; inhibits DNA synthesis	Hepatic	Renal	Myelosuppression, hemorrhagic cystitis; pulmonary fibrosis, inappropriate ADH‡ secretion, bladder cancer, anaphylaxis
Ifosfamide	Similar to cytoxan	Hepatic	Renal	Similar to cytoxan; CNS† dysfunction, cardiac toxicity
Antibiotics				
Doxorubicin (Adriamycin) and Daunorubicin (Cerubidine)	Binds to DNA, intercalation	Hepatic	Biliary, renal	Cardiomyopathy, red urine, tissue necrosis on extravasation, myelosuppression, conjunctivitis, radiation dermatitis, arrhythmia
Dactinomycin (actinomycin-D)	Binds to DNA, inhibits transcription	—	Renal, stool, 30% excreted unchanged drug	Tissue necrosis on extravasation, myelosuppression, radiosensitizer
Bleomycin	Binds to DNA, cuts DNA	Hepatic	Renal	Pneumonitis, stomatitis, Raynaud's phenomenon, pulmonary fibrosis, dermatitis

Vinca Alkaloids				
Vincristine (Oncovin)	Inhibits microtubule formation	Hepatic	Biliary	Local cellulitis, peripheral neuropathy, constipation, ileus, jaw pain, inappropriate ADH‡ secretion, seizures, ptosis, minimal myelosuppression
Vinblastine (Velban)	Inhibits microtubule formation	Hepatic	Biliary	Local cellulitis, leukopenia
Enzymes				
L-Asparaginase	Depletion of L-asparagine	—	Reticuloendothelial system	Allergic reaction; pancreatitis, hyperglycemia, platelet dysfunction and coagulopathy, encephalopathy
Hormones				
Prednisone	Unknown; lymphocyte modification?	Hepatic	Renal	Cushing's syndrome, cataracts, diabetes, hypertension, myopathy, osteoporosis, infection, peptic ulceration, psychosis
Miscellaneous				
BCNU (carmustine, nitrosourea)	Carbamylation of DNA; inhibits DNA synthesis	Hepatic; phenobarbitol increases metabolism, decreases activity	Renal	Delayed myelosuppression (4–6 wk); pulmonary fibrosis, carcinogenic, stomatitis
Cis-platinum	Inhibits DNA synthesis	—	Renal	Nephrotoxic; myelosuppression, ototoxicity, tetany, neurotoxicity, hemolytic-uremic syndrome; aminoglycosides may increase nephrotoxicity, anaphylaxis
Etoposide (VP-16)	Topoisomerase inhibitor	—	Renal	Myelosuppression, secondary leukemia
Etretinate (vitamin A analogue) and Tretinoin	Enhances normal differentiation	Liver	Liver	Dry mouth, hair loss, pseudo tumor cerebri, premature epiphyseal closure

Modified from Behrman RE, Kliegman RM: *Nelson's essentials of pediatrics*, Philadelphia, 1994, WB Saunders.

*Many drugs produce nausea and vomiting during administration, and many cause alopecia with repeated doses.

†CNS, Central nervous system.

‡ADH, Antidiuretic hormone.

20

TREATMENT AND PROGNOSIS (Disease-Free Survival)

		Favorable histology	Anaplastic
I	Surgery + chemotherapy	95%	90%
II	Surgery + chemotherapy	95%	50%
III	Surgery, chemotherapy, radiation	90%	50%
IV	Surgery, chemotherapy, radiation	75%	50%

PROGNOSTIC FACTORS

- Unfavorable: anaplastic, sarcomatous (rhabdoid, clear cell)

BRAIN TUMORS

- Second most common group of malignant tumors (20%)
- Most infratentorial (70%), except in teens and those <1 yr
- Infratentorial: cerebellar astrocytoma, medulloblastoma
- Brainstem: gliomas
- Supratentorial
  - Cerebral hemisphere: astrocytoma, ependymoma
  - Sella: craniopharyngioma, optic nerve glioma
- Age
  - Ependymomas: soon after birth
  - Medulloblastomas, brainstem glioma: 2-12 yr
  - Astrocytoma: increase with age

SIGNS AND SYMPTOMS
Infratentorial

- Raised intracranial pressure: vomiting, headache, cranial enlargement, papilledema, head tilt, VI nerve palsy
- Other cranial nerves, incoordination, ataxia

Supratentorial

- Focal abnormalities, seizures, long tract signs
- Parinaud's syndrome (pineal tumor): failure of upward gaze and pupillary reaction to light
- Diencephalic syndrome

Dissemination to Spinal Cord

- Medulloblastoma, germ cell: back pain, radicular pain, bowel and bladder symptoms

DIAGNOSIS

- CT
- MRI: better for posterior fossa
- MRI + gadolinium: delineate cystic/solid, blood brain barrier breakdown
- CSF exam: at OR or postop for tumor cells
- Biopsy

CHAPTER 21

OPHTHALMOLOGY

Aʟᴇx Vᴀɴ Lᴇᴠɪɴ ᴀɴᴅ Sᴛᴇᴘʜᴇɴ P. Kʀᴀғᴛ

ROUTINE PROCEDURES AND SCREENING

PERINATAL
Red Reflex

- All infants should be screened in newborn nursery for abnormalities in their red reflexes
- Examiner should use direct ophthalmoscope and stand approximately 0.5 m away from child; while viewing through ophthalmoscope, illuminate both eyes simultaneously using largest circle of white light provided by instrument; focus ophthalmoscope so that face is in focus; reflex may be red or orange-yellow or any combination but must be symmetric between two eyes; test may be easier if child is held close to upright by assistant, this position often causes reflex opening of eyes (see Pupil and Iris for abnormalities of red reflex)

Ophthalmia Neonatorum

- Prophylaxis consists of erythromycin ointment, tetracycline ointment, or silver nitrate 1% drops to both eyes in immediate perinatal period; *Chlamydia* conjunctivitis and gonococcal conjunctivitis may occur despite prophylaxis

PREMATURE NEONATES

- Neonates < 1500 g and/or < 32 wk gestation should have first retinal examination at 4-6 wk postpartum to begin screening for retinopathy of prematurity (see p. 307)
- Neonates > 1500 g or > 32 wk exposed to high doses of oxygen or long-term oxygen may also be at increased risk

INFANTS AND TODDLERS

At time of routine pediatric care visits, all newborns and older infants should have periodic external eye exams for anatomic eye defects, ocular movements, ocular alignment, injected conjunctivitis, and ability of each eye individually to fixate on and follow objects at close range; infants should be able to fixate on face of caretaker while feeding

- Assessment of red reflex should be performed at each routine postnatal visit

>4 YEARS

- In general, children should be seen by ophthalmologist if there are systemic risk factors, ocular signs, family history of significant ocular disease, or visual symptoms; otherwise, when able to do so, visual acuity screening by letter, picture, or E game chart should be conducted by primary care physician or school annually until 10 yr of age, after which screening should continue every 2-3 yr

BASIC PRINCIPLES

- When patient has glasses, visual acuity should be tested when patient is wearing glasses
- Abnormal vision corrected by viewing through pinholes indicates need for glasses as opposed to nonglasses-related ocular pathology; pinhole test useful on patients who have no glasses or have not brought glasses to examination; with glasses on, useful improvement of vision through pinhole indicates need for recheck of glasses prescription; pinhole device can be made by placing several 18-gauge needle holes in piece of paper, which child then holds up to his or her eye
- When testing vision, test one eye at a time, being sure that eye not being tested is securely covered; preferable to tape nontested eye shut rather than making use of hand to cover eye
- Amblyopia refers to subnormal vision in eye, not caused by internal eye disease; it may or may not be associated with strabismus; amblyopia can be unilateral or (less commonly) bilateral; usually due to arrest of visual development of unpreferred eye since it is "ignored" by the brain; causes of amblyopia include any ocular abnormality that makes one eye less preferred (e.g., unequal glasses prescription, ptosis, strabismus)
- If there is high suspicion of ruptured globe either by history or exam (see Cornea), exam should be *stopped, no drops* instilled, eye *shielded* (not patched), and patients referred immediately to ophthalmologist
- If ruptured globe has been ruled out, there is virtually no contraindication to dilating pupils for maximum visibility on retina examination (phenylephrine 2.5%, cyclopentolate 1%, and/or tropicamide 1%); if concern about impaired pupillary reactivity for neurologic assessment, use only short-acting mydriatic, phenylephrine, or dilate one eye at time
- Only contraindication to using drop of topical anesthetic (proparacaine or tetracaine) on intact globe is known allergy to this class of anesthetics; if patient feels better after drop instillation, then pain is coming from eye surface (cornea or conjunctiva) problem
- Direct ophthalmoscope may be used as hand-held illuminated magnifier to view ocular surface and iris by dialing in higher black/green numbers as one gets closer to patient
- Ophthalmology consultation is recommended in all cases of decreased visual acuity [poor fixation of eye during preverbal years, <20/40 [6/12] in verbal preschool child, <20/20 [6/6] in school-aged child)
- Topical steroids, atropine or homatropine, miotics, glaucoma treatments, or antivirals should not be used without ophthalmologic consultation

EYELIDS

HORDEOLUM (STYE) AND CHALAZION

- Obstruction of eyelid glands; on eyelid margin (stye) or within body of lid (chalazion); stye may have discharge; chalazion may be chronic, mobile, noninflamed lump

- Treatment: baby shampoo eyelash scrubs; erythromycin or Polysporin ointment for 1 wk may be helpful; refer if nonresolving, symptomatic, chronic chalazion on lid scrubs for 4-6 wk

TRAUMA

- May result in ptosis, ecchymosis, edema, or laceration
- Upper lid eversion and complete dilated eye examination should be performed to rule out foreign body or injury to globe; may require radiologic studies (see discussion on blowout fractures)
- Ophthalmologic consultation required for ptosis that persists after ecchymosis and swelling have resolved, laceration of eyelid margin or extending obliquely into canthus, deep lacerations with or without ptosis

PTOSIS

- Drooping of upper eyelid; can be unilateral or bilateral, congenital or acquired; can be isolated abnormality or associated with neurologic or orbital disease
- Severe ptosis (covering pupil) can cause amblyopia in young children
- Hemangiomas of lids can cause ptosis and result in amblyopia

NASOLACRIMAL DUCT OBSTRUCTION

- Generally from congenital failure of complete canalization of lower end of nasolacrimal duct
- Recurrent mild discharge with or without tearing, without conjunctival injection; worse on waking, when outdoors, and during upper respiratory infection; often associated with crusting on lid margins and chronic changes in lower lid skin

Treatment

- Massage several times per day; place index finger in sulcus between eye and side of nasal bridge (medial to medial canthus), apply pressure in posterior direction (toward occiput) or in circular motion; discharge may be expressed on to surface of eye
- May administer 1-week courses of antibiotic drops during periods of increased discharge
- Majority of cases resolve spontaneously by 12 mo of age after minimum of 3 mo of massage; otherwise, refer to ophthalmologist

21

CONJUNCTIVA

NEONATAL CONJUNCTIVITIS
Chemical

- Purulent conjunctivitis, lid edema; occurs in first 24 hr usually following instillation of silver nitrate prophylaxis; treatment involves frequent saline lavage and erythromycin or Polysporin ointment

N. Gonorrhea Conjunctivitis

- Marked purulent discharge and lid edema
- Vision-threatening emergency; usually occurs in first week of life but may occur any time in first few mo

- Gram stain shows intracellular gram-negative diplococci; must have culture confirmation to rule out nonpathogenic diplococci but begin treatment based on Gram stain
- Requires IM ceftriaxone with or without topical treatment with erythromycin or Polysporin; frequent ocular lavage with normal saline may be beneficial
- Evaluate child for other sexually transmitted diseases, including syphilis and *Chlamydia;* arrange for culture and treatment of mother and her partner(s)

Chlamydia

- Milder conjunctivitis; less discharge and edema
- Usually occurs in first or second week of life but chronic carriage with delayed symptoms may occur
- Culture should be performed, but rapid immunologic tests on eye swab are acceptable; Gram stain negative; giemsa stain of conjunctival scrapings
- Treat with *oral* erythromycin 40-50 mg/kg/day divided into four doses for 14-21 days, in addition to topical erythromycin, to prevent subsequent pneumonitis
- Arrange for culture and treatment of mother and her partner(s)

Other

- Conjunctivitis may be caused by various other bacteria and viruses in neonatal period; herpetic keratoconjunctivitis is diagnosed with dendritic ulcer on fluorescein stain and should be referred to ophthalmology; bacteria should be treated with appropriate antibiotics

CONJUNCTIVITIS BEYOND NEONATAL PERIOD (Table 21-1)

- Antibiotics are only indicated when bacterial conjunctivitis proven or strongly suspected
- Avoid sulfa agents (risk of Stevens-Johnson syndrome), aminoglycosides (corneal toxicity and selection of prevalent resistant organisms), combined steroid-antibiotics, fluoroquinolones, and products containing neomycin (high allergy rate)
- Recommend erythromycin (ointment), Polysporin (ointment or drop), Polytrim

Chemical

- Early management at home: tap water or shower
- In emergency room, immediate copious lavage (saline or any available variation) is essential; use 2 L or continue for 20 min; topical anesthetic before lavage only if readily available
- Monitor pH of affected eye if test strip is available; lavage should continue until pH is equal to that of nonaffected eye; upper lid eversion and if required, eyelid speculum and restraint; do not wait for sedation
- After lavage, treat as corneal abrasion; all alkali or acid burns require urgent ophthalmologic consultation

Table 21-1 Differential Diagnosis of Conjunctivitis

	Bacterial	Viral (nonherpetic)	Herpetic	Chlamydial	Allergic
Discharge	Purulent	Clear or mildly purulent	Clear	Mildly purulent	Clear
Lid swelling	Moderate to severe	Mild to severe	Mild	Mild	Mild to severe
Onset	Subacute	Subacute	Acute	Subacute or chronic	Hyperacute (exposure) or chronic (seasonal)
Injection	Severe	Moderate to severe	Moderate (focal)	Moderate	Mild to severe
Cornea fluorescein staining	Nonspecific	Nonspecific	Dendrite	Nonspecific	None
White corneal infiltrates	—	Adenovirus (late)	Possible	Multiple peripheral	—
Unilateral/bilateral	Uni/bi	Uni/bi	Uni	Usually bi	Usually bi
Contact history	Common	Common	No	Common; STD*	Rare
Preauricular node	Common	Common	Occasional	Occasional	None
Other associations	Otitis media	Otitis media, pharyngitis	History of skin lesions	Genital discharge	Chemosis

*STD, Sexually transmitted disease symptoms or contact.

21

Chemosis

- Blisterlike swelling of conjunctiva from conjunctival inflammation, allergy, generalized systemic edema, or venous obstruction (e.g., cavernous sinus thrombosis)
- Treatment: artificial tear ointments to avoid desiccation

TRAUMA
Subconjunctival Hemorrhage

- Caused by blunt trauma, Valsalva maneuver, severe forceful cough, severe vomiting, bleeding diathesis, severe hypertension, or suffocation
- Infants and young children with large (180°-360°) hemorrhages should have full ocular examination to search for nontraumatic causes
- Following trauma, 360° hemorrhage should prompt ophthalmology consult to assess scleral integrity especially if accompanied by chemosis
- Treatment is generally limited to artificial tears for comfort; blood resorbs over 7-14 days and turns dark red, green and yellow before disappearance

Foreign Body

- May be hidden in recesses of fornices; have patient look in all directions to expose; upper lid eversion may be needed; remove with forceps or cotton swab

CORNEA

FOREIGN BODY

- Lies on or may be embedded in cornea
- Diagnosis by examination with light, magnification, and fluorescein staining
- High-velocity foreign bodies (e.g., hammering metal on metal) may require ophthalmologic consultation and radiologic investigation, even with minimal external evidence of injury to rule out penetration into eye or orbit; ophthalmologic consultation generally recommended
- After removal, patient is treated as for corneal abrasion

ABRASION

- Area of absent corneal epithelium
- Symptoms are pain and photophobia relieved by topical anesthetic
- Corneal fluorescein stain shows area of absent epithelium
- If vertical linear abrasion(s), suspect conjunctival foreign body under upper lid and perform lid eversion, facilitated by having patient look down during procedure
- Treat with Polysporin or erythromycin ointment plus cycloplegic agent (cyclopentolate 1%); patch affected eye for 24 hr; refer if still symptomatic after 24-48 hr, large central abrasion, or poor healing

LACERATIONS OR RUPTURED GLOBE

- Requires immediate ophthalmologic consultation
- May be caused by blunt trauma, as well as penetration by sharp objects;

clinical features are oval pupil, hyphema, iris prolapsing through cornea, black/blue/brown tissue protruding from sclera, 360° subconjunctival hemorrhage, or posttraumatic chemosis
- If high index of suspicion on history alone and marked lid edema or noncompliant patient, refer or use nonpressure techniques to gently open lids (speculum, pressure with thumbs on orbital bones to draw lids apart)
- Stop eye examination immediately; shield eye; no pressure on eye; no eyedrops

ENLARGED OR CLOUDY CORNEA

- May indicate glaucoma or systemic disease; refer promptly

ANTERIOR CHAMBER

HYPHEMA

- Blood in anterior chamber (behind cornea and in front of iris)
- Almost always sign of severe ocular trauma; requires urgent ophthalmologic consultation
- Treatment may include bed rest, shielding, oral antifibrinolytics, topical steroids, and/or cycloplegics; recurrent hemorrhage and secondary glaucoma may occur; sickle cell anemia patients at higher risk

IRITIS

- Inflammation in aqueous humor
- Causes include trauma, collagen vascular disease, JRA, sarcoid, Lyme disease, leukemia, retinoblastoma, intraocular infection; may be acute or chronic and asymptomatic, as in some forms of juvenile arthritis
- On inspection, ring of conjunctival injection behind edge of corneal scleral junction may represent ciliary flush of iritis, but slit-lamp examination is required for diagnosis
- Traumatic iritis may be delayed 24-48 hr following trauma
- Treatment: topical cycloplegics and steroids after ophthalmologic consultation; orbital injections, oral steroids, or IV steroids may be needed in severe cases

HYPOPYON

- Collection of white cells in anterior chamber
- Causes include internal ocular infection, tumors, or severe inflammation; refer promptly

PUPILS AND IRIS

AFFERENT PUPIL DEFECT (APD) (MARCUS-GUNN'S PUPIL)

- Diagnosed by swinging-flashlight test of consensual pupil responses
- Indicates visual pathway pathology anterior to optic chiasm (e.g., severe vitreous hemorrhage, retinal detachment, optic nerve disease) and requires thorough ophthalmic and neurologic assessments

ANISOCORIA

- Must first ascertain which pupil is abnormal
- Each pupil should be examined for reactivity; nonreactive pupil is abnormal but if both react briskly, examine size of pupils under very dim and bright illumination; if anisocoria is worse in dim light, then smaller pupil is abnormal one (Horner's syndrome or scarring following intraocular inflammation); if anisocoria is enhanced by bright illumination, then larger pupil is abnormal (third nerve palsy, traumatic mydriasis, or Adie tonic pupil)
- Most common cause is physiologic anisocoria, which occurs in 20% of population; in this case, relative difference in pupil size will be same in light or dim illumination

COLOBOMA

- Inferior-nasal defect in iris (keyhole pupil)
- May be associated with microphthalmia or visually significant coloboma involving retina and/or optic nerve

LEUKOCORIA

- White pupillary reflex; causes can be congenital (e.g., cataract) or acquired (e.g., retinoblastoma tumor)
- Requires prompt ophthalmologic consultation

ABSENT RED REFLEX

- Black reflex caused by inability of light to pass into eye because of obstruction from corneal opacity, hyphema, cataract, vitreous hemorrhage
- Requires ophthalmologic consultation
- Most common cause is small pupils, especially in neonates; repeat red reflex test (see Routine Procedures and Screening) after pharmacologic dilation of pupils; if normal, then no referral needed

RETINA

RETINAL HEMORRHAGES

- May be caused by birth, vasculitis, meningitis, cyanotic congenital heart disease, endocarditis, sepsis, blood dyscrasias, severe life-threatening accidental head trauma, and shaken baby syndrome
- These entities can usually be distinguished based on history and dilated exam by ophthalmologist
- CPR is extremely rare cause and then is only associated with few hemorrhages in posterior retina
- Child abuse team consultation may be important diagnostic test, particularly when no obvious cause is found (see p. 26)
- Sickle cell disease and diabetes *do not* cause retinal hemorrhages in young children

INTRAOCULAR CANDIDIASIS

- Appears as fluffy white intraretinal, preretinal, or vitreous opacities
- Ophthalmology exam required only when *Candida* isolated from sys-

temic site, representing true infection (not colonization) in immunocompromised child
- Treatment: IV amphotericin; sometimes requires intraocular intervention

RETINAL CYTOMEGALOVIRUS INFECTION (CMV)
- Necrotic hemorrhagic retinitis; may involve optic nerve
- More common in immunosuppressed children, especially HIV; screening eye exam recommended only when such children have active systemic CMV, positive urine, or nasopharyngeal CMV

OPTIC NERVE

PAPILLEDEMA
- Characterized by blurred optic disc margins, peripapillary splinter hemorrhages, disc elevation, loss of optic nerve central cup, dilation and tortuosity of veins at optic nerve, and possibly retinal exudates; presence of spontaneous venous pulsations does not rule out diagnosis
- Papillitis may look similar on clinical examination; vision usually preserved in papilledema, decreased in papillitis
- Bilateral papilledema usually from increased intracranial pressure; papillitis may be from vasculitis; optic nerve infiltration with neoplastic cells (e.g., leukemia) is main differential diagnosis
- Treatment depends on underlying cause

OPTIC ATROPHY
- Can be congenital or acquired
- Requires thorough ophthalmic and neurologic investigations

OPTIC NERVE HYPOPLASIA
- Congenital anomaly with varying degrees of severity
- Mild forms may be compatible with good vision
- Most cases are unilateral; bilateral cases may require neurologic assessment because of association with CNS abnormalities such as septo-optic dysplasia

21

STRABISMUS (Figs. 21-1 and 21-2)
- Strabismus refers to any kind of abnormal eye alignment
- Esotropia (crossed eyes) may be infantile (congenital) or from need for glasses to correct farsightedness (accommodative esotropia); in latter, eyes will still cross with glasses off
- Esotrophia and exotropia (turned-out eyes) may be treated with patching, glasses, and/or surgery
- Hypertropia (one eye higher) may be seen in children with congenital strabismus or may be suggestive of more serious underlying orbit or neurologic problem
- Alignment can be assessed by Hirschberg (light reflex) test (see Fig. 21-1)
- Pseudoesotropia is appearance of crossing because of wide nasal bridge

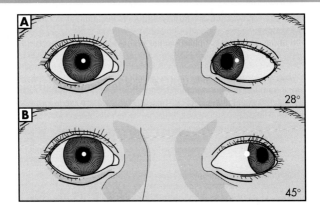

Fig. 21-1 Hirschberg's Test. Light reflection on cornea is observed by examiner. **A,** Left esotropia; resulting from in-turning of left eye, light reflex appears to be lateral to center of pupil. **B,** Left exotropia; resulting from out-turning of left eye, light reflex appears medial to center of pupil.

and/or epicanthal folds; Hirschberg light reflexes will be central and symmetric in each eye
- Strabismus may cause amblyopia in eye that is misaligned, but in many cases eyes retain equal vision despite strabismus; if amblyopia is present, and child is less than 6-10 yr old, patching of good eye may help brain to redevelop vision in amblyopic eye
- Children with strabismus usually have no symptoms (e.g., no diplopia)
- Refer child with strabismus after 4 mo of age, as eyes should be straight and more in tandem by this age, sooner if eyes extremely misaligned
- Children with neurologic problems, such as cerebral palsy or after head trauma can show various abnormalities of eye alignment
- Strabismus is only emergent when eye(s) cannot move fully in all directions; may indicate paretic muscle or restriction (see the following discussion)
- Test each eye independently up, down, and to either side; active following movements are equivalent to passive doll's head maneuver eye movements

BLOWOUT FRACTURE

- Results from blunt trauma pushing eye into socket and causing one or more bones of orbital wall to fracture; fractures involving inferior or medial wall are most common
- Restriction of eye movement may occur; eye may appear sunken or proptotic; hypoesthesia of inferior orbital skin may occur in inferior floor fracture

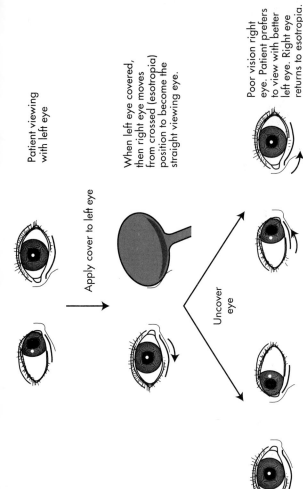

Patient viewing with left eye

Apply cover to left eye

When left eye covered, then right eye moves from crossed (esotropia) position to become the straight viewing eye.

Uncover eye

Poor vision right eye. Patient prefers to view with better left eye. Right eye returns to esotropia.

Equal vision. Right eye able to continue viewing, leaving the left eye esotropic.

Fig. 21-2 Use of cover-uncover test to evaluate strabismus.

21

- CT scan with coronal views for diagnosis; many cases of eye movement restrictions will resolve spontaneously
- Ophthalmologic consultation often helpful; surgical intervention for severe enophthalmos, orbital roof fracture, failure of conservative management

CHAPTER 22

ORTHOPEDICS

Fatima Roshanali Kamalia

LOWER LIMB

INTOEING (Fig. 22-1)

- Establish torsional profile (Fig. 22-2)
  1. Foot progression angle
  2. Measure range of internal and external rotation at hip
  3. Measure thigh-foot angle
  4. Measure degree of metatarsus varus
- Establish coordination profile
  1. Jumping by age 2 yr
  2. Hopping by age 4 yr

Differential Diagnosis

- Metatarsus varus
- Internal tibial torsion: thigh-foot angle $< -10°$
- Internal femoral torsion: external rotation of hip $<20°$

Management

- Metatarsus varus: neonate, if flexible, observe 3-9 mo, and if rigid, refer to orthopedic surgery for casts, Wheaton splints, or articulated boot; 9 mo-2 yr, ignore; >2 yr, surgical correction
- Internal tibial torsion: 9-18 mo, observe, rarely consider Denis Browne night splints $\times$ 3-4 mo or counter-rotation splints
- Internal femoral torsion: splints and shoes ineffective; correct sitting habits (encourage lotus position); if severe, consider osteotomy at 10 yr for exceptional cases

OUTTOEING

- Usually external femoral torsion; self-correcting when child begins to roll over

FOOT SHAPE CONCERNS (Table 22-1)

- Must do full neurologic examination (including gait and arch assessment)
- Examine hips carefully

KNEE PAIN

- May be referred pain from hip (e.g., slipped epiphysis)
- Meniscal injury rare in children

Text continued on p. 403.

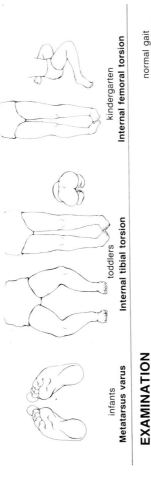

infants
Metatarsus varus

toddlers
Internal tibial torsion

kindergarten
Internal femoral torsion

normal gait
angle is + 10°

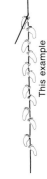

This example
shows—30°

EXAMINATION

1

Assess
Gait
Angle

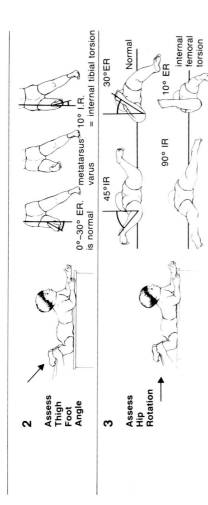

Fig. 22-1 Intoeing varieties (From *Easter Seal guide to children's orthopaedics: prevention, screening, and problem solving*, Ontario, 1982, The Easter Seal Society.)

22

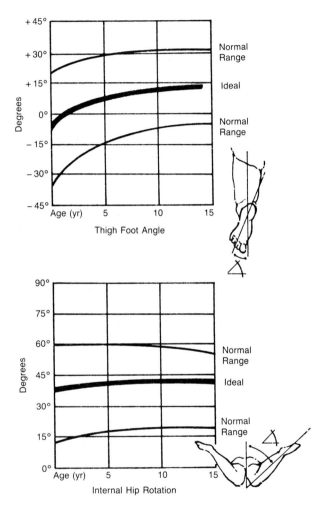

Fig, 22-2 Torsional profile. (Modified from Stahill LT, et al: Lower extremity-rotational problems in children: normal values to guide management, *J Bone Joint Surg* 67A: 41-43, 1985.)

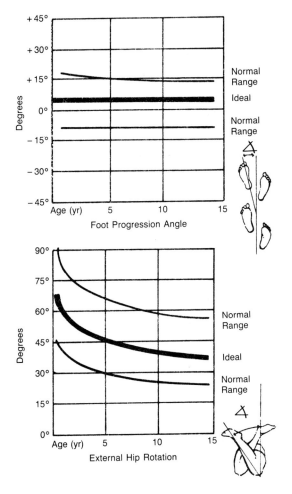

Fig. 22-2, cont'd. See opposite page for legend.

Table 22-1 Differential Diagnosis and Management of Foot Shape Abnormalities

	Age of presentation	Frequency	Main feature	Treatment
Clubfoot	Birth	1:700	Fixed equino varus	Serial casts at birth; operate on 80% at 3 mo
Calcaneovalgus foot	Birth	1:300	Top of foot rests on shin	Always recovers; advise stretching
Metatarsus varus	Birth-3 mo	1:100	Forefoot adduction	Brace at 3 mo; after 2 yr, requires operation
Vertical talus	Birth-3 mo	1:100,000	Rocker bottom sole	Usually requires surgical correction
Hypermobile flat foot	2 yr+	1:10	Arch appears on tiptoeing	Ignore; unaffected by attempts to treat
Pes cavus	10 yr+	1:10,000	Fixed high arch	Investigate: spinal x-ray; nerve conduction studies; possibly myelogram; idiopathic, usually symmetric; often requires surgery
Toe walking	3 yr+	1:700	Short calf muscle	Exclude dystrophy and cerebral palsy; if persistent, grow muscle with stretching casts

OSGOOD-SCHLATTER DISORDER

- Chronic stress fracture of tibial tubercle
- X-ray necessary to rule out other conditions; shows enlarged and fragmented tibial tubercle
- Treatment consists of explanation, quadricep and hamstring stretching, and reassurance (lasts ~18 mo); continue sports using basketball knee protector

PERIPATELLAR PAIN SYNDROME

- Most frequent source of knee pain, probably results from overuse
- Pain reproduced by compressing patella against femur
- X-ray normal
- Anticipate protracted course; quadriceps-strengthening exercises may help

OSTEOCHONDRITIS DISSECANS

- Aching knee pain and "giving way"
- Characteristic x-ray findings: notched lateral aspects of medial femoral condyle
- Refer to orthopedic surgeon
- Observe, occasionally immobilize; rarely drill or pin back; tends to heal spontaneously in those still growing

RECURRENT DISLOCATION OF PATELLA

- May dislocate spontaneously
- Axial x-ray film of patella with knee flexed 40° shows shallow groove
- Treat with quadriceps-strengthening exercises first; usually requires surgical repair

HIP PROBLEMS (Table 22-2)

CONGENITAL DISLOCATION OF HIP

- More common in girls, firstborn, left hip, breech presentation
- Stage 1: Dislocatable, hip stays in joint but can be pushed out on Barlow test (Fig. 22-3, *B*); usually recovers spontaneously after few wk
- Stage 2: Dislocated but reducible, positive Ortolani's test (Fig. 22-3, *A*); lasts few wk before stage 3
- Stage 3: Fixed dislocation irreducible; abduction is limited and thigh looks short (Galeazzi sign, Fig. 22-4); seen after age 3 mo

Differential Diagnosis

- Synovial click: noise from hip resembling cracking knuckles; positive Ortolani's sign is not noise but feeling of femoral head jumping into joint; clicks require continued follow-up
- Congenital adduction contracture in child with "windswept" hips (i.e., adduction contracture of one hip and abduction contracture of other hip)
- Congenital femoral hypoplasia
- Fixed dislocation in arthrogryposis

22

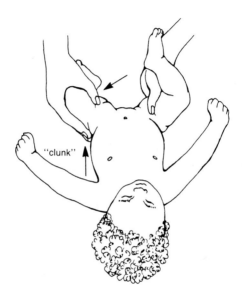

Fig. 22-3 Recognition of congenital dislocation of hip (CDH). (Modified from Shelov MD, Mezey AP, Edelmann CM Jr, Barnett HL: *Primary care pediatrics: a symptomatic approach*, Norwalk, Conn, 1984, Appleton-Century-Crofts.)

Investigations

- US (investigation of choice <3 mo) or x-ray (AP + frogleg) >3 months

Treatment

- Pavlik harness: 0-8 mo
- Traction and closed reduction: 8-18 mo
- Traction, open reduction, innominate osteotomy: 18-30 mo
- Traction, open reduction, innominate osteotomy and femoral shortening: 30 mo-5 yr

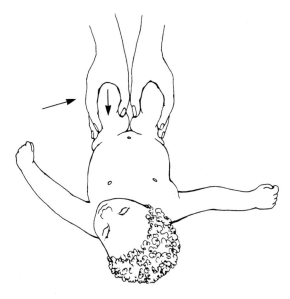

Fig. 22-3, cont'd. See opposite page for legend.

LEGG-CALVÉ-PERTHES DISEASE

- Idiopathic avascular necrosis of femoral head
- Diagnosis made by x-ray (AP and frogleg); changes usually obvious by time patient symptomatic
- "Containment" and maintenance of full range of motion (ROM) are underlying principles of treatment; varies from simple observation to bracing or surgery, depending on age of child and extent of disease
- Bone scan, MRI helpful in occasional cases in which diagnosis is unclear

TRANSIENT SYNOVITIS

- May be difficult to differentiate from early "septic" hip
- Usually afebrile or low-grade fever, and child looks well
- Usually able but reluctant to bear weight; limited and painful hip ROM

22

Table 22-2 Clinical Features of Some Common Hip Disorders

	CDH*	Transient synovitis	Legg-Calvé-Perthes	SFCE	Septic arthritis
Age	0-4 yr	4-8 yr	3-10 yr	8-15 yr	Any (0-1 yr most common)
ROM	↓ Abduction	↓ at extremes	↓ Abduction in flexion	↓ Flexion and internal rotation	↓ With slight movement
Pain	None	+ → + + +	0 → +	+ Ext. rotation in flexion	+ + + +
X-ray	Dislocation	Normal	Abnormal, varies with stage	Abnormal: slip	Frequently normal
Leg size	Normal	Normal	Shorter	Shorter	Normal
Body temperature	Normal	Normal	Normal	Normal	↑
ESR	Normal	Can be ↑	Normal	Normal	↑: Can be normal in early cases
Treatment	External splint early; surgery late	Rest, gentle ROM exercises	Observation, brace, or surgery, depending on age and extent	Surgery	Surgery and antibiotics

CDH, Congenital dislocated hip; *SFCE,* slipped femoral capital epiphysis; *ROM,* range of motion.

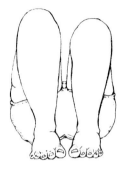

Fig. 22-4 Allis' or Galeazzi's sign. Knee is lower on affected side when knees and hips are flexed because femoral head lies posterior to acetabulum in this position. (Modified from Shelov MD, Mezey AP, Edelmann CM Jr, Barnett HL: *Primary care pediatrics:a symptomatic approach,* Norwalk, Conn, 1984, Appleton-Century-Crofts.)

Investigations

- WBC, ESR usually normal; help to distinguish from septic hip or osteomyelitis; x-ray to exclude Legg-Calvé-Perthes
- If unable to differentiate from septic hip, refer to orthopedic surgery for joint aspiration

Treatment

- Bed rest (at home in most cases) ± nonsteroidal antiinflammatory agent (e.g., naprosyn)
- ± Gentle ROM exercises; gradual resumption of activity
- Careful observation to rule out early septic arthritis
- If recurrent or persistent, need to rule out Legg-Calvé-Perthes, especially if persists beyond two wk with bed rest (~1% are Legg-Calvé-Perthes)

SLIPPED FEMORAL CAPITAL EPIPHYSIS (SFCE)

- 30% bilateral; 90% chronic and 10% acute
- Presents most commonly as insidious ache in groin or knee; often mistaken for "pulled" muscle; diagnosis frequently delayed
- May present as acute severe pain and inability to bear weight following trauma

Investigations

- Lateral frogleg of both hips most useful x-ray in mild degrees of slip
- Previous history of SFCE in contralateral hip requires orthopedic consultation even in absence of x-ray abnormalities

DIAGNOSTIC APPROACH TO THE LIMPING CHILD

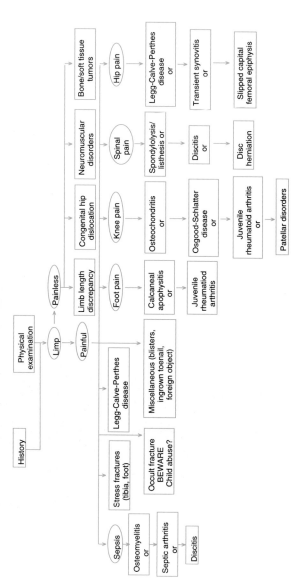

Fig. 22-5   Diagnostic approach to limping child. (From Baxter MP: Evaluating the limping child, *Diagnosis* Jan: 168-169, 1988.)

Treatment

- Urgent surgical pinning of hip
- Association with delayed bone age; rule out endocrine abnormality

SPINE

SCOLIOSIS

- Many minimal curves noted in school screening are nonprogressive
- Early presentation (infancy and early childhood) suggests underlying skeletal or neuromuscular disorder
- All children should have forward-bend test as part of routine physical exam (Fig. 22-6); prominence of one side (ribs or lumbar area) indicates scoliosis

Investigations

- Three-foot *standing* PA x-ray of spine: single film is all that is required to confirm and quantify using Cobb angle (Fig. 22-7); Risser stage refers to stage of skeletal maturation based on degree of ossification of iliac crest

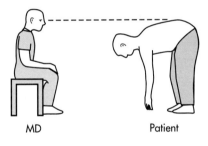

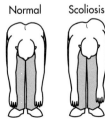

22

Fig. 22-6 Forward-bend test. Seven percent of rotation using scoliometer is nominal value for requesting x-ray of spine.

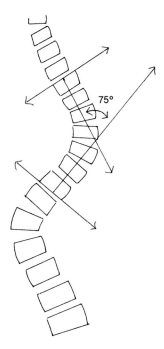

Fig. 22-7 **Measurement of Cobb angle in scoliosis.** Cobb angle is angle between perpendiculars intersecting superior surface of top and inferior surface of bottom vertebrae of curve.

Treatment

- Still growing
    1. 10°-25°: Check every 6 mo using x-ray exam
    2. 25°-45°: Brace
    3. 45°+: Spinal instrumentation and fusion
    - Growth complete
    1. <45°: Ignore
    2. 45°: Spinal instrumentation

KYPHOSIS
Investigations

- Standing lateral x-ray to measure angle of kyphosis between T-3 and T-12

Treatment

- Still growing
  1. <30°: Normal
  2. 30°-45°: Mild; monitor
  3. 45°+: Consider brace
- Growth complete and 50°+: consider surgical correction

BACK PAIN

- More likely to be definite cause in children than in adults, however, 70% have no demonstable cause

Differential Diagnosis

- Mechanical: spondylolisthesis, Scheuermann's, thoracolumbar osteochondritis
- Infection: osteomyelitis, diskitis
- Tumors and tumorlike conditions: eosinophilic granuloma, aneurysmal bone cyst, osteoblastoma, osteoid osteoma
- Injury

Investigations

- X-ray exam, ESR, bone scan
- Consider CT scan or MRI

UPPER LIMB

PULLED ELBOW

- Common in children 2-5 yr of age
- Produced by tug on outstretched arm; radial head is abruptly pulled distally to become trapped by annular ligament
- Child will not use arm (pseudoparalysis)
- Fracture is main differential diagnosis

Investigations

- X-ray normal; rule out other injury, fracture

Treatment

22

- On supination of forearm, "click" felt; represents radial head reducing through ligament
- Pain disappears within few min
- Occasionally requires second attempt next day

NECK

CONGENITAL MUSCULAR TORTICOLLIS

- Contracture of sternomastoid
- Physiotherapy to stretch (Fig. 22-8); surgical release in neglected cases
- Examine hips carefully; may be associated with hip dislocation

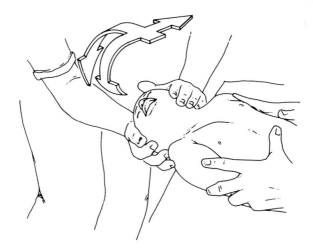

Fig. 22-8 Exercises to stretch out tight sternomastoid muscle in congenital torticollis. Motion is combination of rotation toward affected (right) side, tilting away from affected side, and extension of neck. (From Behrman RE, Vaughan VC, Nelson WE, editors: *Nelson textbook of pediatrics,* ed 13, Philadelphia, 1987, WB Saunders.)

INJURIES

- Sprains rare in children; usually greenstick, buckle, or epiphyseal fractures requiring x-ray diagnosis
- Fractures in infant <18 mo: high index of suspicion for nonaccidental injury (see p. 26)

Management

- Check circulation and nerve function
- Look for skin wound or puncture wound
- NPO in case of potential surgery
- Cover open wounds with sterile dressings, splint, then x-ray
- Undisplaced metaphyseal or diaphyseal fractures: immobilize
- Displaced metaphyseal/diaphyseal fractures: reduce under anesthesia
- Fractures into joint (types 3 and 4) require open reduction (Fig. 22-9)
- Open fractures (including fractures associated with puncture wounds) require tetanus prophylaxis (see p. 434), antibiotic treatment, and urgent debridement

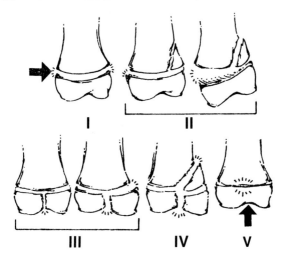

Fig. 22-9 Classification of growth plate injuries. (From Salter RB, Harris WR: Injuries involving the epiphyseal plate, *J Bone Joint Surg* 45A:587, 1963.)

INFECTIONS

SEPTIC ARTHRITIS
Clinical

- Neonatal: nosocomial infection, often multifocal, may be subtle (i.e., pain on moving hip to change diaper; fever)
- Childhood type often solitary
- Acute onset pain, decreased ROM; hot, swollen joint held flexed

Investigations

- US for effusion
- Joint aspiration (hip requires general anesthetic) for WBC and differential, glucose, Gram stain, latex agglutination, culture
- CBC, ESR, blood cultures (only 70% positive)
- X-ray examination to exclude fracture; usually normal
- Bone radionuclide scan (technetium, gallium) may be useful if adjacent osteomyelitis suspected
- Osteomyelitis must be ruled out before antibiotic therapy discontinued

Treatment

- Prompt joint drainage (consult orthopedics) and institution of IV antibiotic treatment are crucial; thick pus does not come out through needle; therefore surgical drainage required in most cases (e.g., hip, shoulder)

22

- Continuous passive movement reduces stiffness and speeds healing; avoid weight bearing during acute illness
- Analgesics for pain control

Antibiotic Therapy

- For empiric therapy, see Table 22-3 (adjust therapy to results of Gram stain and culture)
- If aspiration for diagnosis is imminent, do not start antibiotics until afterward to increase diagnostic yield
- Antibiotics should be given by IV initially; once signs of acute inflammation have resolved, one can switch to equivalent dose of antibiotics if following conditions are met:
  1. Patient can tolerate oral medications, and strict compliance is ensured
  2. Follow-up can be maintained with weekly monitoring of clinical condition and ESR; follow-up x-ray examination before discontinuing therapy if osteomyelitis suspected
- Duration (dependent on clinical response)
  1. Antibiotics should be given for minimum of 2 wk
  2. Shorter courses (1 wk) can be given for gonococcal arthritis
  3. Longer courses (3-4 wk) advised for *S. aureus* arthritis of hip joint, neonates, immunocompromised patients, gram-negative arthritis, or underlying osteomyelitis (4-6 wk)
- Intraarticular instillation of antibiotics is unnecessary and frequently causes chemical arthritis

OSTEOMYELITIS
Clinical

- Neonate: *S. aureus*, gram-negative bacilli, group B *streptococci*
- Infants and children: *S. aureus;* less commonly *S. pneumoniae, H. influenzae,* group A *streptococci*

Table 22-3   Etiologic Organisms and Empiric Antibiotic Selection for Septic Arthritis/Osteomyelitis*

Age	Potential organisms	Empiric antibiotic therapy
Neonates	Group B *Strep, S. aureus,* coliforms	Cloxacillin + gentamicin
Children <5 yr	Group A *Strep, S. aureus, S. pneumoniae, H. influenzae*	Cefazolin†
Children >5 yr	*S. aureus, S. pneumoniae,* Group A Strep	Cefazolin‡
Sickle-cell disease*	As above; also *Salmonella*	Cefotaxime ± cloxacillin
Puncture wound of foot	As above; also *Pseudomonas*	Piperacillin + aminoglycoside
Immunocompromised	*S. aureus, S. pneumoniae,* gram-negative organisms	Cloxacillin + aminoglycoside *or* cloxacillin + cefotaxime

*In children with hemoglobinopathies, consider *Salmonella* and *H. influenzae* in addition to usual pathogens; in sexually active adolescents, consider *N. gonorrhoeae* in addition to usual pathogens.
†If *H. influenzae* is possible (e.g., incompletely vaccinated), use cefuroxime.
‡If allergy to penicillin, use clindamycin.

- Hemoglobinopathies or other asplenic conditions: consider *Salmonella*
- Puncture wound of foot: *P. aeruginosa*
- May be acute, subacute, or chronic (gradual onset of pain, x-ray changes may resemble osteosarcoma)
- Recurrent, multifocal: bone pain in several sites; x-rays show wide growth plates

Investigations

- WBC, ESR (increased), blood cultures (positive in 70%)
- US: subperiosteal abscess
- X-ray: soft-tissue swelling, subperiosteal elevation (bone changes not evident for first 10 days)
- Bone scan ± gallium scan only if further information on localization or multiple sites required; early stage shows increased uptake; may show decreased uptake in late stages
- MRI or CT scan if further imaging warranted by clinical course/x-ray (useful for vertebral, sacroiliac osteomyelitis)
- Needle aspiration or incision and drainage if point tenderness, focal swelling, or x-ray, US, or scan suggestive of subperiosteal pus collection

Treatment (see Table 22-3)

- Analgesia, immobilization
- Antibiotic therapy after sample for culture obtained (see Table 22-3)
- Once organism and sensitivities identified, switch to appropriate antibiotic
- Route: IV; when switching to oral therapy, observe same guidelines as outlined in section on septic arthritis
- Note: For oral treatment of *S. aureus* osteomyelitis, cephalexin suspension has several advantages over cloxacillin (tastes better, can be given with food, and costs same)
- Duration of antibiotic treatment
  1. Acute osteomyelitis: minimum 4 wk, until all clinical signs have resolved, and ESR is normal
  2. *Pseudomonas* osteomyelitis secondary to puncture wound of foot: 1-2 wk after surgical debridement
  3. Chronic osteomyelitis requires long-term treatment (minimum 6 mo)
- Surgical therapy (drainage): if poor response within 72 hr, delayed diagnosis (>4 days), subperiosteal pus, sequestrum, femoral head osteomyelitis with hip joint involvement, or vertebral osteomyelitis with neurologic signs; puncture wound of foot may require debridement

22

OTOLARYNGOLOGY

Vito Forte

ADENOTONSILLECTOMY

INDICATIONS FOR ADENOTONSILLECTOMY
Absolute or Relative

- Obstructive sleep apnea, with or without cor pulmonale
- Dysphagia (tonsillectomy only warranted)
- Possible malignancy (unilateral hypertrophy)
- Peritonsillar abscess (quinsy): 1 episode (because of tendency to recur)
- Nasal obstruction (hypertrophied adenoids) producing discomfort in breathing, severe speech distortion, or dentofacial maldevelopment

Possible (Controversial)

- Chronic or recurrent suppurative otitis media
- Conductive hearing loss (serous otitis media)
- Chronic or recurrent tonsillitis: at least three episodes in each of 3 yr, or four in each of 2 yr or five episodes in 1 yr, associated with temperature ($> 101°$ F or $38.3°$ C), tonsillar or pharyngeal exudate, cervical lymphadenitis, positive culture for group A β-hemolytic *streptococci*
- Rheumatic fever in poorly compliant patients
- Mouth breathing, snoring, or halitosis

Contraindications

- Medical contraindications to surgery (e.g., bleeding, cardiovascular disease)
- Velopharyngeal insufficiency (adenoidectomy should not be performed)

COMPLICATIONS

- Hemorrhage
  1. Primary: occurring within 24 hr postop
  2. Secondary: occurring between 5 and 8 days postop; usually secondary to infection
- Avoid ASA in postop period

MANAGEMENT

- Admit patient for at least 1 day for observation in secondary hemorrhage
- Assess fluid status, and consider cross-matching and starting IV after CBC
- Make paste of bismuth subgallate in epinephrine (1:1,000) (yellow powder mixed with epinephrine until pasty), and apply it to pack
- Remove clot, and insert pack in nasopharynx or tonsillar fossa for 10 min; postnasal pack may also be required

- Check CBC again at 8 hr after control of hemorrhage
- If bleeding persistent or difficult to control, consider checking PT, PTT, and platelets
- Start antibiotic therapy

FOREIGN BODY (FB) IN EAR

- Visualize with head mirror or headlamp, and attempt removal
- Soft material: use loop
- Hard, smooth object: use hook or loop
- Insect: kill it before removal by instilling rubbing alcohol; general syringing with warm water is helpful (if FB is vegetable matter, foam, or paper, it may swell)

FOREIGN BODY IN NOSE

- Foreign body is most common cause of unilateral (usually foul-smelling) nasal discharge
- Visualize with head mirror or light
- Anesthetize nasal mucosa, and shrink it by inserting cotton packs soaked with cocaine 4%-5% (max dose = 3 mg/kg) or 0.25% phenylephrine-3% lidocaine solution
- Suction off discharge surrounding FB
- Attempt removal of soft material (e.g., paper, cotton) with forceps or of solid object with hook

FOREIGN BODIES IN LARYNX, TRACHEOBRONCHIAL TREE

- Keep possibility of FB in mind when assessing any child with enigmatic chronic cough, wheeze, chest disease, and/or dysphagia
- Usually history of choking or cyanotic episode, but may not have history of acute presentation
- Aphonia + airway distress = laryngeal FB
- Stridor or wheeze, unequal expansion of chest, decreased air entry unilaterally; may also have normal exam

Radiology

- Order inspiratory and expiratory chest films, at least two views
- Collapse suggests complete obstruction
- Hyperinflation suggests ball-valve obstruction
- Tracheal FB (e.g., coin) may be seen head-on in lateral view, as opposed to esophageal FB, seen head-on in PA view because of diameters of respective tracts
- Fluoroscopy may show unequal diaphragmatic movement

23

Management

- See the following discussion

FOREIGN BODY IN ESOPHAGUS

- History of ingestion, dysphagia, regurgitation, vomiting, or drooling; may be several months' duration
- Examination may be normal, or stridor may be present if trachea compressed

Radiology

- AP and lateral views (see earlier discussion)

Management

- Remove FB endoscopically under general anesthesia
- FB in larynx may cause complete obstruction and require immediate or urgent removal; if bronchoscopist not immediately available, direct laryngoscopy and removal with McGill's forceps followed by endotracheal intubation may be lifesaving
- Cricothyroidotomy is last resort
- Use only for laryngeal/pharyngeal obstruction

EXTERNAL OTITIS

- Localized infection usually furuncle in outer third of ear canal; diffuse infection occurs following aggressive cleaning of canal, trauma, or swimming
- *Staphylococcus aureus* commonly causes localized infection, while *Pseudomonas aeruginosa* and *Candida* most commonly cause diffuse infection

Management

- Cleansing canal is single most important part of therapy
- Furuncle may require incision and drainage
- Debridement: gently remove infective and epithelial debris from ear canal (by wet swabbing, gentle irrigation, and suctioning)
- Topical antibiotic drops (e.g., those containing polymyxin, neomycin, Garamycin with or without steroid) for up to 10 days only
- If ear canal occluded by circumferential inflammatory edema, use aluminum acetate 1% solution; insert moist cotton or self-expanding (Pope) wick into ear canal; keep it wet with solution until canal has expanded sufficiently to permit debridement after 1-2 days; then use topical antibiotic drops
- If periauricular swelling, regional adenopathy, and signs of systemic infection present, systemic antibiotics should be used (e.g., cefuroxime or cloxacillin)
- If difficulty exists differentiating from furuncle of ear canal or mastoiditis with subperiosteal abscess formation, ENT referral indicated

EPISTAXIS

- Bleeding is usually from Little's area (anterior septum)
- Bleeding is more common during acute URIs and in allergic rhinitis

Management

- Mild cases often respond to firm, persistent pressure to nose between fingers for 10 min
- Following application of pressure, insert cotton plug with petroleum jelly into nose and leave 3-4 hr
- More persistent cases are managed as follows:
  1. May be facilitated by sedation prn, visualization (head mirror or light), and suction
  2. Control bleeding with pressure and cotton pledgets moistened with cocaine 4%-5% (max 3 mg/kg) or 0.25% phenylephrine-3% lidocaine solution
  3. Cauterize with silver nitrate stick behind bleeding point of vessel followed by dry cotton pack for approximately 5 min
  4. Pack nostrils (Oxycel, Gelfoam, Vaseline gauze) only if cautery ineffective
  5. If bleeding persistent, recurrent, or originating posteriorly, request ENT consult
- Persistent bleeding may rarely represent bleeding diathesis; these children should not have cautery with silver nitrate; control bleeding with Oxycel gauze, topical thromboplastin, and pressure

FRACTURED NOSE

Management

- Examine nose for septal hematoma or dislocation (causes nasal obstruction and/or pain and may result in late nasal deformity); septal hematoma requires urgent surgical drainage
- Nasal x-rays not necessary; even if negative,may still be serious pathologic condition
- ENT should be contacted to reduce deformity early (within 2-3 hr of injury) if no swelling
- If swelling, may observe 3-4 days; all cases should be referred to ENT clinic for 3-7 day follow-up to check for late septal hematoma, abscess formation, or deformity (noted after swelling subsides)

CORROSIVE BURNS OF UPPER GI TRACT

- Alkaline corrosives common in drain and oven cleaners
- Esophagus may be damaged by time child arrives in ER
- Degree of visible burns in mouth and pharynx may not be indicative of degree of esophageal involvement
- Presence of two or more symptoms and signs (e.g., dysphagia, oral burns) correlates with esophageal burns

Management

- Notify ENT immediately
- Determine nature (acid/alkali/other) and form (solid/liquid) of ingested material, if possible

- Do not give emetic
- Do not attempt gastric lavage
- Promote ingestion of appropriate fluids if early, unless drooling or signs of mediastinal leak (chest or back pain, dyspnea, etc.) present:
  1. If alkali ingested, give milk or water
  2. If acid ingested, give milk or water
  3. If bleach ingested, give water (first choice) or milk; ages 1-5, give 250-500 ml (1-2 cups); > 5 yr, give up to 1 L (qt)
- Observe for respiratory distress secondary to laryngeal involvement (hoarseness, stridor, dyspnea)
- Observe for shock; monitor vital signs carefully
- Severe chest and abdominal pain are ominous signs; may be indicative of visceral perforation
- Esophagoscopy usually performed after oral burns improve (3-5 days) to assess extent of esophageal burn
- Esophageal stricture develops in approximately 15% of cases of caustic ingestion
- Prophylactic use of systemic steroids and antibiotics following early endoscopy is done in some centers (controversial)

FACIAL NERVE PARALYSIS

- Fairly common in children: may be secondary to Bell's palsy, trauma (also birth), otitis media, aural neoplasm, or intracranial tumor; Bell's palsy (does not always resolve spontaneously in children) is diagnosis of exclusion

Management

- Investigations may include
  1. Audiogram
  2. Impedance studies
  3. Nerve-conduction test
  4. Mastoid tomograms/CT
  5. Schirmer's test (lacrimation)
  6. Salivary-secretion tests

Therapy

- Refer to ENT; may need immediate myringotomy if secondary to acute otitis media
- Treat underlying condition
- Steroids may be useful in Bell's palsy

ACUTE (SUPPURATIVE) OTITIS MEDIA

- Major organisms include *Streptococcus pneumoniae, Haemophilus influenzae, Moraxella catarrhalis,* and *Streptococcus pyogenes*
- See p. 254 for assessment and criteria for treatment
- Treatment is initially for 10 days minimum (Table 23-1), follow-up essential

Table 23-1 Management of Acute Otitis Media

Antibiotic	Advantages	Disadvantages
Amoxicillin/pivampicillin	First choice	
Trimethoprim-sulfamethoxazole	Effective, cheap alternative when penicillin sensitivity	Hepatitis Stevens-Johnson syndrome
Cefaclor	Effective against β-lactamase-producing organisms	Rash, diarrhea 1% risk *erythema multiforme* and serum sickness Expensive
Amoxicillin-clavulinate	Effective against β-lactamase-producing organisms	Expensive 15% diarrhea
Cefixime	As cefaclor, once-a-day dosage	
Clarithromycin	As cefaclor	

- In infants < 6 wk, early myringotomy may be warranted for culture
- For perforation with discharge, antibiotic otic drops tid × 10 days, in addition to systemic antibiotics, are usually recommended
- Analgesics and antipyretics as indicated
- Decongestants or antihistamines are of no proven efficacy
- Myringotomy indicated for
  1. Severe pain: immediately
  2. Bulging drum and severe pain after 48-72 hr of therapy
  3. Otitis media with complication (e.g., meningitis, mastoiditis, facial nerve paralysis)
  4. Residual serous otitis causing hearing loss > 12-16 wks after acute otitis, despite apparently adequate medical therapy
  5. Immunosuppressed (e.g., chemotherapy)
- If discharge persists after > 1 wk of adequate therapy, obtain swabs from deep in external canal for culture
- Mastoid radiographs usually obtained only if disease present for > 3 wk or if acute mastoiditis present (admission for parenteral antibiotics ± surgery required if air-cell coalescence)
- If symptoms or discharge persist for > 1 wk, check cultures for resistant organism, and treat appropriately; daily microdebridement by ENT may be necessary
- Tympanometry may be useful pretreatment and posttreatment to assess presence of and follow-up effusion

23

RECURRENT OTITIS MEDIA

Management

- Choice of prophylactic antibiotic (long-term or seasonal) or myringotomy and tympanostomy tube insertion (M&T)
- Amoxicillin or sulfisoxazole are usual choices for chemoprophylaxis; failure of this method, despite compliance, is indication for M&T
- If < 6 wk of age, rule out immunodeficiency

SEROUS OTITIS MEDIA

- Most common cause of hearing loss in children
- Common accompaniment of adenoidal hypertrophy, atopy, and cleft palate
- If undiagnosed or left untreated, may result in delayed onset of speech and learning problems and lead to chronic ear disease

Management

1. Asymptomatic: follow until disappears (tympanometry useful)
2. Medical
   - First choice unless
     a. Symptoms present for > 6 mo at time of diagnosis
     b. Bilateral hearing loss > 20 dB
     c. Behavior or speech problem secondary to hearing loss
   - Treat with antibiotics (see Table 22-1) PO × 3-4 wk
   - Autoinsufflation: Valsalva's maneuver
3. Surgical: as above, and if medical therapy fails
   - Assess each patient individually for required surgical procedure (e.g., adenoidectomy ± tonsillectomy, if indicated with myringotomy with or without insertion of middle-ear ventilation tubes has been frequently performed versus insertion of ventilation tube only)
   - Note that these procedures are not free of complications (e.g., tympanostomy tubes may cause permanent structural damage to TM and perforation and may rarely themselves induce cholesteatoma formation)
   - Drainage from tympanostomy tubes can be treated with antibiotic ear drops (e.g., Garamycin)

TRAUMATIC PERFORATION OF TYMPANIC MEMBRANE

Management

- Notify or consult ENT service immediately; emergency exploration and repair may be required
- Water must be kept out of ear

MASTOIDITIS

Management

- Consult ENT
- If subperiosteal abscess formation, surgical drainage may be required; if erythema behind ear and no radiographic evidence of coalescence, give parenteral antibiotics (e.g., cefuroxime)
- Wide myringotomy usually necessary
- Chronic mastoiditis with chronic otorrhea may be demonstrated by mastoid air cell loss and coalescence on x-ray; surgery may be necessary to stop otorrhea

HEARING LOSS

- May be congenital or acquired (conductive or sensorineural, unilateral or bilateral)
- Early, accurate diagnosis critical for effective rehabilitation and genetic counseling
- Investigations may include soundfield audiometry, auditory brainstem responses, acoustic emissions, CT head and temporal bones (inner ear dysplasia)
- Early referral to otolaryngologist necessary

Congenital

- Hereditary sensorineural most common; most are recessive
- Often related to consanguinity

Acquired

- May be related to antenatal infection (TORCH), perinatal asphyxia (prematurity), neonatal sepsis (ototoxic medications, such as gentamycin), hyperbilirubinemia, meningitis, or temporal bone injury

CHAPTER 24

PAIN

David Fear, Sheila Jacobson, and Jennifer Stinson

PAIN MANAGEMENT IN CHILDREN

- Good pain control contributes to enhanced quality of life and may also decrease morbidity and mortality
- Although there are age-related differences in children's behavioral responses to pain, there is no evidence that infants' and children's sensitivity to pain is different from that of adults
- However, children have often been undermedicated or not given analgesia before, during, or after painful procedures or surgery or for disease-related pain
- Recently, much attention has been directed to improvement of pain management in children

ASSESSMENT OF PAIN IN CHILDREN

- Many variables may influence child's pain experience; Fig. 24-1 outlines some factors that should be explored with child and family

GENERAL PRINCIPLES OF PAIN ASSESSMENT

- Obtain pain history from child and/or parents at time of admission
- Measure child's pain using self-report and/or behavioral observation tools that have established reliability and validity
- Use self-report measures whenever possible; self-report tools are appropriate for most children 4 yr and older and provide most accurate measure of child's pain; children over age of 7 or 8 can use numeric rating scale
- Use behavioral observation tools with preverbal and nonverbal children and as adjunct to older child's self-report; these tools include such factors as vocalizations, verbalizations, facial expression, motor response, body posture, activity, and appearance
- Use physiologic measures (e.g., heart rate, respiratory rate, blood pressure) as adjuncts to self-report and behavioral observations; physiologic measures are not sensitive or specific indicators of pain
- Tailor assessment strategies to child's developmental level and situation
- Assessment tools should be used routinely and at regular intervals to determine effectiveness of pain management techniques; tools used and results must be documented on chart

PAIN ASSESSMENT SCALES

- Many scales available to measure pain in children; consist of combinations of behavioral, cognitive, and physiologic parameters

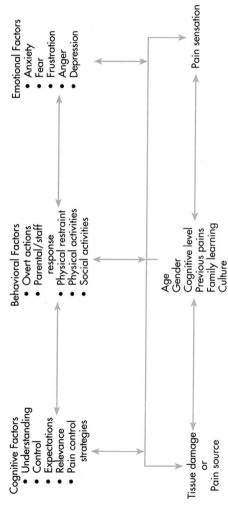

SITUATIONAL FACTORS

Cognitive Factors
• Understanding
• Control
• Expectations
• Relevance
• Pain control
  strategies

Behavioral Factors
• Overt actions
• Parental/staff
  response
• Physical restraint
• Physical activities
• Social activities

Emotional Factors
• Anxiety
• Fear
• Frustration
• Anger
• Depression

Age
Gender
Cognitive level
Previous pains
Family learning
Culture

Tissue damage
or
Pain source

Pain sensation

Fig. 24-1 Pain Assessment Model (From McGrath PA, Hillier LM: Controlling children's pain. In Gatchel RJ, Turk DJ, editors: *Psychological approaches to pain management: a practitioner's handbook,* New York, 1996, Guilford Press.)

24

Self-Report Scale

- Verbal numeric self-report scale is used with school-aged children and adolescents; children are asked to rate their pain on scale of 0 (no pain) to 10 (worst pain)

Objective Behavioral Pain Scales

- For example, Children's Hospital of Eastern Ontario Pain Scale (CHEOPS) was developed to measure postoperative pain in infants and children; it rates six behaviors: crying, facial expression, verbal expression, torso position, touch, and leg position

Oucher Scale (Fig. 24-2)

- Combines numeric and faces scales, making it appropriate to use for children 3 to 15 years old

GENERAL PRINCIPLES OF PAIN MANAGEMENT

- Prevent pain, where possible
- For procedures that will have to be repeated, provide maximum relief of pain and anxiety during first procedure to minimize anticipatory anxiety before subsequent procedures
- Nonpharmacologic interventions can be useful adjuncts to conventional pharmacologic methods
- Doses of analgesics should be individualized and administered at regular intervals; patients should be reassessed frequently so that necessary dosage adjustments can be made; prn dosing should only be used if pain is truly intermittent
- Appropriate dosage of analgesic provides pain relief with minimal or no side effects; additional "rescue" dosages should be available to treat breakthrough pain
- Use oral or intravenous routes; avoid intramuscular injections, which may cause pain and can result in unpredictable drug absorption
- Although many new analgesics are available, morphine remains most effective drug for many children with pain when given in appropriate doses
- Meperidine (Demerol) offers no advantages over codeine or morphine and has greater degree of toxicity
- All patients given opioids should be closely monitored for level of consciousness and respiratory status; naloxone should always be available for treatment of significant respiratory depression
- Addiction is extremely rare in children given opioids for treatment of acute pain; however, dependence may occur, especially if duration of treatment is greater than 2 wk; therefore to avoid withdrawal symptoms, dosage should be tapered by about 10%-20% per day

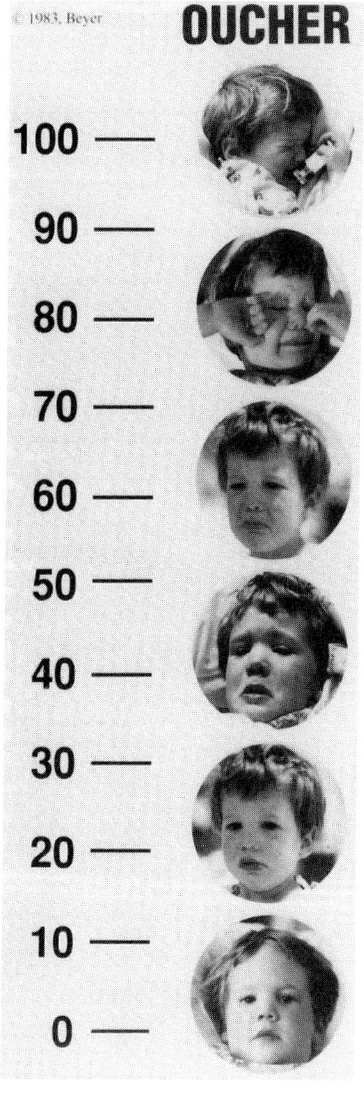

Fig. 24-2 Caucasian version of Oucher. (Developed and copyrighted by Judith E. Beyer, RN, PhD, 1983, University of Missouri, Kansas City. Used with permission.)

Table 24-1   Systemic Dosing Guidelines

Medication	Dosage	Route	Frequency
Nonopioid			
Acetaminophen	10-20 mg/kg	PO/PR	q4h
NSAIDs			
(e.g., Naproxen)	5-10 mg/kg	PO/PR	q12h
Opioid*			
Codeine	1-1.5 mg/kg	PO	q4-6h
Morphine†‡	0.15-1.5 mg/kg	PO/PR	q3-4h
	0.05-0.1 mg/kg	IV bolus	q2-4h
	0.01-0.04 mg/kg/hr	**IV infusion**	**Continuous infusion§**
Meperidine	1.5 mg/kg	PO	q4-6h
	0.5-1 mg/kg	IV bolus	q2-4h

*For nonintubated infants younger than 3 mo of age, initial opioid dose should be reduced to ⅓-¼ of doses recommended above.

†Dosages recommended are initial doses: may be repeated q15-30 min until child is comfortable, and dose increased as necessary after steady-state levels have been achieved (i.e., q8-12h) in increments not greater than 25% of previous dosage.

‡For breakthrough pain: 0.02-0.05 mg/kg IV q2-4h prn should be prescribed when round-the-clock or continuous morphine is ordered.

§Morphine infusion: ½ body weight = # of mg morphine; dilute to 50 cc in syringe; 1 cc/hr = 0.01 mg/kg/hr.

Table 24-2   Adverse Effects of Opioid Analgesics*†

Adverse effect	Management
Nausea/vomiting	Antihistamine (e.g., dimenhydrinate) 1 mg/kg/dose q6h prn
	Neuroleptics (e.g., chlorpromazine) 2 mg/kg/24 hr PO/IV ÷ q4-6h 4 mg/kg/24 hr PR ÷ q6-8h
Constipation	Stool softeners (e.g., docusate sodium) 5 mg/kg/24 hr q6-8h
Pruritis	Antihistamines (e.g., diphenhydramine) 1 mg/kg IV q6h
Somnolence	Reduce dose if possible
	Naloxone: titrate at 1-2 µg/kg/dose
Respiratory depression	Stop opioid
	Mild: stimulation and oxygen
	Severe
	• Respiratory support
	• Naloxone: titrate at 1-2 µg/kg/dose

*Routine close monitoring of all patients taking opioids will permit early recognition and management of any adverse effects.

†At equipotent analgesic doses, all opioids produce similar degrees of nausea, constipation, biliary tract spasm, sedation, and respiratory depression.

PHARMACOLOGIC METHODS OF PAIN CONTROL
(Tables 24-1 to 24-3)

MONITORING OF PATIENTS WHILE TAKING OPIOIDS

- To minimize adverse effects of opioids, important to monitor patients on regular basis; as well as assessment of pain every 4 hr, following should be monitored and recorded on chart:
  - Respiratory rate: hourly
  - Pulse and BP q2h
  - Sedation score: hourly
  - Oximetry should be used for children under age of 1 yr

LOCAL ANESTHETICS (Table 24-3)

- Local anesthetics can be administered by soaking cotton pledget and placing in wound; when injecting, use 27-30 gauge needle to infiltrate around wound; allow 10 min for onset of adequate analgesia

NONPHARMACOLOGIC METHODS OF PAIN CONTROL

- Following are some suggested developmentally appropriate sensorimotor and cognitive-behavioral nonpharmacologic strategies for management of pain and anxiety in children:

Developmental stage	Strategy
Infant	Pacifiers, rapid rocking, patting, singing, holding
Toddler	Holding, rocking, bubble blowing, distracting with music, videos or pop-up books, having child act out procedure in play after own experience
Preschooler	Stroking, talking, storytelling, using distraction objects (e.g., magic wands, pop-up books, toys with movable parts), bubble blowing, having child act out procedure in play before and after own experience
School age	Breathing and blowing, stroking or massage, using distracting objects (e.g., videos, Nintendo), using guided imagery, practicing the "child's job" before procedure
Adolescent	Using breathing and blowing to relax each body part, massage, listening to favorite music on personal stereo, guided imagery

- For children who are extremely anxious or need more intensive therapy, consider seeking consultation and advice from Psychiatry, Clinical Nurse Specialists, and Child Life Specialists

24

Table 24-3 Local Anesthetic Dosing Guidelines

Medication	Dose	Route
Lidocaine plain 1% or 2%	5 mg/kg	Subcutaneously
Lidocaine with epinephrine 1:100,000	7 mg/kg	Subcutaneously
Bupivacaine 0.25% or 0.5%	Up to 2-3 mg/kg	Subcutaneously
Tetracaine, adrenaline, and cocaine (TAC)	1 ml per cm wound length up to 4 ml (0.9 mL/kg)	Not for mucous membranes
Topical anesthesia (e.g., EMLA)	2.5 g	Under occlusive dressing for 90 min
		Not for abraded skin
		Not for mucous membranes

FOR DIFFICULT PAIN MANAGEMENT PROBLEMS

- Department of Anaesthesia at HSC provides acute anesthesia pain service; major responsibility is in area of postoperative pain control using patient-controlled analgesia (PCA) pumps or continuous epidural analgesia; pain service can be contacted to provide consultation and advice

CHAPTER 25

PLASTIC SURGERY

TOMMY KWOK LEUNG HO

TYPES OF WOUNDS

ABRASIONS

- Scrub area to remove embedded dirt and prevent tattooing; use saline or povidone-iodine to avoid irritation caused by stronger detergents; mechanical debridement most important aspect; consider scrub brush; general anesthesia if extensive

CONTUSIONS

- Ice in early stages to minimize swelling (24-48 hr); warm compresses afterward to help speed absorption of blood; consider need to evacuate if collection present

LACERATIONS
Hand Lacerations

- Examine position of fingers; note if any abnormal sweating patterns (sympathetic nerve damage); note anatomic structures in area of injury
- Vascular supply: assess both radial and ulnar arteries separately
- Sensory testing (Fig. 25-1): test median, ulnar, and radial areas with sterile needle or paper clip; test both sides of each finger
- Motor testing: *profundus,* stabilize PIP joint, ask to flex fingertip; *superficialis,* stabilize other fingers in extension and have patient flex finger at PIP (Index finger may need to be tested differently); *median nerve (motor branch),* palmar abduction of thumb (use resistance) and simultaneously palpate thenar eminence (muscle belly of abductor pollicis brevis); *ulnar nerve,* abduction and adduction of fingers; *extensor tendons,* with wrist flexed, all fingers should fully extend (Fig. 25-2)
- Flexor tendon laceration in zone II or "no-man's-land" (area between distal palmar crease and PIP area) (Fig. 25-3) should be repaired by trained hand surgeon; splint hand always in "safe" position (wrist at 45°, MCP joints at 60°, IP joints straight, and thumb abducted and in apposed position)

Facial Lacerations

- Use small bites of subcuticular suture to avoid stitch marks; sutures should be removed 5 days later; consult appropriate surgical specialty for free borders of mouth, nose, eye or eyelids, ears

MANAGEMENT

- Cleanse adjacent skin and infiltrate area with 1% lidocaine (Xylocaine); do not use epinephrine in appendages; flush with normal saline only

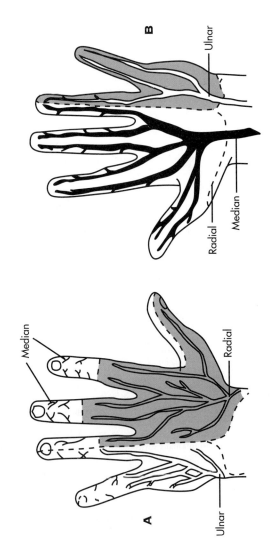

Fig. 25-1   Nerves of hand. **A,** Dorsal surface; **B,** palmar surface.

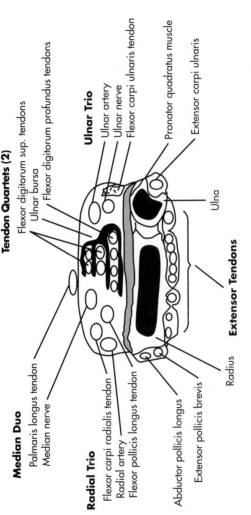

Tendon Quartets (2)
Flexor digitorum sup. tendons
Ulnar bursa
Flexor digitorum profundus tendons

Ulnar Trio
Ulnar artery
Ulnar nerve
Flexor carpi ulnaris tendon

Pronator quadratus muscle

Extensor carpi ulnaris

Ulna

Median Duo
Palmaris longus tendon
Median nerve

Radial Trio
Flexor carpi radialis tendon
Radial artery
Flexor pollicis longus tendon

Abductor pollicis longus

Extensor pollicis brevis

Radius

Extensor Tendons

Fig. 25-2   Wrist anatomy. Proximal to flexor retinaculum.

25

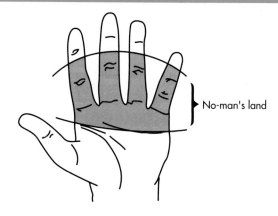

Fig. 25-3 No-Man's Land.

Table 25-1 Tetanus Immunization Guidelines

| | Wound classification/susceptibility to tetanus | | |
Clinical scenario	Clean/none	Moderate	High
Fully immunized and < 5 yr since booster	—	—	—
Fully immunized and 5-10 yr since booster	—	Td*	Td
Fully immunized and > 10 yr since booster	Td	Td	Td
Incompletely immunized or uncertain	Td	Td + TIG†	Td + TIG

*Td, Adult-type tetanus and diptheria toxoids.

†TIG, Tetanus immune globulin; should not be given if known to have two primary doses of Td.

- Close fascia and deep dermal layers of mucosa with 4-0 or 5-0 absorbable sutures (e.g., catgut or Dexon)
- Close skin using 5-0 or 6-0 nonabsorbable sutures (e.g., nylon or polyethylene); use 6-0 suture to close skin on face; use small bites to avoid large stitch markers
- Remember tetanus immunization (Table 25-1)
- Removal of skin sutures: face, 5 days; elsewhere, 7-10 days

AVULSION

- Partial: suture after revision
- Total: do not replace tissue totally; may replace as skin graft after fat is removed

PUNCTURE

- Must check underlying damage; exploration may be necessary, because of possible foreign body (FB)

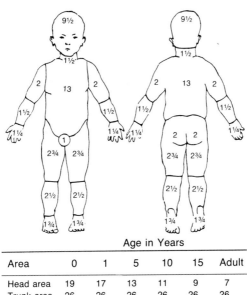

			Age in Years			
Area	0	1	5	10	15	Adult
Head area	19	17	13	11	9	7
Trunk area	26	26	26	26	26	26
Arm area	7	7	7	7	7	7
Thigh area	5½	6½	8½	8½	9½	9½
Leg area	5	5	5	6	6	7

Total 3rd degree burn_____
Total 2nd degree burn_____ TOTAL BURNS_____

Fig. 25-4 Estimation of burn area.

BURNS (Fig 25-4, Table 25-2, and Box 25-1)

- Prevent severe immersion burns by keeping home water at recommended setting of between 49° C (120° F) and 54° C (130° F)
- Cold water immersion of burned area may be helpful immediately after burn or within first hr
- Careful history (including social) and physical examination noting degree, location, and extent of burn; beware of nonaccidental injury (see p. 26)

MANAGEMENT
Outpatient

- Diagram burn area, noting degree (Fig. 25-4 and see Table 25-2)
- Cool part; eliminate agent (copious irrigation with water if chemical burn)

25

Table 25-2   Severity of Burn

Degree	Level of burn	Characteristics
First	Epidermis	Erythema, painful
Second		
Superficial	Superficial dermis	Blisters, painful
Deep	Deep dermis	Eschar, painful
Third	Subcutaneous tissue	Leathery eschar, painless

- Cleanse with saline (use sterile gloves); leave intact blisters alone
- Debride broken blisters and loose debris; apply Polysporin and then Sofra-Tulle
- Dress with dry gauze and secure with Kling bandage
- Review tetanus immunization status (see Table 25-1); analgesics prn for pain and reevaluate in 2-5 days

Inpatient (see Box 25-1)

- Resuscitation
    1. Establish airway and ventilation (see p. 2) especially if flame burn and patient confined to smoke-filled space (see p. 18 for management of smoke inhalation)
    2. Start large-bore IV in unburned area
    3. CBC, urea, electrolytes, protein, and albumin
    4. Ringer's lactate IV: 4 ml/kg/% BSA of burn over first 24 hr, replacing half in first 8 hr postburn and half in subsequent 16 hr postburn; colloids (e.g., albumin, plasma) may be used as part of replacement fluid after first 8 hr
    5. In addition to above, in children under 2 yr of age, give maintenance fluids as 3.33% dextrose and 0.33% saline ($\frac{2}{3}$-$\frac{1}{3}$)
    6. Above formula is only a guide and must be reassessed and adjusted according to hourly urine output (> 2-3 ml/kg/hr), general hydration state, hemoglobin, urea, serum electrolytes
    7. Insert urinary catheter
    8. Record accurate hourly input and output
    9. NPO, nasogastric tube in severe burns, H_2 blocker
- Burn management
    1. Evaluate and document burn size, location, and depth
    2. Cleanse in burn bath (lukewarm salt water: 38° C or 100° F) and debride loose tissue and broken blisters; leave intact blisters alone
    3. Take swabs for culture and sensitivity from nose, throat, and burn wound
    4. Apply silver sulfadiazine cream to burn areas on body and Polysporin ointment to burns on face
    5. Consider IV penicillin (controversial)
    6. Review tetanus immunization status (see Table 25-1)
    7. May require high environmental temperature (i.e., 28°-30° C [82°-86° F]) to prevent heat loss; observe for hypothermia with large burns
    8. After 24 hr
        a. Adjust IV rate according to clinical status

BOX 25-1 Criteria for Hospitalization of Patients with Burns

Extent
    Under 2 yr: ≥ 6% of body surface area (combination of 2nd and 3rd degree)
    Over 2 yr: ≥ 10% of body surface area (combination of 2nd and 3rd degree)
Location: burns of face, neck, hands, feet, perineum
Type: chemical, electrical
Associated injuries: smoke, head injury, fractures, soft tissue trauma
Complicating medical problems: diabetes
Social situation: abuse, self-inflicted, psychologic

---

   b. Continue albumin, plasma, or blood prn
   c. Observe carefully for sepsis
   d. Start feeds (e.g., PO or NG) on second postburn day; may require parenteral nutrition support
   e. Beware of ileus

CIRCUMFERENTIAL BURNS

- Loss of capillary integrity leads to massive swelling with resuscitation
- Circumferential eschar constriction may compromise distal circulation
- Consider immediate escharotomy

FACIAL FRACTURES

- Examine for contour deformity, pain on deep palpation or mastication, areas of anesthesia, crepitus, malocclusion, subconjunctival hemorrhage, eye movement, visual acuity
- Radiographic assessment includes skull and cervical spine x-rays; specialized views include *Waters' view,* and *Panorex* if mandibular fracture suspected; CT scan may be needed for complex fractures
- Caution: x-ray may be negative

CLEFT LIP AND PALATE

- Require immediate consultation with multidisciplinary team, including plastic surgeon
- Examine child carefully to rule out other malformations (especially cardiac)
- Lip repair at 3 mo, palate repair at approximately 1 yr; may require revision of lip or nasal deformity at 5 yr
- Special attention to airway and feeding difficulties

25

CHAPTER 26

POISONING

CANDICE ROWE

GENERAL MANAGEMENT

- Ensure adequate initial resuscitation and stabilization of every overdose patient (see p. 2 for ABCs of resuscitation)

INGESTED POISON
Dilute Poison

- Dilute nondrug poison by giving water PO
- Do not use milk
- Do not attempt to neutralize poison
- Clinical benefit not demonstrated in studies

Gastric Decontamination

1. Emesis
   - Do not use salt water as emetic
   - Syrup of ipecac:
     - GI irritant: stimulates central chemoreceptors
     - Onset: 95% have emesis within 30 min
     - Duration of nausea: 2 hr
     - Indications: substantial amount of toxin ingested up to 1 hr previously
     - Contraindications:
       a. Age < 6 mo
       b. Airway: loss of airway protective reflexes
       c. Coma
       d. Convulsions (or potential to seize)
       e. Caustics
       f. Petroleum-distillate hydrocarbons unless contains CHAMP:
          C: camphor
          H: halogenated hydrocarbons
          A: aromatic hydrocarbons
          M: metals
          P: pesticides
     - Dose
       6-9 mo: 5 ml; no repeat
       9-12 mo: 10 ml; no repeat
       1-12 yr: 15 ml; can repeat once after 20 min
       >12 yr: 30 ml; can repeat once after 20 min
     - Efficacy
       Given <30 min after ingestion, 50%-60% toxin removed
       Given >30 min after ingestion, 33% toxin removed
       Given >60 min after ingestion, negligible toxin removed

2. Gastric lavage
   - No longer routinely used
   - Indications: as for ipecac; preferred if patient comatose
   - Contraindications:
     a. Coma (unless cuffed endotracheal tube placed)
     b. Caustics
     c. Petroleum-distillate hydrocarbons unless contains CHAMP (see above)
   - Protect airway if patient is comatose
   - Aspirate stomach contents first
   - Use large-bore orogastric tube
   - Efficacy
     15 min after ingestion, 38% toxin removed
     60 min after ingestion, 13% toxin removed
3. Activated charcoal
   - Binds many toxins, making them unavailable for GI absorption
   - Weigh risk of delaying charcoal use against benefit of gastric emptying (ipecac or lavage)
   - Do not give charcoal until ipecac-induced vomiting has subsided
   - Dose: ≥ 1 g/kg; mix appropriate amount in 120-240 ml fluid and give PO or by nasogastric (NG) tube
   - Contraindications: caustics, hydrocarbons, inability to protect airway
   - Charcoal does not bind GAME
     G: glycols
     A: alcohols
     M: metals (e.g., iron, lead, lithium, mercury, arsenic)
     E: electrolytes (e.g., sodium, potassium)
   - Administration of half-doses q4-6h may be beneficial for some toxins (e.g., theophylline, phenobarbital); contact poison information center before administration
4. Cathartics
   - Routine administration of cathartics with activated charcoal is not recommended; clinical benefit from cathartics has not been demonstrated, and use of osmotic cathartics is associated with significant fluid and electrolyte shifts
5. Whole bowel irrigation
   - Polyethylene glycol/electrolyte lavage solution
   - Indications:
     Toxins poorly absorbed by activated charcoal (iron, lead, lithium)
     Sustained-release or enteric-coated products
     Body packers of illicit drugs (cocaine, heroin)
   - Procedure: GoLytely/PegLyte via NG tube
     <6yrs use 0.5 L/hr
     6-12 yr use 1.5-2 L/hr
     >12 yr use 2 L/hr
   - End point when rectal effluent clear ($\geq$2-4 hr)

26

Enhance Elimination

- Diuresis: forced diuresis not indicated
- Urinary alkalinization (salicylates, phenobarbitol)
- Hemodialysis (methanol, ethylene glycol, salicylates, lithium)

INJECTED POISON

- If treatment can be started within a few minutes after injection:
  1. Apply a venous tourniquet proximally
  2. Do not release tourniquet until patient in intensive-care setting (shock may occur)

POISON BY RECTAL ROUTE

- Give enema

INHALED POISON

- Remove from source of contamination
- Maintain clear airway; support ventilation and oxygenation, if necessary (see p. 3)

POISON IN CONTACT WITH SKIN OR EYE

- Wash with copious amounts of water for 10-15 min
- Do not use chemical neutralizers
- If eye contamination, obtain ophthalmology consultation for further evaluation and treatment

UNKNOWN POISONING

- Support vital functions
- Proceed as for ingested poison unless poisoning was by another route
- Save vomitus or lavage aliquots and blood and urine samples for toxicology analysis
- Identify symptom complex (if possible) so that specific diagnosis can be made (Table 26-1)

TOXICOLOGY LABS

- Toxicology screens are different at different centers
- Know drugs tested for and turnaround time of tests (For testing at HSC, see p. 507)

Information to give to Lab

- Suspected agent or class of agent
- Suspected dose
- Time of ingestion and sampling
- Clinical presentation: toxidrome, neurologic, Glasgow coma score

Specimen Type

- Gastric contents if available
- Blood (see p. 507)
- Urine for drug screen (see p. 553)
- If not certain, save 10 cc blood in 2 red-topped tubes and 50-100 cc urine in toxicology lab; ask lab personnel to save in refrigerator
- If testing for barbiturates, blood is better sample
- If testing for antidepressants, urine is better sample

Table 26-1 Common Signs and Causes of Poisoning

System	Sign	Causes
Cardiovascular	Bradycardia	Digitalis compounds
		β-blocking agents
	Tachycardia	Sympathomimetics
		Anticholinergic agents
		Theophylline
	Hypertension	Sympathomimetics
		Phencyclidine
	Hypotension	Hypnotic-sedatives
		Narcotic analgesics
	Arrhythmias	Theophylline
		Digitalis compounds
		Tricyclic antidepressants
Respiratory	Bradypnea	Narcotics
		Ethanol
		Hypnotic-sedatives
	Tachypnea	Salicylates
		Carbon monoxide
		Methanol
Temperature	Hyperthermia	Salicylates
		Anticholinergic agents
		Theophylline
	Hypothermia	Ethanol
		Phenothiazines
Neurologic	Ataxia	Ethanol
		Barbiturates
		Phenytoin
	Miosis	Narcotics
		Barbiturates
		Phenothiazines
		Clonidine
		Benzodiazepines
	Mydriasis	Sympathomimetics
		Anticholinergic agents
	Nystagmus	Phenytoin
	Convulsions	Sympathomimetics
		Anticholinergic agents
		Camphorated oil
		Lindane (γ-benzene hexachloride)
		Strychnine
		Theophylline
	Coma	CNS depressants
		Anticholinergic agents
		Narcotics
		Asphyxiant gases
		Salicylates
	Psychosis	Anticholinergic agents
		Sympathomimetics
		Hallucinogens
		Salicylates
Oral cavity	Dryness	Sympathomimetics
		Anticholinergic agents
		Narcotics

26

Continued.

Table 26-1 Common Signs and Causes of Poisoning—cont'd

System	Sign	Causes
Oral cavity—cont'd	Acetone smell	Acetone
		Methanol
		Isopropyl alcohol
		Phenol
		Salicylates
	Alcohol smell	Ethanol
	Almond smell	Cyanide
	Garlic smell	Arsenic
		Phosphorus
		Organophosphate insecticides
		Thallium
	Wintergreen smell	Methylsalicylate
	Petroleum smell	Hydrocarbons
Skin	Cyanosis	Methemoglobinemia
Gastrointestinal	Emesis, hematemesis	Iron
		Arsenic
		Colchicine
		Salicylates
		Theophylline

- Urine immunoassays better for "drugs of abuse" (cocaine, opiates, cannabinoids)
- For general screen, send urine general toxicology screen

SALICYLATE INTOXICATION

- Toxic dose of ASA: >150 mg/kg
- Lethal dose of ASA: >500 mg/kg
- Oil of wintergreen (methylsalicylate): 1 ml = 1.4 g ASA
- Hyperventilation, vomiting, pyrexia, tinnitus, lethargy, confusion, dehydration (rare); may progress to convulsions, coma, pulmonary edema
- Lab: ↑ or ↓ glucose, ↑ PTT (clinical bleeding is unusual)
- Chronically intoxicated patients generally are sicker than their serum salicylate level would indicate

GENERAL MANAGEMENT

- Gastric emptying (see p. 438) if toxic or unknown dose has been ingested within 1 hr
- Give activated charcoal (see p. 439) once any lavage or ipecac-induced vomiting has stopped
- Blood for salicylate level on presentation and 6 hr postingestion; nomogram (Fig. 26-1) used only for acute ingestion; should not be used for delayed-release salicylates or chronic ingestion; not useful on levels less than 6 hr postingestion

Blood

- Electrolytes, urea, glucose, calcium
- CBC, PT, PTT

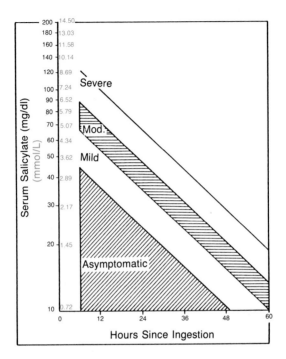

Fig. 26-1 "Done" nomogram for salicylate poisoning. (Modified from Done AK: Salicylate intoxication, *Pediatrics* 26: 805, 1960.)

- Acetaminophen and salicylate level
- Blood gases: mixed acid-based picture predominates (metabolic acidosis, respiratory alkalosis); infants and young children tend to be acidemic, whereas older children and adults tend to be alkalemic

Urine

- pH, ketones, dip for blood (myoglobinuria if dipstick positive and no red blood cells on microbiology)

SPECIFIC MANAGEMENT

- Correct acid-base, electrolyte abnormality, hypoglycemia

Fluids

- Manage shock with normal saline, albumin, or plasma (see p. 6)
- Allow for daily maintenance, replacement of estimated deficit (see p. 100) and ongoing losses; fluid diuresis not necessary
- Add KCl 40 mmol/L to IV solution after patient has voided

26

Urinary Alkalinization

- Use D5W with $NaHCO_3$ infusion (see p. 3)
- Keep urine pH 7.5-8.0
- To prevent paradoxic aciduria, essential to give adequate KCl also
- Keep arterial pH < 7.5
- Indications
  1. Marked decrease in plasma HCO_3 (respiratory alkalosis not contraindication to bicarbonate use)
  2. High serum salicylate level: "Done" nomogram in toxic range (see Fig. 26-1)
  3. Do not give sodium bicarbonate if arterial pH > 7.5
- Indications for hemodialysis
  1. Renal failure
  2. Aspiration pneumonia or pulmonary edema
  3. Salicylate level > 7 mmol/L (100 mg/dl)
  4. Rising or steady salicylate level
  5. Refractory acid-base imbalance
  6. Persistent CNS manifestations

ACETAMINOPHEN POISONING

- Toxic dose > 150 mg/kg
- Hepatotoxic dose > 10-12 g in adults; less if alcoholic enyzme induction, glutathione stores depleted, liver disease
- Toxicity from acetaminophen metabolite (causes hepatocellular damage)
- Glutathione converts toxic metabolite to nontoxic one

CLINICAL PRESENTATION
Phase I (2-24 hr)

- Nausea, vomiting, anorexia, lethargy, pallor
- No change in level of consciousness

Phase II (24-72 hr)

- Initial symptoms resolve
- Hepatic damage
- ↑ Liver enzymes, hepatomegaly, liver tenderness, abnormal liver function

Phase III (72-96 hr)

- Peak liver abnormality
- Jaundice, coagulation defects, hypoglycemia, encephalopathy

Phase IV (7-10 days)

- Enzyme abnormalities resolve
- Renal failure

MANAGEMENT

- Activated charcoal if within 4 hr of ingestion

N-acetylcysteine (NAC)

- Indications
    1. Ingested dose > 150 mg/kg and no level available
    2. Acetaminophen level in hepatotoxic range (Fig. 26-2)
- Dosage
    1. 72 hr oral protocol
        a. Loading dose 140 mg/kg PO
        b. Subsequent doses 70 mg/kg PO q4h × 17 doses
        c. Double loading dose if within 1 hr of activated charcoal
    2. 48-hr IV protocol: Contact poison control center

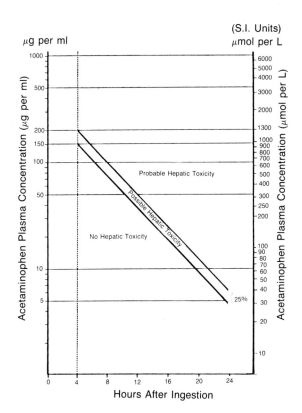

Fig. 26-2 Semilogarithmic plot of plasma acetaminophen levels versus time. (Modified from Rumack BH, Matthew H: Acetaminophen poisoning and toxicity, *Pediatrics* 55:871-876, 1975. The adapted form presented here is used with the permission of Micromedex, Inc, Englewood, Colorado.)

26

- Outcome: Excellent if NAC started within 10 hr of ingestion; NAC treatment initiated >10 hr postingestion is beneficial but diminishes with time

PETROLEUM-DISTILLATE HYDROCARBONS (PDHs)

- Gasoline, kerosene, charcoal lighter fluid, naphthas, mineral seal oils (furniture polish), benzine (not benzene)
- PDHs are not significantly absorbed through GI tract; systemic or pulmonary disease occurs only as result of aspiration

MANAGEMENT OF INGESTION

- Do not induce vomiting or perform gastric lavage unless following are present (CHAMP):
  Camphorated products
  Halogenated products (methylene chloride, carbon tetrachloride)
  Aromatic hydrocarbons (benzene, toluene)
  Metals: heavy (arsenic, mercury, iron, lead)
  Pesticides
- Do not give activated charcoal, oils, or cathartics
- Observe for 2 hr; if no respiratory symptoms, may discharge home

MANAGEMENT OF ASPIRATION

- For patients not *severely* ill but who are coughing, choking, gagging, or vomiting:
  1. History and physical exam
  2. Observe for 6 hr (repeat chest exam and respiratory rate periodically)
  3. CXR at end of 6 hr
  4. If both exam and CXR are normal, may discharge home
  5. If either exam or CXR is abnormal, consider admitting for further observation and treatment
  6. Symptomatic and supportive care
  7. No prophylactic antibiotics or corticosteroids

NONPETROLEUM DISTILLATE HYDROCARBONS (NPDHs)

- Turpentine, xylene, benzene (not benzine), and toluene are only four NPDHs
- Significant GI absorption
- Gastric decontamination using ipecac or gastric lavage
- Minimum toxic amounts are not well established; call poison control center for advice

BARBITURATES AND ANTICONVULSANTS

- CNS depression (especially barbiturates): drowsiness, ataxia, slurred speech, nystagmus may occur

- Respiratory depression, hypothermia, aspiration pneumonia, bullous skin lesions, hypotension may occur in severe cases

MANAGEMENT

- If no decreased level of consciousness, give ipecac (If less than 1 hr after ingestion) followed by activated charcoal
- If depressed level of consciousness, consider activated charcoal (ensure airway protection)
- Support ventilation and circulation
- Urinary alkalinization only effective for phenobarbital intoxication
- Multiple-dose activated charcoal for phenobarbital and carbamazepine (Tegretol) overdoses

PHENOTHIAZINES

- As for barbiturates
- Extrapyramidal reaction: give diphenhydramine 1-2 mg/kg/dose (maximum 50 mg/dose) IV, IM, or PO
- Cardiac arrhythmias: (see p. 60)

TRICYCLIC ANTIDEPRESSANTS

- Examples: imipramine, amitriptyline
- Central and peripheral anticholinergic effects within 6 hr of ingestion

Anticholinergic Effects

- Fever, mydriasis; ↑ HR; dry, flushed skin; ↓ bowel activity; urinary retention
- Does not predict more serious complications

CNS Effects

- Altered mental status (delirium, agitation, coma); muscle twitching, hyperreflexia, seizures, hallucinations

Cardiovascular Effects

- Sinus tachycardia, conduction delays, hypotension
- Atrial and ventricular arrhythmias
- Hallmark ECG pattern suggestive of TCA overdose: rightward shift of terminal 40 ms of QRS (lead I, negative deflection of terminal 40 ms; lead AVR, positive deflection of terminal 40 ms)
- QRS widening frequent

MANAGEMENT

- Immediate evaluation
- ABCs (see p. 3)
- Gastric emptying
  1. Activated charcoal
  2. Ipecac or gastric lavage not recommended
- Cardiac monitor until no arrhythmias for 24 hr

26

- 12 lead ECG hourly until 6 hr after ingestion
  1. QRS > 0.10 sec: risk of convulsions
  2. QRS > 0.16 sec: risk of arrhythmias and convulsions
- Treat seizures with diazepam or phenobarbital
- Arrhythmias
  1. Na HCO$_3$ 1-2 mmol/kg IV bolus; keep pH 7.45-7.55
  2. If refractory, lidocaine or phenytoin
- Correct acidosis and hypoxia, because these conditions worsen cardiac toxicity

ETHANOL

- In children <6 yr, 1 cc/kg of absolute ethanol produces serum concentration of approximately 22 mmol/L (100 mg/dl) 2 hr after ingestion
- Beer: 4%-5% ethanol (4-5 g/100 ml)
- Wine: 10%-12% ethanol (10-12 g/100 ml)
- Liquor: 40%-50% ethanol (40-50 g/100 ml)
- Hypoglycemia may occur within 6 hr of ingestion
- Watch for hypothermia

MANAGEMENT

- Gastric emptying
  1. Ipecac if less than 30 min after ingestion
  2. If obtunded, no emptying because significant absorption has already occurred
- Monitor blood glucose
- Avoid CNS respiratory depressant drugs
- Consider dialysis if ethanol level > 110 mmol/L (500 mg/dl); contact poison control center

IRON

- Toxicity based on amount of elemental iron ingested
  1. Ferrous fumarate: 33% elemental iron
  2. Ferrous gluconate: 12% elemental iron
  3. Ferrous sulfate: 20% elemental iron
- Nontoxic dose   <20 mg/kg
- Potentially toxic dose   20-60 mg/kg
- Highly toxic dose   >60 mg/kg
- Lethal dose   200-300 mg/kg

CLINICAL
Early Phase (½-6 hr)

- Nausea, vomiting, bloody diarrhea, abdominal pain, lethargy, hypotonia, hypotension, shock, ↑ WBC, ↑ glucose

Quiescent Phase (4-48 hr)

- Patient may appear to improve; in very ill patients, this phase may not be evident

Delayed Phase (12-48 hr)

- Acidosis, hypoglycemia, shock, hepatic failure, pulmonary edema, coma

Fourth Phase (2-6 wk)

- Late sequelae, GI scarring ± obstruction, hepatic damage, and cirrhosis

MANAGEMENT

- ABCs (see p. 3)
- GI decontamination
  1. Ipecac preferred if within 60 min
  2. Whole bowel irrigation if tablets seen on AXR
- Labs
  1. CBC, electrolytes, glucose, ABGs, urea, creatinine
  2. Serum iron level (STAT)
  3. Abdominal x-ray (AXR)
- Correct fluid, electrolyte, acid-base abnormalities
- Monitor urine output and renal function closely
- If asymptomatic, normal labs, and ingested < 20 mg/kg, may discharge home
- Others observe for at least 8 hr
- Iron level q4h

Deferoxamine

- Use depends on iron level 4-6 hr after ingestion; contact poison center for treatment regimen
  1. <53 μmol/L (<300 μg/dl): supportive measures only
  2. 53-90 μmol/L (300-500 μg/dl): brief chelation therapy
  3. >90 μmol/L (<500 μg/dl): vigorous chelation therapy
- If iron level not available, deferoxamine indicated if >60 mg/kg elemental iron ingested or if iron tablets on AXR
- Hemodialysis if serum iron level > 180 μmol/L (>1000 μg/dl) or if anuric

THEOPHYLLINE

- Severity of theophylline toxicity is directly related to serum concentrations
- Chronic overmedication results in severe toxicity at lower serum concentrations
- GI symptoms: nausea, vomiting, abdominal pain, GI bleed
- CNS symptoms: restlessness, irritability, seizures
- Cardiovascular effects: arrhythmias
- Fever (hypermetabolism)

26

MANAGEMENT

- ABCs (see p. 3)
- Cardiac monitor
- Activated charcoal (AC) 1g/kg; if level in toxic range, give AC 0.5g/kg q4h until symptoms resolve or level < 20-25 mg/L

- Monitor theophylline level
- Treat seizures aggressively: use diazepam, lorazepam, and barbiturates, not phenytoin
- Treat arrythmias (p. 60)
- Charcoal hemoperfusion indicated if
    1. Severe toxicity > 440 μmol/L (>80 mg/L) in children; consider hemoperfusion at lower levels if theophylline clearance reduced (e.g., neonates, premature infants, hepatic disease, cardiac failure, or chronic toxicity)
    2. Refractory arrythmias or seizures

ALKALINE CORROSIVES

- See p. 419 for management of ingestion
- Emesis and gastric lavage *contraindicated*
- Eye contact: wash eyes thoroughly with water
- Skin contact: wash with running water

NARCOTICS

- Heroin, morphine, pethidine-meperidine, methadone, diphenoxylate, propoxyphene, codeine
- Pinpoint pupils, respiratory depression, coma
- Cyanosis, bradycardia, hypotension

MANAGEMENT

- Maintain ventilation and circulation (see p. 3)
- Naloxone 0.03 mg/kg IV; if no response (and diagnosis is certain), naloxone 0.1 mg/kg IV; doses may be repeated as needed to maintain reversal of narcotic signs; contact poison center or anesthesia department for continuous naloxone infusion

SNAKE BITES

- Rattlesnakes are the only poisonous snakes in Canada and one of several in United States
- Proper identification of snake is important
- Bites are more serious in children than in adults
- The majority of bites are not serious
- Characteristics include:
    1. Fang marks
    2. Local pain (or numbness) and edema; develop within 4 hr after bite
    3. Local bleeding, ecchymosis
    4. Lymphangitis
    5. Severe pain and swelling; indicate serious envenomation
    6. Paresthesias, diaphoresis
    7. Nausea, vomiting
    8. Bleeding diathesis, hemolysis, disseminated intravascular coagulation

9. Arrhythmias
10. Renal failure, convulsions

MANAGEMENT

- First aid
  1. Suction (without cutting) over fang marks within 30 min after bite
  2. Immobilize extremity
  3. Loose superficial venous-lymphatic tourniquet
  4. Transport to hospital
- Wound therapy
  1. Clean and dress wound
  2. Tetanus prophylaxis (see p. 434)
  3. Observe for gram-negative infection
- Systemic therapy (for severe pain or swelling or systemic symptoms)
  1. Measure and record bite area
  2. IV access
  3. CBC, platelets, type and cross-match, PT, PTT, fibrinogen, electrolytes, Ca, urea, creatinine, glucose, albumin
  4. Urinalysis, ECG
  5. Antivenin: polyvalent Crotalidae antivenin is available; contact poison center for management advice

SPIDERS

BROWN RECLUSE

- May be no pain on envenomation
- Local vesicles may progress to ulcerations
- Hematologic, cardiovascular, and renal effects may occur
- No antivenin available
- Many treatment regimens have been proposed, some of which need to be started early after bite; contact poison center for recommendations

BLACK WIDOW

- Mild to moderate pain on envenomation
- Muscle spasms within 2 hr, calcium gluconate may help
- May cause abdominal pain and rigidity
- Symptomatic and supportive care
- Tetanus prophylaxis (see p. 434)
- Antivenin is available; contact poison center for advice

INSECTICIDES (Organophosphate Type)

- Examples: malathion, diazinon
- Cholinergic signs (SLUDGE):
  Salivation, secretions
  Lacrimation
  Urination
  Diarrhea
  Gastrointestinal cramps
  Emesis

26

- Nicotinic signs: weakness, muscle fasciculations, coma, convulsions, respiratory insufficiency

MANAGEMENT

- Airway management: suction ± assisted ventilation (see p. 3)
- Gastric lavage if ingested < 30 min previously
- Activated charcoal preferred
- If skin contamination, remove clothes and wash skin with soap and water
- If increased bronchial secretions:
  - Atropine sulfate 0.05 mg/kg IV (max dose 2 mg)
  - Repeat every 5 min until secretions dry
- Notify poison center if respiratory insufficiency
- Pralidoxime chloride 25-50 mg/kg up to 2 g IV slowly; repeat in 1 hr if no improvement; used if respiratory muscle weakness, as evidenced by respiratory insufficiency

LEAD POISONING

- Most serious poisonings are associated with housing renovations or with ingestion of leaded paint (and putty) from housing built before 1950
- Present in moonshine whiskey, earthenware, ceramic food containers, leaded pipes
- Increased GI absorption of lead if iron deficiency; dietary protein deficiency; calcium, zinc, copper deficiency; excessive dietary fats and oils

CLINICAL FEATURES

- Symptoms and signs depend on age and blood lead concentrations
- No pathognomonic signs or symptoms; most have minimal or no clinical symptoms
- Mild to moderate poisoning may cause detectable neuropsychiatric deficits

Severe Poisoning (Rare)

- Insidious onset of anorexia, apathy, poor coordination, sporadic vomiting, loss of newly acquired skills (especially speech)
- Hypochromic, microcytic anemia, elevated blood erythrocyte protoporphyrin (EP) levels, and radiodensity of metaphyseal lines ("lead lines")

Lead Encephalopathy (Rare)

- Gross ataxia, persistent forceful vomiting, periods of lethargy or stupor, coma, convulsions
- Anemia and convulsions strongly suggest lead encephalopathy
- Encephalopathy constitutes true medical emergency

MANAGEMENT

- GI decontamination in acute overdose with whole bowel irrigation if AXR positive (AXR positive indicates ingestion within 24-36 hr)
- Screening tests are blood lead and EP levels; elevated capillary blood lead levels should be confirmed on venous sample

- Check CBC and iron level
- Chelation decision based on venous lead concentration:
  - <10 μg/dl (0.5 μmol/L); no treatment
  - 10-15 μg/dl (0.5-0.7 μmol/L); remove environmental lead sources
  - 15-20 μg/dl (0.7-1.0 μmol/L); treat with supplemental iron, remove environmental lead sources; consider oral chelators (penicillamine, DMSA [2, 3-dimercaptosuccinic acid])
  - >20 μg/dl (>1.0 μmol/L): treat with oral chelators and iron supplements, and remove lead sources
  - >70 μg/dl: treat with BAL 50 mg/m^2 IM q4h × 3 days or Ca EDTA 1000 mg/m^2/day as continous infusion for 5 days

Symptomatic Patients

- Acute lead encephalopathy
  1. ABCs (see p. 3)
  2. Chelation: BAL 75 mg/m^2 IM q4h then
  3. Ca EDTA 1.5 mg/m^2/day continuous infusion or second dose of BAL; continue for 5 days
  4. Further treatment depends on lead level
- No encephalopathy
  1. Remove from source; admit for chelation
  2. Chelation BAL 50 mg/m^2 IM q4h then
  3. Ca EDTA 1000 mg/m^2/day continuous infusion for 5 days
- Repeat lead level 7-10 days to check for rebound

26

CHAPTER 27

RESPIROLOGY

MELINDA SOLOMON

ALVEOLAR-ARTERIAL (A-a) GRADIENT

- Normal A-a gradient $(PAO_2 - PaO_2) \leq 16$ mm Hg
- $PAO_2 = \%$ inspired $O_2 \times$ (P barometric − vapor pressure mm Hg) − $PaCO_2/R$
  - $PAO_2 = 0.21 \times (760\text{-}47) - PaCO_2/0.8$
- In room air, $PAO_2 \sim 100$ mm Hg
- PaO_2 is measured in arterial blood
- If patient is hypoxemic and retaining CO_2, relative contribution of hypoventilation versus impaired gas exchange can be determined by knowing A-a gradient (i.e., normal A-a gradient, correct hypoxemia by ensuring adequate ventilation; all other causes of hypoxemia will ↑ A-a gradient)
- Oxyhemoglobin dissociation curve is illustrated in Fig. 27-1

PULMONARY FUNCTION TESTING (PFTs)

- (Fig. 27-2; Table 27-1)

PATTERNS OF PFTs OBSERVED (Fig. 27-3)
Obstructive

- Forced vital capacity (FVC) normal or decreased
- Forced expiratory volume in 1 sec (FEV_1) decreased
- Forced expiratory flow (FEF) at 25%-75% lung volume ($FEF_{25\text{-}75}$) decreased
- Ratio of FEV_1 to FVC (FEV_1/FVC) < 80% (normal: >80%)
- Total lung capacity (TLC) normal or increased
- Functional residual capacity (FRC) normal or increased
- Residual volume (RV) normal or increased
- RV/TLC normal or increased (normal: 20%)

Restrictive

- FVC decreased
- FEV_1 decreased
- FEV_1/FVC ≥ 80%
- TLC decreased
- RV normal or decreased (RV may be slightly increased in some neuromuscular disorders)
- FRC normal or decreased

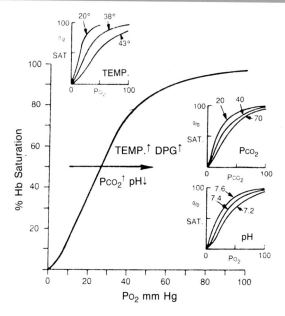

Fig. 27-1 Oxyhemoglobin dissociation curve. (From West JS: *Respiratory physiology: the essentials,* ed 5, Baltimore, 1995, Williams & Wilkins.)

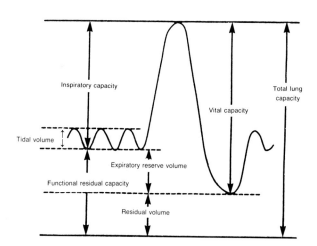

Fig. 27-2 Lung Volume Subdivisions.

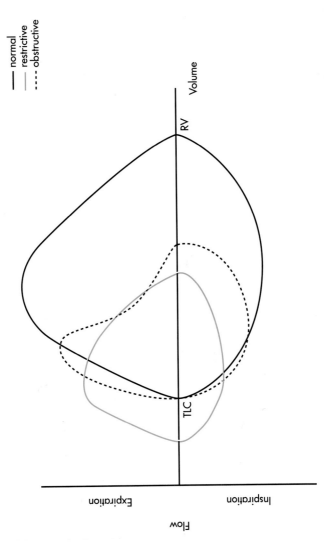

Fig. 27-3 Flow Volume Curves.

Table 27-1 Normal Values for Peak Flow FVC and FEV*

	Male			Female		
Height (cm)	FVC (L)†	FEV$_1$ (L)†	PEFR (L/min)†	FVC (L)	FEV$_1$ (L)	PEFR (L/min)
110				1.146	0.976	145
115	1.311	1.134	160	1.268	1.078	157
120	1.452	1.250	175	1.403	1.191	170
125	1.609	1.378	191	1.552	1.316	184
130	1.782	1.519	208	1.718	1.454	199
135	1.975	1.674	226	1.901	1.606	216
140	2.188	1.845	247	2.104	1.774	234
145	2.424	2.034	269	2.328	1.960	253
150	2.685	2.241	293	2.576	2.165	274
155	2.975	2.470	319	2.851	2.392	296
160	3.296	2.723	348	3.155	2.642	321
165	3.652	3.001	379	3.491	2.919	347
170	4.046	3.308	414	3.864	3.225	376
175	4.482	3.645	451	4.276	3.562	407
180	4.966	4.018	491	4.732	3.936	441
185	5.502	4.428	536	5.236	4.348	477
190	6.095	4.881	584	5.794	4.803	517

*Values obtained with Roxon portable battery-operated turbine spinometer at Hospital for Sick Children.

†*FVC*, Forced vital capacity; *FEV$_1$*, forced expiratory volume in 1 sec; *PEFR*, peak expiratory flow rate.

RESPIRATORY DISTRESS

- Consider pulmonary and extrapulmonary disease (e.g., cardiac, neurologic, sepsis) in differential diagnosis of respiratory failure; treat underlying cause

CLINICAL FEATURES

- Tachypnea or bradypnea/apnea
- Grunting, retractions, use of accessory muscles
- Cyanosis
- Decreased or absent breath sounds
- Drooling, stridor (upper airway obstruction)
- Wheeze (lower airway obstruction)
- Restlessness, stupor, obtundation
- Decreasing PaO_2, increasing $PaCO_2$

MANAGEMENT

- ABCs (see p. 3)
- IV access: In certain clinical situations (i.e., severe upper airway obstruction), risk of exacerbation of respiratory distress by anxiety and pain must be weighed against need for IV access; adequate hydration important, but use caution in cardiac or renal conditions in which fluid overload may exacerbate respiratory distress

27

- Consider pneumothorax if sudden onset of respiratory distress; in life-threatening situations, may be indication for intrapleural needle aspiration on clinical grounds alone (see p. 494).
- Avoid pharyngeal suctioning in upper airway obstruction
- Position head up at 45° C
- CXR, lateral neck x-ray should not delay above management strategies
- ABG; avoid reliance on venous blood gas in respiratory abnormalities; useful only if CO_2 normal

UPPER AIRWAY OBSTRUCTION

- Prolonged inspiration
- Subcostal, suprasternal, and supraclavicular retractions
- Increased respiratory rate
- Stridor
- Barking cough suggestive of subglottic or tracheal obstruction
- Aphonia suggests obstruction at level of cords

MANAGEMENT

- Foreign body (see p. 417) and infection (Table 27-2) are major differential diagnoses in acute situation
- Investigations may include CXR (PA and lateral) and lateral soft tissue x-rays of neck; which should be performed only if highest supervision in radiology suite available; investigations should *never* delay establishment of artificial airway in severe airway obstruction
- Laryngoscopy and bronchoscopy may be required

Table 27-2 Upper Airway Infection

Factor	Epiglottitis	Croup	Bacterial tracheitis
Age	Usually older (2-6 yr)	Usually younger (6 mo-4 yr)	Any age
Sex	M = F	M > F	M = F
Agents	Bacterial: *H. influenzae* type B (+++), β-hemolytic strep (+)	Viral: Parainfluenza 1 (+++), RSV, parainfluenza 2,3 (+), influenza	Bacterial: *S. aureus* pneumococcus, *H. influenzae*
Seasons	Year-round	Late spring, late fall	Any time
Recurrence	Rare	Fairly common	Rare
Clinical	Toxic	Nontoxic: may be restless, cyanotic	Toxic
	Severe airway obstruction	Not drooling	Crouplike cough
	Drooling, sitting forward	Stridor common	Stridor
	Stridor	Sternal recession common	
	Sternal recession	Barking cough, hoarseness, coryza	
Progression	Rapid	Usually slow	Moderately rapid

- Barium swallow useful in detecting vascular compression in nonacute situation; CT scan for other extrinsic causes of airway obstruction

EPIGLOTTITIS (Table 27-2)

MANAGEMENT

- Pediatric emergency
- Diagnose on clinical grounds; "the four Ds": dysphagia, dysphonia, drooling, and distress
- Do not obtain x-ray or blood work (child may deteriorate while procedures are being done)
- Do not try to examine throat or upper airway
- Do not agitate child; keep npo; minimal handling
- Contact ENT and anesthesia personnel immediately
- Controlled intubation done in OR or if necessary, emergency room
- Once child is intubated: IV fluids and antibiotics appropriate for coverage against *Haemophilus influenzae* (cefuroxime usually first line)
- Continue IV antibiotics until child is over acute phase, then continue with oral antibiotics for 7 to 10 days total
- Rifampin prophylaxis recommended for patients and family
- Other *H. influenzae* infections may coexist (e.g., septic arthritis and meningitis)

CROUP (ACUTE LARYNGOTRACHEOBRONCHITIS)

CLINICAL FEATURES (see Table 27-2)
MANAGEMENT

- Avoid agitation as much as possible
- Mild croup may be managed at home with PO fluids and humidity (bathroom with shower on)
- Warn parents that croup may be worse at night; may clear in cold air outside
- Stridor at rest; moderate chest wall retractions; decreased air entry; and anxious, restless child are all indicators of moderate-to-severe disease and signal need for hospitalization
- Rising respiratory rate correlates well with falling PaO_2
- Hypercapnia occurs late in upper airway obstruction and is sign of increasing respiratory failure
- If concerned about degree of respiratory failure, ABG indicated
- Keep in O_2 and humidity
- Racemic epinephrine, 0.5 ml of 2.25% solution in 3 ml normal saline, by nebulizer may provide relief; effect may last 30-60 min; may repeat q1-2h or rarely, up to q20min, if necessary; a child who has received racemic epinephrine must be admitted for observation
- If not responding to racemic epinephrine, should be observed in ICU setting and may require intubation
- Recommend use of dexamethasone in moderate to severe croup (0.6 mg/kg PO/IM)

27

BRONCHIOLITIS

CLINICAL FEATURES (see Table 27-2)

- Prodrome: upper respiratory tract infection ± fever, poor feeding, and irritability
- Physical signs include fever, dehydration, wheezing, dyspnea, tachypnea (rate, 50-80/min), intercostal indrawing with use of accessory muscles, and tachycardia; wheezing and crackles on auscultation
- May see hyperinflation with increased AP diameter and hyperresonance
- Increasing severity indicated by apnea, decreasing PaO_2 (≤65 mm Hg), increasing $PaCO_2$ (≥45 mm Hg), tachycardia or bradycardia, increasing tachypnea, cyanosis progressing to respiratory arrest

INVESTIGATIONS

- CXR: shows hyperinflation, increased linear markings, and areas of atelectasis
- ABG: if clinically indicated; initially shows hypoxemia and hypercapnia in more severe cases
- Nasal swab for rapid detection of RSV antigen

MANAGEMENT

- Transcutaneous O_2 monitoring
- Humidified O_2 to maintain O_2 saturation > 92%
- Trial of Salbutamol (0.5% solution), 0.01-0.03 ml/kg in 3 ml normal saline, by inhalation
- Intubation and ventilation rarely required
- Ribavirin used only in consultation with infectious disease specialist in treatment of hospitalized children with severe RSV infections; indications for ribavirin include congenital heart disease, bronchopulmonary dysplasia, chronic lung disease, immunosuppression (chemotherapy, transplant), immunodeficiency, age <8wk; additional indications dictated by clinical situation
- Ribavirin given by small-particle aerosol generator (SPAG-2); possible teratogenicity, therefore warn pregnant women; particles may precipitate on contact lenses
- Mortality < 1%; 30% of patients may have subsequent recurrent wheezing episodes; recurrent wheeze likely because of asthma

PNEUMONIA

ETIOLOGY (Table 27-3)

- Viruses most common overall (RSV, parainfluenza, influenza A and B, adenovirus)
- Newborn: group B *streptococci, Escherichia coli, Listeria*
- 0-4 mo: consider CMV, *C. trachomatis, S. pneumonia*
- 0-5 yr: *S. pneumoniae;* in sick child < 2 yr of age consider *S. aureus,* especially if pneumatocele, empyema; *H. influenzae* (decreased incidence because of immunization)

Table 27-3 Epidemiologic, Clinical, and Laboratory Features of Acute Pneumonia in Normal Infants and Children According to Etiologic Agents

	Bacteria	Virus	Mycoplasma
Temperature	Majority ≥ 39° C	Majority < 39° C	Majority < 38° C
Onset	Abrupt; may follow URI	Gradually worsening URI	Gradually worsening cough (days-wk)
Others in home ill	Infrequent	Frequent, concurrent	Frequent; wk apart
Associated signs, symptoms	Respiratory distress common; meningitis and septic arthritis occasionally co-exist; pleuritic chest pain common	Frequent: myalgia, rash, conjunctivitis, pharyngitis, mouth ulcers, diarrhea	Frequent: Headache, sore throat, myalgia Occasional: rash, conjunctivitis, myringitis, enanthem, hacking paroxysmal cough (sometimes productive)
Toxicity	+++	+	+
X-ray	Usually infiltrate in distribution of lobe or subsegment of lobe	Interstitial pattern; may be diffuse	May be lobar or diffuse
Pleural fluid	May occur	Infrequent; majority small	Infrequent; majority small

Modified from Long SS: Treatment of acute pneumonia in infants and children, *Pediatr Clin North Am* 30:299, 1983.

27

- >5 yr: *M. pneumoniae* (most common cause in school-age child); *S. pneumoniae*
- Aspiration: oral bacteria (anaerobes); may be associated with pleural effusion and lung abscesses
- Nosocomial: aspiration (oral bacteria), *S. aureus,* enteric bacilli

INVESTIGATIONS

- CBC, differential count
- Blood culture
- Sputum culture (nasopharyngeal cultures not representative)
- ABG if patient in respiratory distress
- CXR
- Tuberculin skin test (see p. 258)
- Cold agglutinin titer, mycoplasma titer, throat swab for *Mycoplasma* culture
- Diagnostic thoracentesis if significant pleural fluid present (see p. 495)

TREATMENT

- General supportive care, including IV or PO fluids
- Humidified O_2
- IV or PO antibiotics (Table 27-4)
- Empyema requires chest tube drainage (see p. 495)
- In immunocompromised patients, broaden coverage to include *S. aureus* (cloxacillin, vancomycin), *P. aeruginosa* (aminoglycosides, piperacillin, ceftazidime), anaerobes (penicillin, clindamycin)
- Flexible bronchoscopy and bronchoalveolar lavage to rule out viral or *P. carinii* infection may be indicated in immunosuppressed patients or in those deteriorating on maximum therapy; open-lung biopsy occasionally necessary
- Most regimens last 10-14 days total; *S. aureus* usually requires minimum of 3 wk of therapy

ACUTE ASTHMA

HISTORY

- Duration and course of attack, triggering factors (may include viral respiratory tract infections, cold air, exercise, chemical irritants, tobacco smoke, stress, and allergens)
- Determine number of hospital admissions, dependency on steroids, history of ICU admissions, family history of asthma, allergies, medication, and adverse drug-reaction history
- Rule out cardiac disease, foreign body (FB) aspiration, gastroesophageal reflux, bronchiolitis

PHYSICAL EXAM

- Assess for fatigue, restlessness, altered mental status, inability to speak
- Level of consciousness is a major indicator of deterioration.
- Beware RR > 30 breaths/min, HR > 110 beats/min in older child
- Look for cyanosis; use of accessory muscles of respiration; asymmetry

Table 27-4 Bacterial Pneumonia*

Age	Bacteria	Inpatient	Outpatient
Neonate	Gr B *strep*, Gram-neg bacilli	Ampicillin + gentamicin ± erythromycin	
1-3 mo	*S. pneumonia, chlamydia, pertussis, S. aureus, H. flu*	Ampicillin± erythromycin or Cefuroxime ± erythromycin	
3 mo-5 yr	*S. pneumoniae, S. aureus, H. influenzae*	Ampicillin ± erythromycin† or Cefuroxime	Amoxicillin
>5 yr	*S. pneumoniae, Chlamydia, Mycoplasma, H. influenzae*	Erythromycin† or Ampicillin or cefuroxime	Erythromycin† or Penicillin
Immunocompromised	Any organism but particularly PCP, CMV, Gram-neg bacilli, *S. aureus* (consider fungi; other organisms)	*Nonneutropenic* Cefuroxime ± cotrimoxazole ± erythromycin *Neutropenic* Piperacillin + gentamicin ± cotrimoxazole‡ ± erythromycin	
Pleural effusion		Cefuroxime	
Lung abscess		Cloxacillin ± clindamycin	
Aspiration		Penicillin or clindamycin	
Sickle cell disease		Cefuroxime	

*Majority of infectious pneumonias are of viral etiology; also consider TB.

†May use clarithromycin.

‡For PCP, atypical interstitial pneumonitis ± hypoxia.

27

of air entry; evidence of subcutaneous emphysema, pneumothorax, or pneumomediastinum
- Significant pulsus paradoxus > 15 mm Hg

INVESTIGATIONS

- O_2 saturation monitoring, if available
- ABG in moderate or severe cases: beware of patient with normal, rising, or elevated $PaCO_2$, or with O_2 saturation <92% in room air
- CXR only if clinically indicated; may show hyperinflation, increased peribronchial markings, atelectasis, or evidence of pneumothorax or pneumomediastinum
- Pulmonary function testing (e.g., peak flow) with portable spirometric device for objective assessment of degree of obstruction; in severe asthma, peak flow rates 20%-30% predicted value (see Table 27-1)
- Obtain theophylline level if child receiving theophylline preparation

TREATMENT

- For management of status asthmaticus, see p. 17
- Humidified O_2 to maintain O_2 saturation > 92%, by mask or nasal prongs
- Correct fluid deficits if dehydration present, and provide maintenance IV fluids and electrolytes; caution: avoid fluid overload
- Sympathomimetic drugs: Salbutamol (drug of choice) (0.5% solution, 5 mg/ml), 0.03 ml/kg/dose (maximum 1 ml) in 3 ml normal saline, by aerosol mask; mild cases, masks q3-4h; moderate-to-severe cases, may give 0.03 ml/kg in 3 ml normal saline up to q20min
- Anticholinergic drugs: Ipratropium bromide (Atrovent) useful in treatment of acute asthma when combined with β_2 agents (e.g., Salbutamol); may give 250 μg (1 ml) ipratropium bromide q4h with Salbutamol mask; up to q20min × 3 in severe cases
- Corticosteroids
  - Use early in management of moderate-to-severe cases, in conjunction with aggressive bronchodilator therapy; prednisone 2 mg/kg/day PO (maximum 60 mg/day) for 5 days; dexamethasone 0.3 mg/kg/dose PO as alternative
  - IV steroids if not tolerating oral steroids or severe exacerbation: IV hydrocortisone 4-6 mg/kg q4-6h (may give 5-10 mg/kg for initial dose if severe/deteriorating)
  - If patient improves, convert to oral steroids
- Use antibiotics only with documented bacterial infection
- In refractory cases, ICU care may be needed for trial of IV Salbutamol or possible intubation and ventilation (rare)

CHRONIC ASTHMA

MANAGEMENT

- Environmental control: eliminate specific environmental allergens or irritants (e.g., cigarette smoke)
- Immunotherapy: not generally useful in asthma, consider only if attacks triggered by specific unavoidable allergens; never sole therapy

- Exercise programs should be encouraged; swimming often well tolerated even in patients whose asthma triggered by exercise-induced bronchospasm
- Pharmacologic strategy (Fig. 27-4): bronchodilators prn to relieve symptoms of cough and wheeze (β_2 agonists, anticholinergics); if patients require bronchodilators > 3-4 ×/wk on frequent basis, consider regular antiinflammatory prophylaxis

BRONCHODILATORS

- Inhalation route preferred
- For infants and young children: Salbutamol metered-dose inhaler (MDI) with aerochamber and mask attachment at 100-200 μg (1-2 puffs) qid prn for symptoms of cough, wheeze, or shortness of breath (if just recovering from exacerbation use 0.2-0.3 puffs/kg/dose qid × 2 days and then above maintenance dose)
- For adolescents, similar dose with MDI or dry powder system

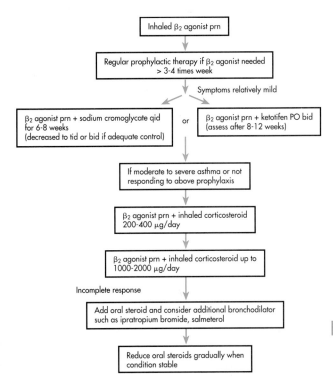

Fig. 27-4 Pharmacologic Management of Chronic Asthma.

27

- Alternative (in selected cases): nebulization, Salbutamol 0.01-0.03 ml/kg (max 1 ml of 0.5% solution in 3 ml of normal saline by aerosol mask q4-6h prn)
- Give 2-3 puffs Salbutamol 5-10 min before exercise for exercise-induced bronchospasm
- Other β_2 agonist: terbutaline (Bricanyl) 1 puff q4-6h prn
- Anticholinergics: ipratropium bromide (Atrovent), available as MDI 1-2 puffs (20 µg/puff) qid

ANTIINFLAMMATORY THERAPY (PROPHYLAXIS)
- Corticosteroids may be used as chronic or intermittent therapy (seasonal)
- Beclomethasone 200-400 µg/day (2 puffs qid, then bid when stable); high-dose beclomethasone (up to 1600 µg/day) in severe asthma
- Budesonide 200-400 µg/day by MDI or 0.25-0.5 mg bid by nebulizer
- Fluticasone (Flovent) 50-100 µg bid (starting dose)
- Side effects of inhaled steroids: oral thrush, dysphonia (suggest rinsing mouth with water after each use); adrenal suppression possible with prolonged high-dose inhaled steroid
- Severe asthma may require oral prednisone; side effects minimized with alternate-day therapy
- Sodium cromoglycate (Intal): for exercise-induced bronchospasm if bronchodilator unsuccessful; 2 puffs (1 mg/puff) or 1 spincap qid, then decrease to bid when stable; should be used up to 6 wk to determine effectiveness
- Nedocromil sodium (Tilade): prevents antigen-challenge and exercise-induced bronchospasm; for use in children >12 yr only; 2 puffs (2 mg/puff) qid
- Ketotifin (Zaditen): oral prophylactic with antihistamine properties; should be used 8-12 wk to determine effectiveness; 1 mg PO bid for age >3 yr; side effects are mild sedation, weight gain (rarely)

CYSTIC FIBROSIS (CF)

CLINICAL FEATURES
- See Table 27-5 and Fig. 27-5

DIAGNOSIS
- Most reliable method of diagnosis: quantitative analysis of sodium chloride content in sweat using urecholine or pilocarpine ionophoresis
- Minimum of 100 mg of sweat should be collected
- May be difficult to obtain enough sweat in first wk of life; limiting factor in testing very young infants
- Sweat chloride > 60 mmol/L in 98% of cases of cystic fibrosis (CF)
- False-positive results seen with poor laboratory technique, nephrotic syndrome, Addison's disease, malnutrition, nephrogenic diabetes insipidus, G6PD deficiency, glycogen storage disease, ectodermal dysplasia, and hypothyroidism
- Pancreatic dysfunction determined by use of 3- to 5-day fecal fat collection and bentiromide test

Table 27-5 Clinical Features Present at Diagnosis of CF

Age and clinical feature	Approximate incidence, %
0-2 yr	
Meconium ileus	10
Obstructive jaundice	
Heat prostration/hyponatremia	
Hypoproteinemia/anemia	
Bleeding diathesis	
Failure to thrive	
Steatorrhea	
Bronchitis/bronchiolitis	
Staphylococcal pneumonia	
Rectal prolapse	20
2-12 yr	
Recurrent pneumonia/bronchitis	60
Malabsorption	85
Nasal polyps	
Intussusception	1-5
13 yr+	
Chronic pulmonary disease	70
Clubbing	
Abnormal glucose tolerance	20-30
Chronic intestinal obstruction	10-20
Recurrent pancreatitis	
Focal biliary cirrhosis	15-25
Portal hypertension	2-5
Gallstones	4-12
Diabetes mellitus	5-7
Aspermia	98

From MacLusky I, McLaughlin FJ, Levison H: Cystic fibrosis, part I, *Curr Prob Pediatr* 15(6):13, 1985.

MANAGEMENT
Respiratory
- Frequent sputum samples for culture and sensitivity
- Physiotherapy: postural drainage bid to tid in conjunction with bronchodilator therapy
- Bronchodilators (Salbutamol) often helpful, especially when given before physiotherapy, because high percentage of CF population has component of hyperreactive airway disease
- Inhalational tobramycin (2 ml=80 mg tid with Salbutamol) is occasionally used in chronic maintenance therapy for up to 1 yr
- Long-term daily oral antibiotics (e.g., cloxacillin, cotrimoxazole, or oral cephalosporins tailored to sputum culture results)
- Antenatal diagnosis now available: gene localized to long arm of chromosome 7; ΔF508 mutation is 3-base-pair deletion present in 70% of CF chromosomes; genetic counseling is available

27

Age-Related Manifestations of Cystic Fibrosis

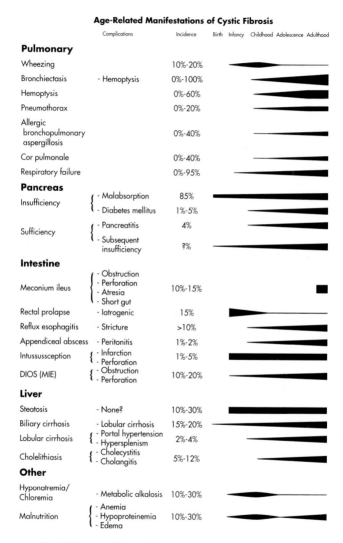

	Complications	Incidence	Birth	Infancy	Childhood	Adolescence	Adulthood
Pulmonary							
Wheezing		10%-20%					
Bronchiectasis	- Hemoptysis	0%-100%					
Hemoptysis		0%-60%					
Pneumothorax		0%-20%					
Allergic bronchopulmonary aspergillosis		0%-40%					
Cor pulmonale		0%-40%					
Respiratory failure		0%-95%					
Pancreas							
Insufficiency	- Malabsorption	85%					
	- Diabetes mellitus	1%-5%					
Sufficiency	- Pancreatitis	4%					
	- Subsequent insufficiency	?%					
Intestine							
Meconium ileus	- Obstruction / - Perforation / - Atresia / - Short gut	10%-15%					
Rectal prolapse	- Iatrogenic	15%					
Reflux esophagitis	- Stricture	>10%					
Appendiceal abscess	- Peritonitis	1%-2%					
Intussusception	- Infarction / - Perforation	1%-5%					
DIOS (MIE)	- Obstruction / - Perforation	10%-20%					
Liver							
Steatosis	- None?	10%-30%					
Biliary cirrhosis	- Lobular cirrhosis	15%-20%					
Lobular cirrhosis	- Portal hypertension / - Hypersplenism	2%-4%					
Cholelithiasis	- Cholecystitis / - Cholangitis	5%-12%					
Other							
Hyponatremia/Chloremia	- Metabolic alkalosis	10%-30%					
Malnutrition	- Anemia / - Hypoproteinemia / - Edema	10%-30%					

Fig. 27-5   Age-Related Manifestations of Cystic Fibrosis.

Acute Chest Exacerbation

- Manifested by fevers, increased cough, shortness of breath, sputum production, anorexia, and weight loss
- Increased WBC and ESR may be seen, especially with *P. cepacia* infection
- Check for deterioration in PFTs, ABGs, and CXR
- Mild exacerbation: 2-3 wk trial of oral antibiotic; if sputum grows *P. aeruginosa* and patient >13 yr, consider ciprofloxacin
- More severe: hospitalization, IV antibiotics appropriate for sputum culture results, inhalational therapy, physiotherapy ± O$_2$, nutritional support

Nutrition

- See Table 27-6

PLEURAL EFFUSION (Table 27-7)

- Send fluid for cytologic examination (cell differential, RBC, WBC, and malignant cells), biochemistry (protein, glucose, pH, LDH, fat content if chylous), microbiology (Gram's stain, culture, acid-fast staining, virology), and immunologic investigations when appropriate (e.g., complement studies)
- Transudates associated mainly with congestive heart failure, nephrotic syndrome, acute glomerulonephritis, cirrhosis, myxedema
- Exudates commonly caused by infection (bacterial, viral, *Mycoplasma,*

Table 27-6   Nutritional Management for Cystic Fibrosis

Calories	120%-150%
Protein	RDA*
Essential fatty acids	3%-5% total calories
Vitamin A	5,000-10,000 IU/day
Vitamin D	400-800 IU/day
Vitamin E	100-300 IU/day (water-soluble form)
Vitamin K	5 mg 2×/wk for infants 5 mg/day for children and older
Vitamin Bs	RDA* × 2
Vitamin C	RDA* × 2
Pancreatic enzymes	
Infants:	Add 1 regular Cotazym capsule or ⅓ tsp powder to 4 oz of formula (8,000 U lipase/120 ml formula)
Children and adults:	Regular capsules = 6/meal (48,000 U lipase/meal); 2/snack (16,000 U lipase/snack); enteric-coated microspheres (Cotazym ECS) = 3/meal (24,000 U lipase/meal); 1/snack (8,000 U lipase/snack)

Note: Enteric-coated capsules should not be used in children who cannot swallow capsules whole, as mucosal ulceration may develop.

Modified from MacLusky I, McLaughlin FJ, Levison H: Cystic fibrosis, part II, *Curr Prob Pediatr* 15(7):11, 1985.

*Recommended daily allowance. See p. 366.

27

Table 27-7 Constituents of Pleural Effusions

Test	Transudate	Exudate
Protein	<3 g/dl	>3 g/dl
Pleural-to-serum ratio, protein	<0.5	>0.5
Pleural-to-serum ratio, LDH	<0.6	>0.6
WBC	<1000/mm^3, usually >50% lymphocyte or mononuclear cells	>1000/mm^3 >50% PMN (acute inflammation) >50% lymphocytes (TB, neoplasm)
pH	>7.3	7.3 (inflammatory)
Glucose	= serum	↓
Amylase		↑ in pancreatitis

    mycobacterial, fungal), collagen vascular diseases, malignancy, pancreatitis, and subdiaphragmatic abscess
- See p. 495 for thoracocentesis; chest tube generally indicated for empyema, severe respiratory distress, or rapid reaccumulation of pleural fluid

PNEUMOTHORAX

- Common causes include asthma, trauma, cystic fibrosis, iatrogenic, hyaline membrane disease, or infection
- Incidence of spontaneous pneumothorax is highest in tall, thin, young adult males (approximately 1 : 10,000); usually caused by rupture of apical pleural blebs

CLINICAL FEATURES

- Dyspnea, chest pain, or shoulder tip pain
- May see marked respiratory distress and cyanosis on physical examination
- Chest wall movement decreased on affected side
- Percussion note on affected side tympanitic
- Larynx, trachea, and mediastinum may be shifted contralaterally
- Cardiac function may be compromised if pneumothorax under tension

MANAGEMENT

- Small pneumothorax (<5%) requires only observation; usually spontaneous resolution within 1 wk
- Small pneumothoraces resolve more quickly with 100% O_2, which will increase N_2 gradient between pleural gas and blood; beware CO_2-retaining patient depending on hypoxic drive; avoid hyperoxia in premature infants
- Larger pneumothoraces require chest tube drainage to underwater seal (see p. 495)
- To prevent recurrences in patients at risk, consider chemical pleurodesis (e.g., quinacrine), possible open thoracotomy, and pleural bleb excision or plication and stripping of apical pleura

CHAPTER 28

RHEUMATOLOGY

BETH GAMULKA

APPROACH TO CHILD WITH ARTHRITIS/JOINT SWELLING

HISTORY
- Early morning stiffness, interference with activity, weakness, heel pain (enthesitis)
- Associated fever, rash, weight loss, fatigue
- Older child: sexual activity
- Family history: psoriasis, inflammatory bowel disease, chronic back pain, ankylosing spondylitis, or SLE
- Travel history, TB exposure, school days missed

PHYSICAL EXAM
- Complete physical exam
- All joints, including spine; muscle wasting, muscle strength, Gowers sign
- Gait: walking and running; limb length discrepancy
- Bony tenderness
- Tenderness at entheses (sites of insertion of tendons and ligaments to bone)
- Tendon thickening

INVESTIGATIONS
- CBC + differential, ESR
- Blood cultures, when indicated
- Antinuclear antibody (ANA); specific autoantibodies if ANA positive: anti-dsDNA, anti-Sm, anti-RNP, anti-SSA(Ro), anti-SSB(La)
- If suspect SLE: C_3, C_4, PT/PTT, antiphospholipid antibodies, baseline liver and renal function, urinalysis, and 24-hour urine studies
- Joint X-rays: if trauma, infection, malignancy, or chronic arthritis suspected
- Slit lamp exam to detect uveitis
- Bone scan/arthrocentesis: if bone/joint infection suspected

JUVENILE ARTHRITIS (JA)(TABLES 28-1, 28-2, and Box 28-1)

DIAGNOSTIC CRITERIA FOR JA
- Arthritis in one or more joints for at least 6 wk
- Onset < 16 yr
- Exclusion of other rheumatic diseases

Table 28-1 Synovial Fluid Analysis

	Normal	Inflammatory	Infectious
Color	Colorless to straw	Yellow	Variable
Turbidity	Clear	Clear to turbid	Turbid
White cell count	$< 0.2 \times 10^9$/L (< 200/mm^3)	2.0-75.0×10^9/L ($2,000$-$75,000$/mm^3)	Often $> 100 \times 10^9$/L ($> 100,000$/mm^3)
Neutrophils, %	< 25	> 50	> 75
Glucose (mmol/L)	Nearly equal to blood glucose	< 2.8	> 2.8
Culture	Negative	Negative	Often positive

Modified from Kelley WN, Harris ED, Ruddy S, Sledge CB: *Textbook of rheumatology*, vol. 1, ed 2, Philadelphia, 1985, W.B. Saunders.

CLASSIFICATION

- Based on clinical presentation within first 6 mo
- Systemic: fever, rash, hepatosplenomegaly, lymphadenopathy, serositis, leucocytosis, anemia
- Polyarticular: ≥ 5 joints
- Pauciarticular: ≤ 4 joints

MANAGEMENT
Goals

- Reduce inflammation, prevent deformity, and maximize growth and development

Multidisciplinary Approach

- Physiotherapy, occupational therapy, social worker, school, orthopedic surgery, ophthalmology, rheumatology, pediatrics

Physical and Occupational Therapy

- Exercise to maintain range of motion (ROM) of joints and muscle strength
- Activities such as swimming and bicycle riding
- Splints to help prevent deformity
- Heat (e.g., warm bath): to help relieve pain and morning stiffness

Drug Therapy

- NSAIDs: monitor CBC, liver function, and renal function every 6 mo
- Intraarticular corticosteroids
- Slow-acting antirheumatic agents: methotrexate, sulfasalazine, IM gold, hydroxychloroquine (frequent CBC, liver-function, renal-function monitoring)
- Systemic corticosteroids (in systemic JRA, severe morning stiffness)
- Cytotoxic/antimetabolite therapy: azathioprine, cyclosporine

Table 28-2 Subgroups of JA*

	Pauciarticular type I	Pauciarticular type II	Polyarticular RF-negative	Polyarticular RF-positive	Systemic onset
% of JRA patients	30	15	25	10	20
Sex	80% girls	90% boys	90% girls	80% girls	Male = female
Age at onset	Early childhood	Late childhood	Throughout childhood	Late childhood	Throughout childhood
Joints	Large joints: knee, ankle, elbow	Large joints: hip girdle	Symmetric: any joints	Symmetric: any joints	Usually polyarticular: any joints
Sacroiliitis	No	Common (late)	No	Rare	No
Eye	~ 20% iridocyclitis (painless)	10%-20% acute iritis (painful)	No	No	No
RF	Negative	Negative	Negative	100%	Negative
ANA	60%-80% (risk factor for eye involvement)	Negative	25%	75%	Negative
Association with HLA-B27	No	Yes: 75%	No	No	No
Ultimate morbidity	Ocular damage	Subsequent spondyloarthropathy	Severe arthritis 10%-15%	Severe arthritis > 50%	Severe arthritis 25%-50%
Other features		Psoriasis, colitis, enthesitis, sausage digits, mouth ulcers, urethritis		Rheumatoid nodules, Sjögren's	Lymphadenopathy, fever, hepatosplenomegaly, rash, serositis, leukocytosis, anemia, thrombocytosis, hypoalbuminemia

Modified from Schaller, JG: Chronic arthritis in children. *Clin Orthop* 182:79-87, 1984.
*Classification based on clinical presentation within first 6 mo after onset of disease.
RF, Rheumatoid factor; *ANA,* antinuclear antibodies.

28

BOX 28-1 Common Differential Diagnosis of Arthritis in Childhood

Juvenile rheumatoid arthritis
    Pauciarticular type I
    Polyarticular RF-negative
    Polyarticular RF-positive
    Systemic
Spondyloarthropathies
    Pauciarticular type II:
        Juvenile ankylosing spondylitis
        Psoriatic
        Reiter's
        Inflammatory bowel disease (IBD)
Connective tissue diseases
    Systemic lupus erythematosis (SLE)
    Juvenile dermatomyositis
    Systemic sclerosis
    Mixed connective tissue disease
Vasculitides
    Henoch-Schönlein purpura (HSP)
Noninflammatory
    Fibromyalgia
    Reflex sympathetic dystrophy
    Growing pains
    Hypermobility syndrome
Infectious
    Primary (bone, joint, systemic)
        Bacterial: *Staphylococcus, H. influenza, Meningococcus, Gonococcus, Borrelia, Mycobacteria*
        Viral: Rubella, hepatitis B/C, parvovirus, EBV
        Mycoplasma
    Secondary (postinfectious)
        Acute rheumatic fever (post-strep arthritis)
        Shigella, Salmonella, Yersinia, Campylobacter
        Chlamydia
Malignancy
    Leukemia
    Neuroblastoma
    Lymphoma
    Bony tumors
Hematologic
    Hemophilia
    Sickle cell disease
Trauma
Orthopedic/Mechanical
    Legg-Calvé-Perthes (hip)
    Osgood-Schlatter (knee)
    Slipped capital femoral epiphysis (hip)
    Transient synovitis

HENOCH-SCHÖNLEIN PURPURA

- *Leukocytoclastic vasculitis*
- Features include purpuric skin lesions; abdominal pain ($\pm$ intussusception, GI bleeding); arthralgia/arthritis; hematuria/proteinuria; subcutaneous edema; rarely testicular, pulmonary, and neurologic changes
- Often have increased IgA
- Clinical diagnosis; most managed as outpatients; admit for severe abdominal pain
- For most, baseline renal function and urinalysis adequate with serial urinalyses needed for 3 mo
- More severe impairment of renal function: 24-hr urine studies for creatinine, protein
- If hospitalized (severe GI, renal, CNS): treatment mainly supportive (hydration, nutrition)
- Steroid use controversial but advocated by some for GI hemorrhage, testicular torsion, CNS; no proven value in renal disease
- Surgical consultation if intussusception or testicular torsion

KAWASAKI DISEASE

- 80% of affected children are $<$ age 4
- Most common in Asian children $>$ black $>$ white
- Most common cause of acquired heart disease in children

DIAGNOSTIC CRITERIA

- Fever $\geq$ 5 days
- Presence of four of following five conditions:
  1. Bilateral nonpurulent conjunctival injection
  2. Oral mucosal changes: may have any one of erythema, dryness, or fissuring of lips, strawberry tongue, erythema of oropharynx
  3. Peripheral extremities: may have any one of edema or erythema of palms or soles, desquamation of skin of tips of fingers or toes (in subacute phase)
  4. Rash: commonly truncal; polymorphic, nonvesicular
  5. Cervical lymphadenopathy $>$ 1.5 cm of one or more nodes
- Illness unexplained by another disease (e.g., streptococcal, staphylococcal, or measles infections)

ASSOCIATED CLINICAL FEATURES

- Irritability, arthritis, aseptic meningitis, hydrops of gallbladder, hepatic dysfunction, anterior uveitis, diarrhea, pneumonitis, urethritis, serous otitis media, skin peeling in inguinal area

CARDIOVASCULAR MANIFESTATIONS
Acute Phase

- Disease onset until resolution of fever, usually 1-10 days
- Myocarditis, pericarditis, endocarditis
- Arrhythmias
- ECG abnormalities

28

BOX 28-2 Classification Criteria of Systemic Lupus Erythematosus (SLE)

Four of eleven criteria needed:
1. Malar rash
2. Discoid rash
3. Photosensitivity
4. Oral and nasal ulcers
5. Nonerosive arthritis
6. Serositis (pericarditis, pleuritis)
7. Renal involvement (active sediment, proteinuria)
8. CNS involvement (seizures, psychosis)
9. Hematologic changes (hemolytic anemia, leukopenia, lymphopenia, thrombocytopenia)
10. Positive ANA
11. Immunologic abnormality: Positive anti-dsDNA, anti-Sm, LE prep, or false-positive VDRL

Modified from Tan EM, Cohen AS, Fries JF, et al: The 1982 revised criteria for the classification of systemic lupus erythematosus, *Arthritis Rheum* 25(11):1271-1277, 1982.

Subacute Phase

- From end of fever until resolution of all clinical features, usually 10-25 days
- Coronary artery aneurysms in approximately 20% of untreated cases

LABORATORY FEATURES

- Nonspecific and nondiagnostic
- Increased WBCs, neutrophilia
- Mild-to-moderate anemia
- Elevated ESR
- Increased platelets in subacute phase
- Mild increase in transaminases

TREATMENT

- Treat in consultation with rheumatologist and cardiologist
- Acute phase (febrile): ASA 100 mg/kg/day and IV gamma globulin 2 g/kg × 1 dose
- Subacute phase (afebrile): ASA 3-5 mg/kg/day ± dipyridamole (depending on results of echocardiogram)

INCOMPLETE (ATYPICAL) KAWASAKI DISEASE

- May not fulfill all diagnostic criteria
- Kawasaki disease difficult to diagnose in very young infants
- Maintain high index of suspicion in any prolonged febrile illness

FOLLOW-UP

- ECG and 2D-ECHO at diagnosis, 2 mo, 6 mo ± 1 yr after disease onset
- Length and mode of treatment depend on extent of coronary artery involvement

CHAPTER 29

SURGERY

Aₛₜᵣᵢ_d Gᵤₜₜₘₐₙₙ

NEONATAL ABDOMINAL EMERGENCIES

- Vomiting of bile-stained fluid in first few days of life indicates intestinal obstruction until proven otherwise
- Must rule out (R/O) sepsis (with paralytic ileus)
- Other suspicious signs and symptoms of surgical problem:
  - Polyhydramnios during pregnancy
  - Large gastric aspirate in delivery room
  - Cyanosis or choking with feeds
  - No meconium in first 24 hr of life
  - Abdominal distension

General Management Principles

- ABCs (see p. 3)
- NPO
- Nasogastric tube insertion (No. 10 if weight >2000 g; No. 8 if <2000 g); open-ended or to low gomco (suction) if obstruction suspected
- Cross-match ~100 cc of packed red cells at time of admission
- Correct electrolyte and acid-base abnormalities (see p. 100)
- Culture blood, urine, CSF if sepsis suspected; ampicillin, gentamycin ± metronidazole (if bowel perforation suspected)
- Chest, abdominal x-rays (AP, lateral decubitus)
- Radiocontrast studies to R/O malrotation, volvulus, and intestinal atresias
- Rule out other congenital anomalies

ESOPHAGEAL ATRESIA

- ~1/4000 live births
- Polyhydramnios, excess salivation, choking with feeds ± cyanotic spells
- Diagnosis made by inability to pass nasogastric tube into stomach and demonstration of its tip in air-filled dilated proximal esophagus (usually T3-T5) on CXR
- Majority associated with tracheal-esophageal fistula (TEF)
- See general management principles above; add penicillin or clindamycin if aspiration pneumonia present 2° to TEF
- Operation to correct atresia with fistula usually done within 24 hr of diagnosis; may be delayed if:
  1. Aspiration pneumonitis
  2. Severe associated cardiac (or other) anomalies (e.g., VACTERL)
- While awaiting surgery, infant should be kept head up, supine or prone, with suction tube in proximal pouch to avoid further aspiration

- Common complications:
  1. Reflux
  2. Esophageal stricture
  3. Anastomotic disruption
  4. Decreased pulmonary function

DUODENAL ATRESIA OR STENOSIS

- ~1/10,000 live births
- History of polyhydramnios
- Not associated with distended abdomen; jaundice may be present; if obstruction proximal to Vater's ampulla, vomitus is not bile stained (<10% of cases)
- 30%-50% associated with malrotation
- See general management principles
- AXR: "double bubble" pattern
- Urgent contrast studies to R/O malrotation, volvulus, and colonic atresias
- Duodenal atresia: ⅓ associated with trisomy 21
- Duodenal stenosis may appear later in childhood

JEJUNOILEAL ATRESIA (JA)/STENOSIS

- ~1/5000 live births
- Bilious vomiting with abdominal distension
- Etiology: secondary to intrauterine mesenteric vascular accident
- ⅓ associated with malrotation
- See general management principles
- AXR: dilated loops (thumb-sized) and multiple air-fluid levels
- Contrast enema: helpful in defining level and cause of obstruction and ruling out more distal second obstruction
- Exclude cystic fibrosis (~10% incidence in JA)

MALROTATION WITH MIDGUT VOLVULUS

- Bilious vomiting ± abdominal distension
- Presentation may be similar to necrotizing enterocolitis ± hematochezia ± peritoneal signs
- Presentation may be delayed or subacute; see general management principles
- AXR: multiple air-fluid levels or relatively gasless abdomen; occasionally, film is compatible with duodenal obstruction
- If diagnosis in doubt and no evidence of compromised bowel, urgent radiocontrast enema and upper GI study necessary to confirm presence of malrotation or duodenal obstruction; otherwise, direct to OR
- Delays associated with high morbidity and mortality 2° to gangrenous small bowel
- Must have radiographic evidence of normal position of stomach, duodenum, ligament of Treitz, and ileocecal region to R/O malrotation

MECONIUM ILEUS (MI)

- >95% associated with cystic fibrosis
- Complicated MI: may present with clinical and radiologic signs of peri-

tonitis (distended bowel with "ground glass" appearance, air-fluid levels absent ± intraabdominal calcifications)
- Uncomplicated MI less systemically ill; AXR shows distended loops of bowel
- Contrast enema: microcolon; reflux into distal ileus showing obstructive concretions
- Gastrograffin or Hypague Muco-myst enema used to relieve obstruction in attempt to avoid surgery; may need to be repeated
- Surgery required in ~50% of all patients
- Cystic fibrosis workup (see p. 466)

NECROTIZING ENTEROCOLITIS
- Most common in premature babies; etiology controversial
- In full-term infants, history of anoxic/asphyxial event
- Presentation ranges from subtle signs such as feeding intolerance to more acute picture of abdominal distension, reddened abdominal wall, bloody stools, bilious aspirates, and systemic signs (shock, thrombocytopenia, neutropenia, anemia)
- AXR: variable, thickened bowel loops +/- ascites; pneumatosis intestinalis or gas in portal vein; pneumoperitoneum; persistently dilated bowel loops
- In acute stages, frequent assessments including abdominal x-rays (to exclude pneumoperitoneum) and blood work (CBC, gas, lytes) q6-8h
- Barium enema contraindicated during acute episode, unless diagnosis is in doubt
- See general management principles, including full septic workup
- IV antibiotics (e.g., ampicillin, gentamicin, and metronidazole) × 7-10 days
- Indications for surgical intervention include
  1. Perforation
  2. Increasing abdominal wall erythema
  3. Failure of medical therapy
  4. Persistent fixed loop on consecutive abdominal films
- May use trial of peritoneal drainage with penrose drain to avoid operative risks in very low–birth weight babies (center-dependent)
- Complications include late strictures (3-4 wk; usually large bowel) and "short-gut" syndrome with malabsorption

HIRSCHSPRUNG'S DISEASE
- ~1/500 live births
- Congenital absence of intramural ganglion cells in distal intestine
- Variable involvement: majority involve rectum/rectosigmoid area only; 25% total colonic
- On history: delayed passage of meconium with subsequent constipation
- On exam: abdominal distension with explosive passage of loose stool and air on rectal examination (may present as neonatal enterocolitis)
- Barium enema may not be diagnostic in first few days of life but is useful in excluding other causes of bowel obstruction; barium is not cleared in delayed film 24 hr later in Hirschsprung's disease
- Rectal biopsy necessary to confirm absence of ganglion cells

- Manage with one-, two-, or three-stage pull-through procedures (Soave, Swenson, Duhamel)
- If clinical picture of gastroenteritis, treat aggressively (IV antibiotics, rectal decompression)

IMPERFORATE ANUS

- ~1/5000 live births

High

- Male > female (2:1)
- 60% associated with genitourinary (GU) anomalies
- Treatment: colostomy, posterior sagittal anorectoplasty (PSARP)

Low

- 15%-20% associated with GU anomalies
- Treatment: anoplasty in neonatal period

DIAPHRAGMATIC HERNIA

- ~1/3000 live births
- Most common on left side
- Presentation variable: respiratory distress worsened with bagging
- On exam: scaphoid abdomen, absent breath sounds on affected side; may hear bowel sounds in chest
- CXR: diagnostic (e.g., bowel loop in thoracic cavity)
- See general management principles
- Preop management: orogastric decompression, mechanical ventilation, paralysis, and optimal cardiorespiratory support
- Poor prognostic signs:
  1. Respiratory distress in first 12 hr of life
  2. Hypoplastic lungs, persistent pulmonary hypertension (PPHN), and high ventilatory requirements

HYPERTROPHIC PYLORIC STENOSIS

- ~1/300 live births
- More common in males (4:1); genetic predisposition
- Present at ~3 wk of age with nonbilious, projectile vomiting; dehydration
- Diagnosis is made by palpating pyloric "tumor;" to facilitate examination:
  1. Insert No. 10 nasogastric tube, and connect to suction to empty stomach
  2. Allow baby to drink solution of warm dextrose water while flexing legs at hips to relax abdominal wall
  3. As baby relaxes, hypertrophied pylorus is felt midway between xiphisternum and umbilicus, slightly to right of midline in upper abdomen
  4. Structures that can be mistaken for pylorus include left lobe of liver and right kidney
- Diagnostic tools: abdominal ultrasound (UGI series, if diagnosis in doubt)

- May have associated electrolyte imbalances ($\downarrow Cl^-$, $\downarrow K^+$, metabolic alkalosis), jaundice
- Correct fluid and electrolyte deficits before operative intervention (useful approach is 0.45% normal saline with 20 mEq KCl/L to correct deficit and to provide for maintenance and ongoing losses)
- Surgery is definitive treatment; early refeeding postop

MISCELLANEOUS EMERGENCIES IN OLDER CHILDREN

INTUSSUSCEPTION

- ~2-4/1000 live births
- Most common in first year of life; male > female (3:2)
- Colicky abdominal pain, currant-jelly stools, and palpable abdominal mass are classic, but often signs more subtle
- See general management principles (neonatal, apply to older children); rehydrate before reduction
- Air contrast enema will confirm diagnosis and can be used to reduce intussusceptions in 85% of cases (barium enema an alternative)
- 10% incidence of recurrence after successful hydrostatic reduction; may need to repeat reduction
- Hydrostatic reduction of intussusception contraindicated when clinical evidence of peritonitis

APPENDICITIS

- Rare in children < 1 yr of age
- With classical presentation and physical exam, no blood work or imaging required for diagnosis
- See general management principles
- Antibiotics (usually ampicillin, gentamicin, and metronidazole) used for all cases of ruptured appendicitis and continued for 5-7 days
- Dose of antibiotic, usually cefoxitin, given preoperatively for prophylaxis in unruptured appendicitis
- When diagnosis is not certain; admit and observe

INGESTED FOREIGN BODY

- Foreign body (FB) in esophagus must be removed endoscopically (see p. 418)
- Once FB is in stomach, 95% will pass without intervention
- Absolute indications for intervention:
  1. Signs of obstruction, fever, vomiting, hematemesis
  2. Battery (may use cathartics like Mg citrate or enema if distal)
- Relative indications:
  1. Long, sharp objects if not past pylorus
  2. FB still in stomach after 4 wk

INGUINAL HERNIAS

- Incidence: ~2%-4% term babies; up to 30% in premature babies
- M > F; ~60% on right side; 30% on left side; 10% bilateral
- On exam: smooth, firm mass emerging through external inguinal ring,

29

increasing with intraabdominal pressure (stretch infant with legs and arms extended; crying will increase pressure; ask older children to cough)
- Must differentiate from retractile testis
- High incidence of incarceration below age 1 yr with danger of testicular artery thrombosis and intestinal obstruction
- Incarcerated hernia: nonreducible, tender mass ± irritability, vomiting, fever
- Reduction of previously incarcerated hernia should be followed by repair within 24-48 hr
- In premature infants, repair usually delayed until weight of 2500 g attained

CRYPTORCHIDISM

- More common in premature infants; genetic component
- Etiology controversial: idiopathic, anatomic abnormality, endocrine disorder
- Bilateral can be associated with anomalies of abdominal wall or renal system
- Most undescended testes will descend during first year of life
- Physical exam: document size compared with other testis and position to which it can be manipulated
- Hormonal challenge (β-HCG 10,000 units IM × 5-6 doses/2 wk) best in retractile/high scrotal testes; not usually successful in true undescended testes but may increase size to facilitate surgery and may predict which testis will descend on its own; side effects related to increased production of testosterone
- Complications: torsion, tumor, trauma, ↓ spermatogenesis, hernia, and psychologic
- Orchiopexy at ~ age 18 mo-2 yr

BILIARY ATRESIA

- ~1/10,000 live births
- Must be ruled out in infant with conjugated hyperbilirubinemia
- Associated developmental anomalies may coexist: situs inversus, dextrocardia, polysplenia
- Differential diagnosis usually includes neonatal hepatitis or metabolic diseases resulting in hepatic dysfunction (see p. 201)
- Liver biopsy and biliary scan (DISIDA) are most useful tests discriminating between neonatal hepatitis and biliary atresia
- Portoenterostomy (Kasai procedure) most successful in relieving jaundice if done before 2 mo and before onset of severe hepatic cirrhosis
- Liver transplantation is treatment of choice if diagnosis made after 3 mo or following unsuccessful Kasai procedure

UMBILICAL GRANULOMA

- Results from chronic infection at site of umbilical cord separation
- Treatment: cautery with silver nitrate sticks or suture ligation
- Must be differentiated from omphalomesenteric duct remnants (look for fecal or serous discharge), which may require excision and abdominal exploration

Table 29-1   Etiology of Gastrointestinal Bleeding by Age and Site

Age	Upper GI	Lower GI
Neonate (0-30 days)	1. Swallowed maternal blood 2. Gastric erosions or peptic ulceration (PUD) 3. Hemorrhagic disease	1. Swallowed maternal blood 2. Anal fissure 3. NEC 4. Malrotation and volvulus 5. ~50% unexplained
Infant (30 day-1 yr)	1. Reflux esophagitis 2. Peptic ulcer disease or gastric erosions	1. Anal fissure 2. Intussusception 3. Volvulus 4. Duplication 5. Gastroenteritis
Child (1-6 yr)	1. Esophageal varices 2. Peptic ulcer disease or gastric erosions	1. Anal fissure 2. Rectal prolapse 3. Gastroenteritis 4. Meckel's diverticulum 5. Juvenile polyps 6. Trauma
Older child (6-18 yr)	1. Esophageal varices 2. Peptic ulcer disease or gastric erosions	1. Polypoid disease 2. Inflammatory bowel disease 3. Hemorrhoids 4. Hemangiomas 5. Arteriovenous malformations 6. Meckel's diverticulum

GASTROINTESTINAL BLEEDING (Table 29-1)

- ABCs (see p. 3)
- Pass NG tube to determine source of bleeding (upper versus lower)
- Investigations may include endoscopy/colonoscopy: labeled RBC isotope scan, angiogram; laparectomy with intraoperative enteroscopy

CHAPTER 30

UROLOGY

DARIUS BÄGLI

ACUTE SCROTUM/TESTICULAR TORSION

- Keep patient NPO: requires urgent referral to urologist in all cases
- Major differential diagnosis is torsion of testis (spermatic cord) versus torsion of appendix testis versus epididymitis versus inguinal hernia
- History very important: acute torsion of testis may show history of precipitating factor, although factor may be mild (e.g., stepping out of bathtub) but can occur spontaneously, even while asleep; often "worst" pain patient has ever felt; cryptorchidism; peripubertal child
- Torsion of appendix more common in 6-7 yr old, less painful overall, more localized to upper pole (may have small "blue dot" visible through thin infant scrotal skin)
- Torsion highly salvageable if less than 6-8 hr duration
- To help differentiate torsion from epididymitis and orchitis (occurs in older and/or sexually active boys ± urethritis): investigate genitourinary tract with color Doppler ultrasonography
- Color Doppler studies: finding flow in testicular parenchyma, not periphery tends to rule out torsion; may be difficult to obtain flow from completely normal testes, especially if testicular volume ≤1cc; standard Doppler unreliable (may pick up signals from surrounding tissues and give false-negative results)
- Nuclear scan for torsion has been gold standard for many years; within first 12 hr after age 8; after 1-2 days, inflammation or even infarction may show increased uptake (i.e., difficult to differentiate epididymitis from torsion)
- Even if manual detorsion performed, patient must undergo bilateral orchiopexy as soon as possible
- Neonatal testicular torsion: generally involves entire scrotal contents: extravaginal versus cord only in older children in whom processus vaginalis obliterated; virtually no chance of salvaging functional testicular tissue; generally explored electively (bilateral neonatal torsion explored immediately) at age 6 mo with contralateral orchiopexy done at that time; always watch for signs of contralateral torsion until then

EPIDIDYMITIS

- Must be differentiated from testicular torsion; true microbial epididymitis rare in prepubertal patient, may be chemical (i.e., due to urine forced retrograde through ejaculatory ducts); should consider ductal or other GU anomaly if no organism documented (IVP or VCUG)
- Etiology: *N. gonorrhoeae, C. trachomatis,* viruses, gram-negative organisms (associated with UTI), and tuberculosis (TB)

- Treat gonorrheal epididymitis as for uncomplicated gonorrhea (see p. 171); must also treat for *Chlamydia* (with 10 days of tetracycline, doxycycline, or erythromycin)
- Follow-up urine cultures 3-7 days after therapy

HYDROCELE

- Fluid collection within potential space derived from peritoneal lining extending into and surrounding testicle; peritoneum passes through internal inguinal ring as processus vaginalis; processus constitutes hernia sac of infant indirect inguinal hernia; if this passage remains patent, fluid moves between hydrocele sac and peritoneum (communicating hydrocele); clearly transilluminates, often revealing testicle that may be otherwise difficult to palpate
- Usually repaired surgically through inguinal approach if not spontaneously resolved by 2-3 yr of age; acute hydrocele (reactive hydrocele) may suggest scrotal pathology (e.g., testicular torsion, torsion of testicular appendix, infection, tumor, trauma); ultrasound (US) useful in these cases to visualize gonad and scrotal contents
- Hydrocele usually asymptomatic; may become painful if full and tense, particularly if fluid forced into sac through sudden bout of coughing, straining; if processus very narrow, fluid may not return easily to peritoneal cavity; patient on peritoneal dialysis may be more predisposed to hydrocele development or delayed/failed resolution

PHIMOSIS

- Most childhood phimosis is physiologically normal and does not mandate circumcision
- Foreskin may not be fully retractable until >10 yr of age; preputial skin should never be forcibly retracted; leads to tearing, scarring, and true acquired phimosis
- Ballooning of foreskin during voiding is acceptable as long as urine stream normal, UTI (documented by culture) absent, and scarring absent

BALANITIS

- Inflammation of glans skin
- Posthitis is inflammation of preputial skin
- Balanoposthitis: inflammation of glans and preputial skin; true balanoposthitis is painful; treat with β-lactam antibiotic or cephalosporin; watch for cellulitis
- Simple reddened foreskin without frank symptoms does not require antibiotic treatment; attention to proper manual evacuation of any residual urine after voiding and drying of foreskin after urination is usually all that is required

HYPOSPADIAS

- Congenital defect resulting in urethra terminating prematurely anywhere along the undersurface (ventral) of penis (glanular, coronal, distal, proximal, scrotal, perineal)
- May include mild, moderate, or severe degree of chordee (ventral curvature) because of skin, ventral fibrous tissue, and/or true ventral corporal disproportion (compared to dorsal aspect of corporal bodies)
- Must always consider intersex in case of hypospadias and bilateral nonpalpable gonads (see p. 95)
- Some genetic predisposition: <10% in father, <15% in brother, <20% in other family member
- Cryptorchidism (10%-30%) and inguinal hernia (10%) may be present
- Hypospadias may accompany more complex constellations of congenital defects
- Low incidence (<5%) of upper tract urologic abnormalities with hypospadias alone; therefore routine screening not done

SURGICAL REPAIR

- Most forms are repaired; indications include normalizing sexual function and ability to void without difficulty; normal genital appearance important in maintaining proper psychosexual development
- Most repairs done in one procedure; preputial foreskin used in repair; do not circumcise newborn; age of repair usually 6-18 mo; goals of surgery include straightening phallus and extending urethra to tip of glans

VESICOURETERAL REFLUX

- Backward ascent of urine up ureter to kidney
- Primary reflux: intramural portion of ureter (tunnel) running within bladder wall is too short
- Secondary reflux: adequate tunnel does not withstand pathologically elevated bladder pressures (e.g., neurogenic bladder, severe dysfunctional voiding); need to address bladder pathology first
- May be unilateral or bilateral; graded from 1-5 (Fig. 30-1)
- Reflux in absence of urine infection considered relatively benign
- Reflux + urine infection = pyelonephritic scarring
- Incidence: <2% in general pediatric population; lower in dark-skinned and higher in light-skinned patients; with UTI (especially febrile), incidence is 30%-50%; indication for radiologic investigation of even first-time UTI

INVESTIGATIONS

- History of fever accompanying urinary symptoms of infection; in infant, new irritability, lethargy, failure to thrive; also consider risk factors for improper voiding (e.g., dysuria, stress, psychosexual trauma, constipation, urgency, urge incontinence, new frequency)
- Urine cultures: never treat positive bagged specimen, always obtain voided or catheter urine; urinalysis, WBC, nitrites, leukocyte esterase support diagnosis of UTI

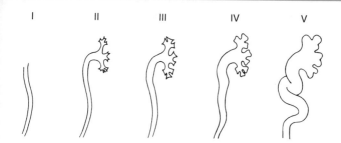

Fig. 30-1 Grades of vesicoureteral reflux (international classification).

- Voiding cystourethrogram (VCUG): first study of choice; defines anatomy, presence, and grade of reflux; degree of renal calyx blunting; post void residual urine
- Ultrasound: Helpful to assess renal cortex, good renal baseline study to assess renal growth
- Nuclear cystogram (RNC; radionuclide cystogram): good follow-up study; not used as initial test because anatomic detail poor

MANAGEMENT
Medical

- May often observe grade 1-3 reflux; place on prophylactic antibiotic (1 ×/day); spontaneous resolution approximately 90% (grade 1), 80% (grade 2), 50% (grade 3); usually within 4 yr; less likely to resolve thereafter; follow yearly; grades 4 and 5 reflux resolution < 15%
- Optimize bladder emptying: timed voiding, double voiding, treat constipation

Surgical

- Indications:
    1. Breakthrough infections on prophylaxis
    2. Poor compliance with prophylaxis
    3. Evidence of progressive scarring, loss of renal function
    4. Prolonged observation without resolution; grade 4 and 5 most likely to come to surgical correction

URINARY TRACT INFECTION (UTI)

- New first-time documented UTI should be evaluated in most cases; need to assess circumstances of UTI in each patient; presence of UTI + fever mandates radiologic evaluation
- Specimen collection: do not treat positive bagged specimens; only really useful if negative; clean catch, catheterized, or suprapubic taps (infants) most reliable
- See also p. 330

HYDRONEPHROSIS

ANTENATAL HYDRONEPHROSIS

- Increasingly detected during prenatal ultrasonography; may occur unilaterally, bilaterally, in isolation, or in association with other congenital anomalies
- Confirm persistence of hydro postnatally with US; do not perform US too early (i.e., hydro may not remanifest postnatally until 7th day of life)

Prophylactic Antibiotics

- ≤2 mo of age: ampicillin 25 mg PO/day; >2 mo of age: trimethoprim-sulfamethoxazole
- Begin prophylaxis at birth and continue until radiologic assessment complete
- Prophylax all reflux, dilated ureters with or without reflux, and very young patients with UPJ obstruction; older UPJ patients being followed can do well without prophylaxis

POSTNATAL HYDRONEPHROSIS

- Obtain VCUG (rule out urinary reflux, posterior urethral valves)
- If reflux absent, obtain DTPA Lasix renogram to assess for antegrade (forward flow) obstruction (i.e., UPJ obstruction)
- Unless urgent, radionuclides (DTPA, DMSA) best handled by neonatal kidney after 2 mo of age

NEUROGENIC BLADDER

- Refers to inability of bladder to relax sufficiently to accommodate (store) urine (hypertonic, poor compliance) or inability to contract sufficiently (hypotonic) and/or incoordination (dysynergy) between bladder detrusor muscle contraction and sphincter relaxation; most common in spinal cord injury or congenital anomaly (neural tube defects)
- Intravesical storage pressure is major predictor of upper urinary tract damage secondary to reflux; generally occurs if pressure > 35 cm H_2O
- Low sphincter tone may be managed with α-adrenergics (e.g., ephedrine) or surgical "tightening" (slings, bladder neck surgery, artificial sphincter)
- Spastic sphincter and unstable detrusor usually managed with anticholinergics (oxybutynin) ± surgery in conjunction with intermittent catheterization protocols
- Concomitant constipation may contribute to high intravesical pressures and significantly exacerbate neurogenic bladder symptoms and dysfunction

GAVIN MORRISON AND ANNE DIPCHAND

TABLE OF CONTENTS

VENOUS ACCESS

- For any procedure involving cannula placement, likelihood of success is increased if physician takes care to optimize conditions under which he or she is working
- Patient positioning, restraint, sedation, and ambient conditions such as lighting can all be manipulated to doctor's advantage

489

- Before skin puncture, skin should be cleaned with appropriate antiseptic or alcohol; consider use of local anesthetic
- Route by which intravascular compartment is accessed will depend on indication for access, urgency with which it is required, ease of patient vascular access, and skill of doctor
- In child with circulatory collapse, access must be attained urgently; for most physicians, choice lies primarily between peripheral venous cannulation and placement of intraosseous (IO) needle; central venous line placement or intravenous cutdowns should only be attempted by experienced personnel
- In emergency situation, attempts at venous cannulation should be restricted to 3 or to time period not exceeding 180 sec before IO needle is sited (unless appropriate personnel is present to attempt central venous access or intravenous cutdown)

INTRAOSSEOUS ACCESS

- Method of choice for gaining access to vascular space in emergency situation when venous access is difficult
- Needle is inserted 2 cm inferior and 1 cm medial to tibial tuberosity
- Before siting needle, create stab wound through skin and subcutaneous tissue down to surface of medial tibial border
- Needle is inserted at 90° angle to surface of bone, using clockwise "screwing" motion until bony cortex has been penetrated; stylet is removed, and needle secured
- Correct siting likely if bloodlike marrow can be aspirated or aliquot of saline solution can be infused without extravasation; through this route colloids, crystalloids, blood products, and common emergency drugs can be administered

CENTRAL VENOUS ACCESS

External Jugular Vein (Figs. III-1 and III-2)

- This vein offers easiest route to access central circulation
- However, especially in small children, correct positioning and restraint are essential if successful cannula placement is to be attained; wrap uncooperative child in blanket so that his or her head and neck are accessible but limbs are controlled; he or she can then be placed in lap of seated assistant so that he or she lies along length of assistant's legs with neck extended as it lies over assistant's knees; alternatively, child may be placed on bed with roll of towels beneath shoulder; in this position, neck is opened up and vein is straightened; needle should penetrate skin in caudal direction where vein crosses sternocleidomastoid muscle (SCM)

Internal Jugular Vein (Fig. III-3)

- Usually right vein is accessed because course to superior vena cava is straight; dome of right lung lies lower than does left (reducing likelihood of iatrogenic pneumothorax); and thoracic duct, left-sided structure, is unlikely to be damaged
- As above, correct patient positioning is important if vein is to be successfully cannulated; patient is positioned supine
- Place roll under shoulders to extend patient's neck; head is turned to

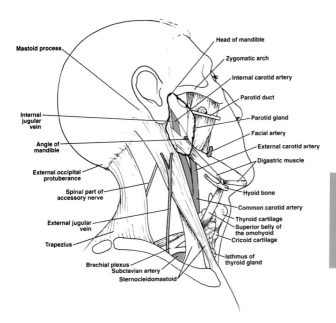

Fig. III-1 Vascular anatomy of neck.

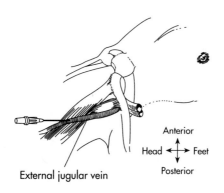

External jugular vein

Fig. III-2 **External jugular vein cannulation.** (See Fig. III-3 for anatomy.) (Adapted from Levin DL, Morriss FC: *Essentials of pediatric intensive care,* St Louis, 1990, Quality Medical Publishing.)

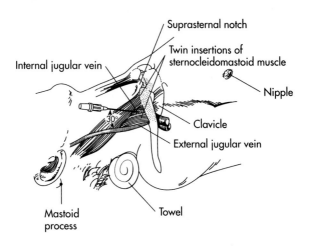

Fig. III-3 Internal jugular vein cannulation. (See text for explanation of technique.) (Adapted from Levin DL, Morriss FC: *Essentials of pediatric intensive care*, St Louis, 1990, Quality Medical Publishing.)

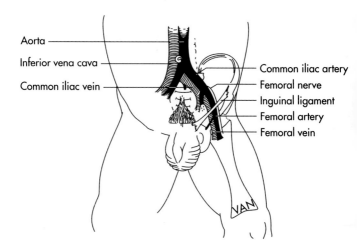

Fig. III-4 Anatomy of femoral region. Vein, artery, nerve (VAN) from medial. (Adapted from Hughes WT, Buescher ES: *Pediatric procedures*, ed 2, Philadelphia, 1980, WB Saunders.)

left to angle of 45° to vertical; operator then imagines straight line between right mastoid process and suprasternal notch
- Needle enters skin at midpoint of this line at 30° angle and is advanced in direction of ipsilateral nipple
- Failure to enter vein is usually due to too-lateral direction of needle advancement
- In older child and teenager, triangle formed by middle third of clavicle and two bellies of SCM forms useful landmark; vein lies under lateral border of medial belly of SCM

Femoral Vein (Figs. III-4 and III-5)

- To access femoral vein, insert needle medial to femoral pulse, 1-2 cm distal to flexion crease of groin
- Aim cephalad and slightly medially (umbilicus is useful target); enter skin at 30° angle and advance until vein is entered
- In neonate, femoral vein lies side by side with artery; in teenager, artery and vein may be 1-1.5 cm apart; adjust techniques used accordingly
- In patients with suspected or proven intraabdominal trauma, avoid using lower limb veins for venous access

Surgically Placed Central Venous Lines

- Generally two types: external (e.g., Roka or Hickman catheter) and buried reservoir (e.g., Port-a-cath)
- Buried reservoir requires needle insertion whenever hook-up is required; otherwise remains "invisible"

Advantages	Disadvantages
External	
• No pain involved in hook-up	• Twice weekly heparin flush
• Double lumen catheters available for large volumes, chemotherapy, dialysis, TPN	• Frequent dressing changes
	• No swimming
	• Risk of pulling out
Buried	
• Little care at home	• Incorrect needle placement
• Heparin flush in hospital when hooking up q4-6wk	• Discomfort with hook-up
• Normal activities, swimming	

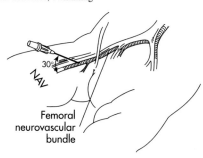

Fig. III-5 Femoral vein cannulation. (See text for explanation.) (Adapted from Levin DL, Morriss FC: *Essentials of pediatric intensive care,* St Louis, 1990, Quality Medical Publishers.)

PROCEDURES

- Complications: infection (especially coagulase negative *Staphylococcus*), blockage, thrombosis, mechanical, breakage

INTRAVENOUS CUTDOWN

- Procedure is not straightforward method of achieving intravenous access in emergency
- Vascular cutdown in hands of unskilled is time-consuming with potential to end in failure
- If all other methods fail, may be attempted by experienced personnel

RESPIRATORY PROCEDURES

- All needles, catheters, and tubes should be inserted over superior surface of rib to avoid damage to neurovascular bundle

NEEDLE ASPIRATION OF PNEUMOTHORAX (Fig. III-6)

- Indicated for immediate management of cardiovascular compromise (e.g., tension pneumothorax), using angiocatheter (IV catheter), 10-cc syringe, and 3-way stopcock
- A 20-23 gauge angiocatheter (attached to syringe and stopcock) is inserted into second interspace in midclavicular line or fifth interspace in anterior or midaxillary line; (in uncommon situation when acquiring

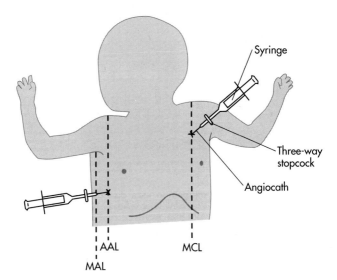

Fig. III-6 Positions for needle aspiration of pneumothorax. (See text.) (*MAL,* Midaxillary line; *AAL,* anterior axillary line, *MCL,* midclavicular line.)

equipment listed above will cause unacceptable delay; merely sticking cannula through chest wall will relieve tension and may be lifesaving)
- Remove air using syringe attached by stopcock to catheter to decrease tension while monitoring hemodynamic parameters; alternatively, attach catheter to IV tubing with distal end under water
- Should always be followed by insertion of chest tube under controlled conditions (see following discussion)

THORACENTESIS

- Sedate patient before undertaking procedure
- Positioning: position infants supine; older, cooperative child can sit upright, leaning forward against pillow or backrest of chair
- Check fluid level by percussion, upright chest x-ray (CXR), or ultrasound (US)
- After appropriate antiseptic and draping, infiltrate with 1% lidocaine to anesthetize skin, muscle, and pleura
- Equipment: 18-gauge needle or angiocatheter attached via tubing to 3-way stopcock and 20-cc syringe
- Insert needle along posterior axillary line at fluid level (generally sixth-seventh interspace appropriate, but will depend on volume, loculation, etc.)
- Aspirate fluid slowly in 20-30 cc aliquots using syringe and stopcock
- Must obtain follow-up CXR postprocedure to exclude pneumothorax

CHEST TUBE INSERTION

- Equipment : 1% lidocaine, chest tube (No. 8 for preterm, 10-12 for infant, 22 for child < 40 kg, 24 for child > 20 kg or adult), scalpel, hemostat, Kelly forceps, 2-0 silk suture, Pleuro-vac or bottle with underwater seal drain (or Heimlich valve)
- Landmarks: fifth interspace in anterior or midaxillary line if chest tube to be placed for relief of pneumothorax (see Fig. III-6); for draining pleural effusion, site of chest tube placement depends on extent of intrapleural fluid
- After antiseptic preparation and appropriate draping, infiltrate skin with 1% lidocaine
- Make 1-1.5 cm incision through skin and subcutaneous tissues; divide underlying intercostal muscle by advancing forceps in opening-and-closing fashion; penetrate pleura with tip of forceps
- Use forceps to grip distal end of chest tube, and guide it through tunnel created and into pleural cavity
- In spontaneously breathing patient, clamp chest tube between time of insertion and connection to underwater seal to prevent inspiration of air into pleural cavity
- Advance chest tube to distance of 4-10 cm, depending on size of child
- Condensation inside tube confirms its location in pleural cavity when draining pneumothorax; if intention is to drain pleural effusion, fluid should appear in chest tube
- Fix chest tube to skin using purse-string silk suture to facilitate subsequent removal of tube and closure of skin defect

- Connect tube to Pleurovac set at suction of 10-20 cm of H_2O or underwater seal
- CXR essential to confirm position of tube and assess effects
- Generally remove after 72 hr if no further escape of free air as evidenced by bubbling in underwater seal and/or no reaccumulation of intrapleural air with suction off or tube clamped for 24 hr
- Postremoval CXR should always be done

TRACHEOTOMY

- Tracheotomy should be performed only by skilled and experienced personnel
- Cricothyroid puncture with 16-gauge IV catheter attached to 3-cc syringe barrel with plunger removed will allow for emergency oxygenation via T-piece until more definitive airway management possible; allows for insufflation; note that patient actually exhales passively through vocal cords (not through catheter); procedure carries significant risk of complications and should only be performed after failure of less invasive techniques to establish airway

ABSCESS INCISION AND DRAINAGE

- Limited effectiveness of topical anesthesia because pH of pus and surrounding tissue inactivates lidocaine; topical ethyl chloride may be optimal form of anesthesia
- Make small incision in overlying skin; after evacuating pus (gentle probing with hemostat for loculated pus), pack abscess cavity with povidone-iodine–soaked gauze ($\times$ 48 hr), and cover with clean dressing

UMBILICAL VEIN CATHETERIZATION

- Indicated for venous access and exchange transfusion
- Appropriate catheter insertion length is calculated using shoulder-umbilicus length (Fig. III-7)
- Apply umbilical tie as loose knot at base of umbilical stump for hemostasis
- After antiseptic preparation and appropriate draping, cut umbilical stump with scalpel to within 1-1.5 cm of abdominal wall
- Identify exposed vessels (two arteries, thick-walled; one vein, thin-walled and larger)
- While maintaining gentle traction on umbilical stump, insert catheter (which should be primed with solution of heparinized saline) into umbilical vein, and carefully advance distance calculated previously
- Check that blood can be freely aspirated through catheter
- Secure catheter with "purse-string" suture around stump, followed by "bridge tape" support (Fig. III-8)
- Confirm position with x-ray (in IVC above diaphragm)
- Main complication is thrombosis/embolism

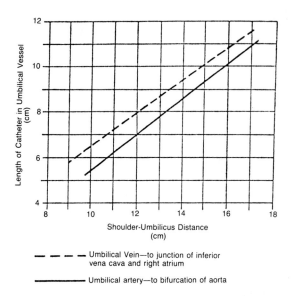

Fig. III-7 Determination of length of catheter to be inserted for appropriate arterial or venous placement. Length of catheter read from diagram is to umbilical ring; add length of umbilical cord stump; shoulder-umbilical distance is perpendicular distance between parallel lines at level of umbilicus and through distal ends of clavicles. (From Klaus MH, Fanaroff AA, eds: *Care of the high risk neonate,* ed 3, Philidelphia, 1986, WB Saunders.)

UMBILICAL ARTERY CATHETERIZATION (Fig. III-8)

- Similar preparation as for UVC
- Because of smooth-muscle content of arterial wall and potential for spasm, use probe or forceps to dilate arterial lumen
- Advance 3.5-5 F catheter primed with solution of heparinized saline to desired length
- Secure as for UVC
- Confirm position (L3-L4) with x-ray; catheter should pass inferiorly before turning back on itself to pass superiorly up aorta
- Use UAC for saline, dextrose-containing solutions; use for TPN or antibiotics if urgent need and no other vascular access

Complications

- Ischemia of
  - Lower limbs

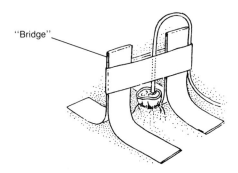

Fig. III-8 Umbilical artery catheterization. (Modified from Klaus MH, Fanaroff AA, eds: *Care of the high risk neonate,* ed 3, Philidelphia, 1986, WB Saunders.)

- • Kidneys (ATN)
- • Bowel (necrotizing enterocolitis)
- • Spinal cord (paraplegia)
- Hemorrhage
- Sepsis
- Aortic aneurysm

Contraindications

- Necrotizing enterocolitis
- Acute tubular necrosis
- Umbilical complications: omphalitis, omphalocele

ENDOTRACHEAL INTUBATION

- For guide to resuscitation, see p. 8
- Emergency intubation should be attempted by most skilled personnel available
- If this skill is not available, most patients can be adequately ventilated and oxygenated using bag and mask
- Essential features of pediatric airway include larynx more anterior, floppy epiglottis, relatively large tongue
- In apneic patient, positive-pressure ventilation by bag and mask with O_2 must be administered before attempts at laryngoscopy
- Airway obstruction that may appear complete often can be partially overcome by bag-and-mask technique allowing correction of hypoxemia and preparation for intubation
- Suctioning equipment should be available
- Muscle relaxant and sedating drugs should not be used in patients with anatomic airway obstruction

Table III-1 Endotracheal Tube Size

Age	Tube size	
Neonate		
< 1500 g	2.5	⎤
> 1500 g	3.0	
1-6 mo	3.5	
7 mo-2 yr	4.0	Uncuffed
2 yr	4.5	
3-4 yr	5.0	
5-6 yr	5.5	⎦
7-8 yr	6.0	⎤
9-11 yr	6.5	
12-13 yr	6.5	Cuffed
14-18 yr	7.0	⎦

- In acute resuscitation situation, oral intubation is preferred until patient stabilized; elective nasotracheal intubation may then be performed
- Nasotracheal intubation is contraindicated in suspected basal skull fracture or severe facial injury
- Selection of appropriate tube size (Table III-1): appropriate ETT is largest one that allows leak of air around tube when 25-30 cm H_2O positive pressure is applied
- Rough guide to ETT size (internal diameter) in children > 1 yr:

$$\frac{\text{age (yr)}}{4} + 4$$

- Use smaller ETT if history of airway obstruction or syndrome known to be associated with anatomic airway abnormality (i.e., Down syndrome)
- For patients with croup, select 3 mm for < 6 mo, 3.5 mm for 6-24 mo, and age (yr)/4 + 3 for older patients
- Introducer may be required for oral intubation; Magill forceps useful for nasotracheal intubation
- Always confirm position with CXR; correct position is ETT tip at midtracheal level (1-2 cm above carina); note that extension of head at time of x-ray will cause tube to advance distally, and flexion will cause tube to rise away from carina
- Check clinically for symmetric chest movement and air entry; if right-sided tube, pull tube proximally
- Complications: trauma, right main stem bronchus intubation with left-sided collapse, bradycardia secondary to pharyngeal vagal stimulation
- Atropine to prevent bradycardia generally used in older children (0.01-0.02 mg/kg/dose)

BLADDER CATHETERIZATION

- Retract prepuce in males if uncircumcised, and swab penis to base with appropriate antiseptic
- In females, separate labia and swab periurethral area with antiseptic

PROCEDURES

Table III-2 Urinary Catheter Sizes

Age	Intermittent catheterization	Indwelling catheters
0-5 yr	3½-5 Fr feeding tube	3½-5 Fr feeding tube
5-7 yr	5 Fr feeding tube	5 Fr feeding tube
7-10 yr	8-10 Fr disposable urinary catheter	8-10 Fr Foley (Silastic)
10-14 yr	10 Fr disposable urinary catheter	10 Fr Foley (Silastic)
> 14 yr	12-14 Fr* disposable urinary catheter	10-14 Fr Foley (Silastic)

*Foleys > 14 Fr are latex.

- Drape sterile towel above and below urethra
- Lubricate catheter
- Apply caudal traction to penis, or separate labia
- Introduce catheter (for size, see Table III-2) into urethral meatus, advancing until urine obtained
- If Foley catheter, inflate balloon with H_2O or saline
- Attach outlet end aseptically to closed drainage system

SUPRAPUBIC BLADDER ASPIRATION

- Infant placed in frogleg position
- Appropriate antiseptic and draping
- Landmark: 1-2 cm (1 fingerbreadth) above symphysis pubis in midline; usually corresponds to transverse lower abdominal crease just above symphysis pubis
- Advance needle (23-25 gauge, 2-3 cm) attached to empty 3-5 cc syringe in caudal direction at 10°-20° from perpendicular to abdominal wall, aspirating gently while advancing

URINALYSIS (Fig. III-9)

- Unspun urine: test for WBCs and bacteria
- Spun urine: look for casts, RBCs (expressed as RBCs/high-power field), bacteria, crystals, debris; method: centrifuge at 2000 rpm for 2 min, look at peripheries of cover slip
- Glucose (dipstick)
- Hematuria: dipstick positive with hemoglobinuria and myoglobinuria (see p. 323)
- Nitrites: screening test for UTIs; only positive with gram-negative organisms
- Clinitest tablets: positive with glucose, fructose, galactose, lactose, ascorbic acid, homogentisic acid, pentose, tyrosine, chloramphenicol, chloral hydrate, sulfonamides, salicylate metabolites; method: add 2 drops urine to 10 drops water, then add tablet
- Dinitrophenylhydrazine (DNPH) test positive (presence of keto acids) in maple syrup urine disease, phenylketonuria, ketotic hypoglycemia, lactic acidosis, methylmalonic aciduria, etc. (see p. 268)
- Cyanide nitroprusside test: screen for cystinuria and homocystinuria (see p. 268)

URINE SEDIMENT

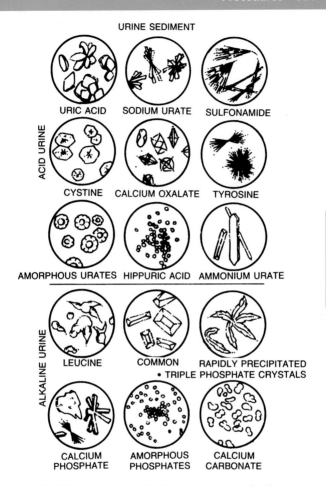

ACID URINE

URIC ACID SODIUM URATE SULFONAMIDE

CYSTINE CALCIUM OXALATE TYROSINE

AMORPHOUS URATES HIPPURIC ACID AMMONIUM URATE

ALKALINE URINE

LEUCINE COMMON RAPIDLY PRECIPITATED
• TRIPLE PHOSPHATE CRYSTALS

CALCIUM PHOSPHATE AMORPHOUS PHOSPHATES CALCIUM CARBONATE

Fig. III-9   Microscopic findings on urine examination.
Continued.

PROCEDURES

LUMBAR PUNCTURE (LP)

- Be sure to exclude ↑ ICP (by examining fundus, palpating sutures and fontanelles, or using computed tomography [CT] scan) before performing LP; consult neurosurgeon if any suspicion
- LP contraindicated in bleeding diathesis, thrombocytopenia (< 50,000), infection over skin or along needle insertion site

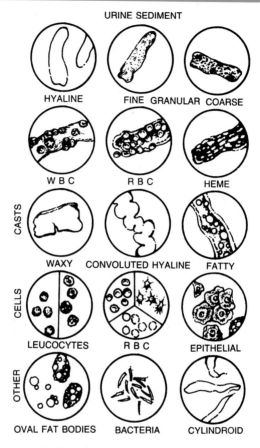

URINE SEDIMENT

HYALINE   FINE GRANULAR COARSE

CASTS

WBC   RBC   HEME

WAXY   CONVOLUTED HYALINE   FATTY

CELLS

LEUCOCYTES   RBC   EPITHELIAL

OTHER

OVAL FAT BODIES   BACTERIA   CYLINDROID

Fig. III-9, cont'd.   For legend see p. 501.

- Proper positioning and adequate restraint of patient absolutely essential to successful tap (Fig. III-10)
- Place patient with back fully flexed and either sitting up or lying on one side with hips, knees, and neck flexed
- Patients with cardiorespiratory compromise need close monitoring during procedure
- Draw imaginary line between two iliac crests and intervertebral space (at L3-L4) or below (L4-5); avoid L2-L3 space in infant (cord lower than in older child)

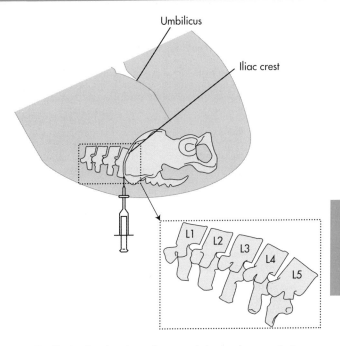

Fig. III-10 Landmarks and approach for lumbar puncture.

- Appropriate antiseptic and draping
- In infants and older children, may infiltrate skin and subcutaneous tissue with 1% lidocaine
- Select appropriate needle (21-23 gauge short needle with stylet for infants, and 20-21 gauge long needle with stylet for older children) and insert in midline, just below spinous process, angle toward umbilicus, and slowly advance until "pop" is felt (except in infant) as dura is penetrated; in infants, stylet must be withdrawn frequently to check for CSF flow
- When fluid appears, attach three-way stopcock and manometer, and measure opening pressure (useless in crying child); normal values 60-160 mm H_2O; do not aspirate fluid
- Collect fluid in appropriate tubes, and send for biochemical (glucose, lactate, protein), bacteriology (culture, Gram stain, antigen detection tests, for example, CIE or latex agglutination), and cytology (count, morphology), as appropriate
- Keep extra specimen refrigerated for later testing (e.g., metabolic tests)

PROCEDURES

ARTERIAL ACCESS (Fig. III-11)

- Preferred sites for arterial puncture in older children are radial, dorsalis pedis, and posterior tibial arteries
- Although femoral artery puncture is generally to be avoided, in child in shock, femoral may be only palpable distal pulse and can be cannulated with low likelihood of subsequent complications (see Figs. III-4 and III-5)
- Use 25-gauge needle and heparinized syringe; alternatively, 23- or 25-gauge butterfly needle may be used while assistant aspirates into syringe
- Insert needle in cephalad direction at 45°-60° angle, bevel up, adjusting position until blood return; then gently aspirate into syringe
- Apply direct pressure after removal for at least 2-3 min
- If patient is likely to require placement of arterial line as part of ongoing management, repetitive arterial sampling by "stabs" should be avoided; damage done makes subsequent line placement more difficult

RADIOLOGIC PROCEDURES

GASTROINTESTINAL/GENITOURINARY

- For barium studies of esophagus, stomach, and small bowel, child should be NPO (4 hr if < age 2; after midnight > age 2)
- Air contrast studies of colon require bowel preparation: generally clear fluids orally for 24 hr before procedure, cathartic and/or enema
- Barium enema, VCUG, IVP, and US studies require no preparation

Computed Tomography (CT)

- Oral contrast (Omnipaque) for abdominal studies (given at time of study; for suspected pelvic pathology may be given earlier, or rectal contrast may be given at time of exam)
- IV contrast (chest, abdomen, head): nonionic contrast generally used; side effects, including nausea, vomiting, flushing, rash, hypotension, and anaphylaxis are uncommon in children; when there is history of allergy/anaphylaxis with previous contrast, future contrast studies should be avoided unless absolutely necessary; premedication with antihistamines and steroids should be considered

NUCLEAR MEDICINE
Bone Scan

- Tc-MDP accumulates predominantly in areas of maximum stress or remodeling; three-phase bone scans, which include flow images, may be used to detect osteomyelitic foci as early as 72 hr after onset of symptoms
- Concurrent gallium scan may be required to differentiate cellulitis or trauma
- Tc-MDP may be used in evaluation of some neoplasms and metastatic disease; false-negative scans may occur with eosinophilic granuloma, neuroblastoma, renal cell and thyroid carcinoma

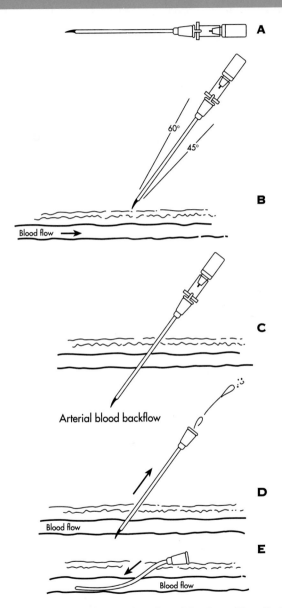

Fig. III-11 Percutaneous insertion of arterial catheter. (From Hughes WT, Buescher ES: *Pediatric procedures,* ed 2, Philadelphia, 1980, WB Saunders.)

Gallium Scan (Ga-67)

- Imaging at 24, 48, and 72 hr used to localize inflammatory processes and some tumors
- Localization mechanism involves binding with WBCs and bacteria; gallium-avid tumors include lymphoma, hepatoma, seminoma, melanoma

Renal

- Tc-DTPA cleared by GFR; used to assess dynamic renal perfusion, GFR, and renal/ureteral obstruction (furosemide study)
- Tc-DMSA cleared by slow tubular secretion; tracer of choice for evaluation of renal parenchymal scarring, morphology, and identification of malpositioned/ectopic kidneys

Hepatobiliary (Tc-DISIDA) Scan

- Used in conjunction with US for diagnosis of biliary atresia; infant requires premedication with phenobarbital 5 mg/kg/day × 5 days to enhance and accelerate biliary excretion of Tc-IDA derivatives

ANNE DIPCHAND, GRAHAM ELLIS, MARTIN PETRIC, AND ANNETTE POON

CONTENTS

HEMATOLOGY

Table IV-1 Hemoglobin, Hematocrit, RBC Count, Reticulocytes

	Hemoglobin (g/L)	Hematocrit	RBC count ($\times 10^{12}$/L)	Reticulocytes ($\times 10^9$/L)
Birth				
28-wk gestation	110-170	0.30-0.40	3.0-4.5	
34-wk gestation	120-180	0.35-0.50	3.0-5.0	
38-wk gestation	140-200	0.40-0.55	3.5-5.5	
40-wk gestation	150-250*	0.52-0.79*	3.5-6.0	200-300
2 days	150-250*	0.46-0.74*	3.5-6.0	<5.0
2 wk	140-200	0.40-0.74*	3.5-6.0	<5.0
1 mo	115-180	0.35-0.54	3.5-5.5	
2 mo	90-135	0.27-0.40	3.5-5.5	
3-6 mo	100-140	0.30-0.42	3.5-5.0	5.0-250.0
1-5 yr	110-140	0.33-0.42	4.0-5.0	10.0-100.0
6-14 yr	120-160	0.36-0.48	4.5-5.5	10.0-100.0

*If capillary value is close to upper limit of normal, venous sample should be obtained; the venous hemoglobin value should be < 220 g/L; venous hematocrit value should be < than 0.65.

Platelet Count

- All ages: 150-450 $\times$ 10^9/L

ESR

- All ages: 1-10 mm/hr

Table IV-2   Red Blood Cell Indices

	MCV	MCH	MCHC
Birth			
28-37-wk gestation	120		
38-40-wk gestation	110		
1 wk	110		
1 mo	90	24-34	320-360
2 mo	80	24-34	
3-12 mo	70	24-31	
Older	80-94	24-31	

MCV, Mean corpuscular volume (fL); *MCH*, mean corpuscular hemoglobin (pg); *MCHC*, mean corpuscular Hb concentration (g/L).

BOX IV-1   Hemoglobin Electrophoresis*

Hb F (%)	
1-30 days	60-95
31-60 days	35-86
61-120 days	11-56
121-180 days	3-14
6-9 mo	1-4
10-12 mo	1-4
13-18 mo	0.5-2.9
19-24 mo	0.2-2.6
> 2 yr	< 2
Hb A$_2$(%)	
1-30 days	0-0.5
31-60 days	0-1.6
61-120 days	0.2-2.6
121-180 days	1.2-2.6
> 6 mo	1.8-2.9

*For full-term newborns and older.

Table IV-3 White Blood Cell Count and Differential ($\times 10^9$/L)

	Birth	1 wk	2 wk	3-12 mo	2-5 yr	6-10 yr	Older
Total WBC	20-40	5-21	5-20	5-15	5-12	4-10	4-10
Differential							
Polymorphs	6-26	1.5-10	1-9.5	1.5-8.5	1.5-8.5	1.5-8	2-7.5
Bands	0-4.5	0-0.8	0	0	0	0	0
Eosinophils	0.02-0.85	0.07-1.1	0.07-1	0.05-0.7	0.02-0.5	0-0.5	0-0.5
Basophils	0-0.6	0-0.2	0-0.2	0-0.2	0-0.2	0-0.2	0-0.2
Lymphocytes	2-11	2-17	2-17	4-10.5	2-8	1.5-7	1.5-4
Monocytes	0.4-3.1	0.3-2.7	0.2-2.4	0.05-1.1	0-0.8	0-0.8	0-0.8

Note: WBC differential counts are reported as absolute numbers.

Table IV-4   Coagulation Values*

	Patient age	Normal value
Antithrombin III (AT-III)	< 1 mo	0.48-1.1 U/ml
	≥ 3 mo	0.80-1.2 U/ml
Bleeding time		2-7 min
D dimer		< 200 ng/ml
Factors V,VIII		0.5-1.5 U/ml
Factors VII, IX, X, XI, XII	< 1 mo	0.2-0.8 U/ml
	≥ 9 mo	0.5-1.5 U/ml
Fibrinogen†		1.6-4 g/L
Partial thromboplastin time (PTT)	< 3 mo	25-60 sec
	≥ 3 mo	25-40 sec
Prothrombin time (PT)	< 3 mo	10.5-18 sec
	≥ 3 mo	10.5-13.5 sec
Ristocetin cofactor		0.5-1.5 U/ml
von Willebrand factor (vWF)		0.5-1.5 U/ml
INR (see p. 191)		

*For full-term newborns and older.
†Fibrinogen is acute-phase reactant.

CLINICAL CHEMISTRY

BLOOD

Blood

Agent or test	Reference values		Notes
	SI units	Traditional units	
Acid-base (blood gases)	**pH (arterial)**	**pH (venous)**	
Birth-6 hr	7.30-7.40 mm Hg	—	Normal values for capillary gas levels range from venous to arterial, depending on how arterialized sample site is
6 hr-adult	7.35-7.45 mm Hg	7.32-7.42 mm Hg	
	pCO$_2$ (arterial)	**pCO$_2$ (venous)**	
Birth-1 hr	30-50 mm Hg	—	
1-6 hr	30-45 mm Hg	—	
6 hr-2 yr	30-42 mm Hg	—	
2 yr-adult	33-46 mm Hg	40-50 mm Hg	
	pO$_2$ (arterial)*	**pO$_2$ (venous)***	*Breathing room air
Birth-1 hr	50-60 mm Hg	—	
1 hr-24 hr	60-70 mm Hg	—	
24-48 hr	70-80 mm Hg	—	
Child-adult	80-100 mm Hg	25-47 mm Hg	
	Actual bicarbonate		
Birth-24 hr	16-22 mmol/L		
24 hr-1 mo	16-24 mmol/L		
1 mo-2 yr	18-24 mmol/L		
2 yr-adult	20-28 mmol/L		
	Base excess		
Birth-24 hr	–8-0 mmol/L		
24-48 hr	–4-+2 mmol/L		
48 hr-2 mo	–4-+4 mmol/L		
>2 mo-adult	–3-+3 mmol/L		

LAB REF VALUES

Continued.

Blood—cont'd

Agent or test	Reference values		Notes
	SI units	Traditional units	
Acid Phosphatase (Total)			
Adults	0-5.4 U/L		Children may have higher values. From:Clin Chem 24:1105-1108, 1978. Source: spleen, liver, prostate, osteoclasts, red blood cells, platelets
Adrenocorticotropic Hormone (ACTH)			
Day1	< 88 pmol/L	< 400 pg/ml	Take blood at 9 AM to use these values; for adequate interpretation, cortisol should be measured in same sample
Over first few wk of life, adrenals mature and values decrease to following: child and adult (9 AM diurnal variation)	< 22 pmol/L	< 100 pg/ml	
Alanine Aminotransferase (ALT, Formerly SGPT)			
At 37° C, with pyridoxal phosphate (Kodak method)			Source: liver, skeletal muscle, kidney, heart
< 1 yr	< 60 U/L		
1 yr-adult	< 40		
Albumin			
0-1 yr	32-48 g/L	3.2-4.8 g/dl	
Child and adult	33-58	3.3-5.8	
Aldosterone			
< 1 yr; free diet; varied time of day	166-2900 pmol/L	6-104 ng/dl	1. Request Na⁺ and K⁺ on same sample 2. 24-hr urine collection for Na⁺ excretion
1-4 yr; free diet; varied time of day	< 940	< 34	Rarely indicated; less useful than urine aldosterone and varies widely over short periods (depends on time of day, posture, Na⁺ and K⁺ intake); to demonstrate hyperaldosteron-

5-15 yr; free diet; varied time of day	< 600	< 22
> 15 yr; normal salt; ambulant; at noon	220-420	8-15
> 15 yr low-salt diet	550-1220	20-44

ism in hypokalemic hypertension, give K+ supplements until K+ is in normal range before aldosterone is measured; diuretics (e.g., furosemide, spironolactone) and several other drugs (especially purgatives and liquorice derivatives, such as carbenoxolone) should be discontinued (if possible) for 3 wk before assessment; indicate any drugs that patient may still be taking

Alkaline Phosphatase
(Kodak method, p-npp at 37° C)

Male

< 1 yr	175-600 U/L
1-8 yr	175-400
9-11 yr	180-475
12-15 yr	200-630
16-17 yr	100-455
18-19 yr	80-210
> 19 yr	60-150

Source: bone, liver, kidney, intestinal mucosa; isoenzymes exist for bone, liver, and intestine

Female

< 1 yr	185-555 U/L
1-2 yr	185-520
3-8 yr	185-425
9-13 yr	160-500
14-15 yr	90-400
16-18 yr	45-140
> 18 yr	25-100

α-1-acid Glycoprotein

(orosomucoid)	0.4-1.3 g/L	40-130 mg/dl	Acute phase reactant

Continued.

Blood—cont'd

Agent or test	Reference values		Notes
	SI units	Traditional units	
α-1-antitrypsin			
Adult	0.9-2 g/L	90-200 mg/dl	Acute phase reactant; protease inhibitor (PI) typing: MM, Normal (89% of population) MS, Normal variant (8%) MZ, Heterozygous for deficiency (< 2% of population) ZZ, Homozygous for deficiency
α-1-antityrpsin Clearance See p. 549			
α-Fetoprotein			Tumor marker, especially gonadal germ-cell or primary hepatic tumor; also raised during rapid liver regeneration (e.g., in acute hepatitis)
Premature	80,000-220,000 µg/L		
Newborn	2000-130,000		
0-2 wk	8000-130,000		
2 wk-1 mo	300-70,000		
1 mo	90-10,000		
2 mo	40-1000		
3 mo	20-300		
4 mo	0-300		
5 mo	0-100		
6 mo	0-40		
7 mo	0-40		
8 mo	0-20		
9 mo-adult	0-10		

Aluminum   < 371 mmol/L   < 11 µg/L

Amino Acids

Purpose: screening done by chromatography to detect genetic-metabolic disease; if screen abnormal, quantitative values should be obtained; reference values are age dependent and should be interpreted by specialist in metabolic disease

Ammonium (NH$_4^+$)
Newborn	< 50 µmol/L
Child and adult	< 35

Amylase
< 1 yr, poorly defined;	
lower than in older child	
1 yr-adult	20-110 U/L

Source: pancreas, salivary glands

Androstenedione

Poorly defined in children

Male
1-5 mo	< 2.8 nmol/L	< 80 ng/dl
5 mo-adrenarche	< 1.6	< 45
Adult	1.7-5.2	50-150

Female
Birth-adrenarche	< 1.6	< 45
Adult	1.7-7.0	50-200

Source: ovaries, adrenals; until puberty in females and from 5 mo of age to puberty in males, can be considered adrenal-specific androgen; in females, values are higher during luteal phase of cycle than during follicular phase, but should still be within range shown

Angiotensin-Converting Enzyme (ACE)
Adult	0-75 U/L

Values not age dependent in children

Antihyaluronidase

See p. 554

Antineutrophil Cytoplasmic Autoantibodies (ANCA)

Normally absent

Continued.

LAB REF VALUES

Blood—cont'd

	Reference values		
Agent or test	SI units	Traditional units	Notes
Antistreptolysin O (ASO)			
See p. 554			
Arginine Vasopressin (AVP, Antidiuretic Hormone)			
Adult	1-10 ng/L	pg/ml	Interpret in relation to plasma osmolality
Aspartate Aminotransferase (AST, formerly SGOT)			
37° C with pyridoxal			
phosphate			Source: Cardiac and skeletal muscle, liver, kidney, erythrocytes
< 1 yr	< 110 U/L		
1-10 yr	< 45		
11-20 yr	< 36		
β-1-C Globulin			
See C3 complement, p. 517			
β-Human Chorionic Gonadotropin (β-HCG)			
Normal adults	< 5 U/L		
β-Hydroxybutyrate (2-Hydroxybutyrate)			
Fasting child	0-0.3 mmol/L		During hypoglycemia, values < 0.6 mmol/L suggest increased insulin or insulin-like activity in absence of metabolic disease
Fasting adult	0-0.42 mmol/L		Ratio of free fatty acids to β-hydroxybutyrate (both in mmol/L) usually < 2
Bicarbonate (Actual)			
See acid-base, p. 511			
Bile Salts (Radioimmunoassay for Glycocholate)			
Fasting	< 1.3 μmol/L		
2-hr after meal	< 5.5		

Bilirubin

Unconjugated

Birth-2 days	< 130 μmol/L	< 8 mg/dl
3-5 days	< 200	< 12
1 mo-adult	< 17	< 1

Conjugated

Neonates	< 10	< 0.6
Others	< 2	< 0.1

Delta

> 14 days	< 3	< 0.2

In general, "physiologic hyperbilirubinemia" clears at approximately 1 wk of age for term neonates and at 2 wk for prematures

Delta-bilirubin is albumin-conjugated (long half-life) and may cause continued hyperbilirubinemia during recovery

Blood Gases

See acid base, p. 511

Blood Urea Nitrogen (BUN)

See urea, p. 539

C-reactive Protein

	0-8 mg/L	< 0.8 mg/dl

C₃ Complement (β-1-c Globulin)

0-5 days	0.39-1.56 g/L	39-156 mg/dl
> 5 days	0.77-1.43 g/L	77-143

C₄ Complement

0-5 days	0.05-0.33 g/L	5-33 mg/dl
> 5 days	0.07-0.40 g/L	7-40

LAB REF VALUES

Continued.

Blood—cont'd

Agent or test	Reference values		Notes
	SI units	Traditional units	
Calcium (Total)			
Premature: birth-3 days	1.8-2.5 mmol/L	7-10 mg/dL	Prolonged venous stasis (e.g., prolonged use of tourniquet) alters result; serum calcium
3 days-2 mo	2.00-2.75	8-11	levels less than previously mentioned range may be normal if hypoalbuminemia present;
Term: birth-2 mo	2.00-2.75	8-11	adjusted calcium should be in normal range
Child	2.25-2.62	9-10.5	For SI units: Adjusted Ca (mmol/L) = $\dfrac{\text{Calcium(mmol/L} - \text{albumin(g/L)}}{40} + 1$
Adult	2.12-2.62	8.5-10.5	For traditional units: Adjusted Ca (mg/dl) = Calcium (mg/dl) − albumin (g/dl) + 4
Calcium (Ionized)			
Capillary	1.18-1.29	4.7-5.2	
Venous or arterial	1.14-1.29	4.6-5.2	
Carboxyhemoglobin	< 0.05		Expressed as fraction of total hemoglobin
Carcinoembryonic Antigen (CEA)			
Adult	< 3 µg/L		
Carnitine			
Total			
0-15 days	23-84 µmol/L		
> 15 days	32-84		
Free			
0-15 days	12-60 µmol/L		
> 15 days	26-60		
Carotene	0.9-3.7 µmol/L	50-200 µg/dl	
Ceruloplasmin			
Male			
1-9 yr	264-473 mg/L	26.4-47.3 mg/dl	
10-13 yr	242-396	24.2-39.6	
14-19 yr	154-374	15.4-37.4	

Continued.

Female

1-9 yr	264-473	26.4-47.3
10-13 yr	253-473	25.3-47.3
14-19 yr	220-495	22-49.5

CH$_{50}$-total Hemolytic Complement

≥ 1:12		Sample must be sent on ice immediately to laboratory

Chloride

		mEq/L
Premature infant	95-110 mmol/L	
Term infant	96-106	
Child	99-111	
Adult	98-106	

Cholesterol

< 3 mo	< 4.5 mmol/L	< 175 mg/dl	Values based on fasting states (before feeds in babies; after 12-hr fast in older children); fasting not essential if total cholesterol requested without any other lipid determinations
3 mo-2 yr	< 4.9	< 190	
2-17 yr	3.2-4.4	124-170	
18-29 yr	3.2-4.6	124-178	

Cholinesterase-Pseudocholinesterase

Cholinesterase	620-1370 U/L
Dibucaine no.	77-83
	(heterozygote, 45-70)
	(homozygote, 15-30)
Fluoride no.	56-68
Chloride no.	4-15
Scoline no.	87-92

Blood—cont'd

Agent or test	Reference values		Notes
	SI units	Traditional units	
Chorionic Gonadotropin			
See β-HCG, p. 516			
Complement			
See C₃, C₄			
Copper			
Child > 6 mo-adult	10.5-23 μmol/L	67-146 μg/dl	
Cortisol			Result at 8 PM is < 50% of the 8 AM value in 88% of cases; diurnal variation of cortisol may not develop until about 1 yr of age; in Cushing's disease or syndrome, cortisol levels may be normal, but diurnal variation lost; other steroids produced in congenital adrenal hyperplasia or tumors cross-react with cortisol assay; only poor diurnal variation may be evident; stress or shock can elevate cortisol levels
Poorly defined during first wk of life			
Child 1-17 yr in hospital			
8 AM-9 AM	190-740 nmol/L	7-27 μg/dl	
8 PM	30-300	1-11	
Healthy adult, 8 AM	140-690	5-25	
Creatine Kinase			Source: skeletal and cardiac muscle, smooth muscle, brain
Male			Elevated CK levels occur after physical activity and intramuscular injections
11 days-1 yr	0-390 U/L		Blacks have significantly higher levels of CK than whites
1-3 yr	60-305		Bedrest for several days may drop CK levels by 20%-30%
4-6 yr	75-230		
7-9 yr	60-365		
10-11 yr	55-215		
12-13 yr	60-330		
14-15 yr	60-335		
16-19 yr	55-370		

Female

11 days-1 yr	0-390 U/L
1-3 yr	60-305
4-6 yr	75-230
7-9 yr	60-365
10-11 yr	80-230
12-13 yr	50-295
14-15 yr	50-240
16-19 yr	45-230

Creatine Kinase Isoenzymes

CK-MB	< 16 U/L or < 4% of total CK

Source: CK-BB, predominately brain; CK-MB, cardiac muscle, type II skeletal muscle fibers; CK-MM, skeletal muscle, cardiac muscle

Purpose: To help differentiate skeletal from cardiac muscle disease or trauma; CK-MB not specific for myocardial damage in first wk or mo after birth

Creatinine

< 5 yr	< 44 μmol/L	< 0.5 mg/dl
5-6 yr	< 53	< 0.6
6-7 yr	< 62	< 0.7
7-8 yr	< 71	< 0.8
8-9 yr	< 80	< 0.9
9-10 yr	< 88	< 1
> 10 yr	< 106	< 1.2

Low concentrations occur in patients with small muscle mass (as with muscle disease or severe malnutrition)

Creatinine Clearance

see p. 543

Cryoglobulins

Normally absent

Continued.

Blood—cont'd

Agent or test	Reference values		Notes
	SI units	Traditional units	
Dehydroepiandrosterone Sulfate (DHAS, DHEA-S)			Source: adrenal glands
Male			
1-5 mo	< 4 µmol/L	< 1500 ng/ml	
6 mo-7 yr	< 0.5	< 180	
8-9 yr	< 3	< 1100	
10-12 yr	< 6	< 2200	
13-19 yr	3-12	1100-4400	
Female			
1-5 mo	< 4 µmol/L	< 1500 ng/ml	
6 mo-7 yr	< 1	< 350	
8-9 yr	< 3	< 1100	
10-12 yr	< 8	< 3000	
13-19 yr	1-12	350-4400	
Dihydrotestosterone			
Child 9 mo-12 yr	31-317 pmol/L		
Male 20-49 yr	217-1650		
Female 13-49 yr	28-616		
1.25 Dihydroxyvitamin D	25-120 pmol/L		
Estradiol			
Male			
Birth	< 370 pmol/L	< 100 pg/ml	
1 yr-adrenarche	< 92	< 25	
Adrenarche-puberty (rising to adult levels)			
Adult	<165	< 45	

Female
  Birth-adrenarche (as in
    males)
  Adrenarche-puberty
    (rising to adult levels
  Adult
    Follicular phase   110-183 pmol/L   30-50 pg/ml
    Luteal phase   550-845   150-230
    Treated with syn-   < 165   < 45
      thetic estrogens

FEP
See free erythrocyte pro-
toporphyrin, p. 524

Ferritin
1-12 mo   14-400 µg/L   ng/ml
12 mo-adult   22-400

α-Fetoprotein
See α-Fetoprotein, p. 514

Folate
RBC folate   > 216 nmol/L   > 96 ng/ml
Serum folate   > 3.5   > 1.6

Follicle-Stimulating Hormone (FSH, WHO 78/549 Standard)
Male
0-4 mo   < 15 IU/L (most <   mIU/ml
                              6 IU/L)
4 mo-2 yr   < 3
2-11 yr   < 4
11 yr-adult   < 7

Blood—cont'd

	Reference values		
Agent or test	SI units	Traditional units	Notes
Follicle-Stimulating Hormone (FSH, WHO 78/549 Standard)—cont'd			
Female			
0-6 mo	< 38 IU/L	mIU/ml	
6 mo-2yr	< 8 (most < 5)		
2-10 yr	< 4		
Puberty (rising to adult level)	< 9		
Adult			
Follicular and luteal values	< 9		
Ovulatory value	< 13		
Free Erythrocyte Protoporphyrin (FEP, Zinc Protoporphyrin)			
0-10 yr	< 0.62 μmol/L	< 35 μg/dl	Investigation of severe lead poisoning, congenital erythropoietic porphyria, erythrohepatic protoporphyria; increased FEP occurs in iron-deficiency anemia and anemia of chronic disease
> 10 yr	< 1.33 μmol/L	< 75	
Free Fatty Acids			
Newborn	0-1.85 mmol/L		
Child and adult	0.22-0.88 mmol/L		
Galactosemia Screen			Qualitative test of RBC galactose-1-phosphate uridyl transferase activity; blood transfusion within 3 mo before this test may invalidate results; other screening tests may be available (depending on center) that may not be invalidated by RBC transfusion, but results may be falsely negative if child not ingesting galactose-containing foods when blood taken

Galactose-1-phosphate Uridyl Transferase

Normal*	300-470 U/kg Hb		Quantitative assessment of RBC galactose-1-phosphate uridyl transferase activity
		18.3-28.6 Beutler and Baluda units/g Hb	
Galactosemia heterozygote*	140-220	8.5-13.4	*Duarte variant enzyme (a normal variant) may distort these ranges; blood transfusion within 3 mo before this test may invalidate the result
Galactosemia homozygote	0-40	0-2.4	

γ-Glutamyl Transferase (GGT)

Kodak method at 37° C		Source: liver, pancreas
< 1 mo	< 385 U/L	
1-2 mo	< 225	
2-4 mo	< 135	
4-7 mo	< 75	
7 mo-15 yr	< 45	
> 15 yr	Male < 75	
	Female < 55	

Gases

See acid-base, p. 511

Gastrin

Fasting	< 90 ng/L pg/ml

Globulin, β-1-C

See C$_3$ complement, p. 517

Continued.

LAB REF VALUES

Blood—cont'd

	Reference values		
Agent or test	SI units	Traditional units	Notes
Globulins			
By electrophoresis			
α_1	1-3 g/L	0.1-0.3 g/dl	
α_2 Birth-6 mo	2-7	0.2-0.7	
> 6 mo	4-11	0.4-1.1	
β Birth-6 mo	3-6	0.3-0.6	
> 6 mo	3-12	0.3-1.2	
γ Birth	6-12	0.6-1.2	
1-6 mo	2-7	0.2-0.7	
6 mo-2 yr	2-9	0.2-0.9	
> 2 yr	4-14	0.4-1.4	
Glucose (Fasting)			
Infant	> 2.5 mmol/L	> 45 mg/dl	
Child < 3 yr	2.5-5	45-90	
Child > 3 yr	2.8-6.1	50-110	
Adolescent-adult	3.3-6.1	60-110	
Glucose-6-phosphate Dehydrogenase (G-6-PD)			
Newborn	1.6-2.8 IU/ml RBC	160-280 IU/100 ml RBC	
> 2 mo	1.2-2.0	120-200	
Growth Hormone			
After stimulation (by clonidine, sleep, exercise, arginine, insulin) peak value shoud be:	> 7 µg/L	> 7 ng/ml	

Haptoglobin

0.32-1.98 g/L   32-198 mg/dl   Acute-phase reactant

HDL Cholesterol

Take blood before feed for neonates and infants and after 12-hr fast for older children

Male		
5-9 yr	0.98-1.91 mmol/L	37.8-73.7 mg/dl
10-14 yr	0.96-1.91	37.1-73.7
15-19 yr	0.78-1.63	30.1-62.9
20-24 yr	0.78-1.63	30.1-62.9
Female		
5-9 yr	0.93-1.89	35.9-73.0
10-14 yr	0.96-1.81	37.1-69.9
15-19 yr	0.91-1.91	35.1-73.7
20-24 yr	0.85-2.04	32.8-78.8

Hemoglobin (Plasma)

< 30 mg/L   < 3 mg/dl

Hemoglobin A$_{1c}$ (Glycosylated Hemoglobin)

Abnormal or variant hemoglobins and hemoglobin F may give falsely elevated levels

Expressed as fraction of total hemoglobin	
Healthy nondiabetic	0.04-0.06
Diabetic with good control	< 0.08
Diabetic with fair control	0.08-0.09
Diabetic with suboptimal control	> 0.09

LAB REF VALUES

Continued.

Blood—cont'd

Agent or test	Reference values		Notes
	SI units	Traditional units	
17-Hydroxyprogesterone			
Infants < 3 mo	< 10 nmol/L	< 3.3 µg/L	Cord blood and samples from neonates 0-48 hr old not satisfactory; values increased in luteal phase of menstrual cycle (up to 14 nmol/L)
Very sick infants < 3 mo	< 30	< 9.9 µg/L	
Children 3 mo-adults	< 6	< 2	
Borderline for nonclassical CAH	6-10	2-3.3	
25-Hydroxvitamin D	25-90 nmol/L	10-36 ng/ml	Values vary seasonally within range because vitamin D produced by skin exposure to sunshine
Immunoglobulins			
IgG			
0-12 mo	2.3-14.1 g/L	230-1410 mg/dl	
1-3 yr	4.5-14.3	450-1430	
4-6 yr	5-14.6	500-1460	
7-9 yr	5.7-14.7	570-1470	
10-13 yr	7-15.5	700-1550	
14-19 yr	7.2-15.8	720-1580	
IgA			
0-12 mo	0-0.8 g/L	0-80 mg/dl	Lower limit of IgA increases progressively in infants from approximately 0.01 g/l at 1 mo to 0.08 g/l at 6 mo
1-3 yr	0.2-1.0	20-100	
4-6 yr	0.3-2.0	30-200	
7-9 yr	0.3-3.1	30-310	
10-13 yr	0.5-3.6	50-360	
14-19 yr	0.5-3.5	50-350	

IgM

0-12 mo	0-1.4 g/L	1-140 mg/dl
1-3 yr	0.2-1.5	20-150
4-6 yr	0.2-2.1	20-210
7-9 yr	0.3-2.1	30-210
10-13 yr	0.3-2.4	30-240
14-19 yr	0.2-2.6	20-260

IgE (values are stated as < mean + 1 standard deviation)

Upper limit of IgE increases progressively in infants from approximately 5.5 μg/L at 6 wk to 17.5 μg/L at 6 mo; after age 10 yr value declines to reach adult levels

0-6 mo	< 17.5 μg/L
6 mo-1 yr	< 31
1-2 yr	< 55
2-5 yr	< 115
5-10 yr	< 204
Adult	< 98

Insulin

Fasting	< 145 pmol/L	< 20 mIU/L

Reference values may be higher in obese patients; hemolysis and insulin antibodies may lower values

Intralipid

See *lipid*

Iron

Newborn	20-48 μmol/L	110-270 μg/dl	Hemolysis elevates result
4 mo-1 yr	5-13	30-70	
> 1 yr	9-27	50-150	
Toxicity (1 yr and older)	> 72	> 408	

Continued.

Blood—cont'd

	Reference values		
Agent or test	SI units	Traditional units	Notes
Iron-binding Capacity (IBC)			
Newborn	11-31 μmol/L	60-175 μg/dl	
> 1 yr	45-72	250-400	
Lactate			
Venous	< 2.5 mmol/L	< 22.5 mg/dl	Delayed separation of serum from RBC and hemolysis both elevate result; transport sample on ice
Lactate Dehydrogenase (LDH)			
At 30° C			Source: highest concentrations in heart, liver, skeletal muscle, erythrocytes, kidney; elevated in hemolyzed samples
Male			
0-5 days	934-2150 U/L		
1-3 yr	500-920		
4-6 yr	470-900		
7-9 yr	420-750		
10-11 yr	432-700		
12-13 yr	470-750		
14-15 yr	360-730		
16-19 yr	340-670		
Adult	310-620		

Female

0-5 days	934-2150	
1-3 yr	500-920	
4-6 yr	470-900	
7-9 yr	420-750	
10-11 yr	380-770	
12-13 yr	380-640	
14-15 yr	390-580	
16-19 yr	340-670	
Adult	310-620	

LDL Cholesterol

5-9 yr	1.63-3.34 mmol/L	62.9-128.9 mg/dl

Take sample before feed for neonates and infants and after 12-hr fast for older children
Desirable/acceptable levels:
2-17 yr: 1.6-2.8 mmol/L
18-29 yr: 1.7-3 mmol/L
(From Canadian Consensus Report and American Academy of Pediatrics)

Male

10-14 yr	1.66-3.41	64.1-131.6
15-19 yr	1.6-3.36	61.8-129.7
>19 yr	1.71-3.8	66-146.7

Female

5-9 yr	1.76-3.62	67.9-139.7
10-14 yr	1.76-3.52	67.9-135.9
15-19 yr	1.53-3.54	59.1-136.6
>19 yr	1.47-4.11	56.7-158.6

Lead

	< 0.5 μmol/L (blood)	< 10.4 μg/dl (blood)

Concentration of lead in whole blood 75 × greater than in serum or plasma

Lipid

During supplementation values should not exceed	1 g/L	

Indication: monitoring for toxicity when exogenous intravenous lipids administered

Continued.

Blood—cont'd

	Reference values		
Agent or test	SI units	Traditional units	Notes
Lipoproteins			
By electrophoresis; descriptive report			Indication: investigation and classification of hyperlipidemia
Luteinizing Hormone (LH, WHO 80/552 Standard)			
Male			Values rise through puberty to adult values
0-3 mo	< 23 IU/L	mIU/ml	
4 mo-2 yr	< 7		
2-6 yr	< 4		
6-10 yr	< 7		
Adult	< 10		
Female			Ovulatory values may reach 100 U/L
1-6 mo	< 20 IU/L	mIU/ml	
6 mo-2 yr	< 7		
2-8 yr	< 6		
8-12 yr	2-13		
Adult			
Follicular and luteal value	< 25		
Magnesium			
Newborn	0.75-1.15 mmol/L	1.5-2.3 mEq/L	
Child	0.7-0.95	1.4-1.9	
Adult	0.65-1.00	1.3-2.0	
Ionized (children and adults)	0.54-0.67		

Methemoglobin
In SI, expressed as fraction of total hemoglobin

< 0.02

< 2%

Alternate value, <5 g/L

5'-Nucleotidase

0-20 U/L

Source: liver

Orosomucoid
(See α₁-glycoprotein, p. 513)

Osmolality

275-295 mmol/kg water

mosm/kg water

May be lower in first 5 days after birth

Parathyroid Hormone

10-65 ng/l

pg/ml

Immunoassay is PTH-intact molecule type (Nichols)

Phenylalanine

< 110 μmol/L

< 1.8 mg/dl

Phenylalanine/tyrosine Ratio

Normal ratio	< 1.0
Equivocal	1.0-1.2
Hetero⁺homozygote	> 1.2

Indication: determination of heterozygosity for phenylketonuria

Phosphate

Birth-1 mo	1.62-3.1 mmol/L	5-9.6 mg/dl
1-4 mo	1.55-2.62	4.8-8.1
4 mo-1 yr	1.30-2.2	4-6.8
1-4 yr	1.16-2.1	3.6-6.5
4-8 yr	1.16-1.81	3.6-5.6
9-14 yr	1.07-1.71	3.3-5.3
> 15 yr	0.87-1.52	2.7-4.7

Reported values vary widely, especially during first mo of life; hemolysis causes elevated value

Continued.

Blood—cont'd

Agent or test	Reference values		Notes
	SI units	Traditional units	
Porphyrins			Purpose: investigation of lead poisoning, erythrohepatic protoporphyria, and congenital erythropoietic porphyria; *see free erythrocyte protoporphyrin*
Porphobilinogen (PBG) Deaminase			Investigation of acute intermittent porphyria, see PBG deaminase
	20-45 nmol porphyrin/ml Erc/h		Formerly uroporphyrinogen-1-synthetase
			Enzyme in RBC decreased in acute intermittent porphyria (during and between attacks)
Potassium			
Newborn infant	4.5-6.5 mmol/L	mEq/L	Hemolysis elevates values
2 days-2 wk	4.0-6.4		
2 wk-3 mo	4.0-6.2		
3 mo-1 yr	3.7-5.6		
1-16 yr	3.5-5.2		
Prolactin			
Birth (mean)	280 µg/L	ng/ml	Level drops to adult range by 12 wk of age (term) and by 20 wk (premature)
Level drops after birth—4 wk (mean)	75		
Children			
1 yr-puberty	3-20		
Adult male	2-15		
Adult female	3-26		

Protein
See total protein, p. 533;
albumin, p. 512, globulins,
p. 526

Protoporphyrin, Free Erythrocyte
See free erythrocyte Pro-
toporphyrin, p. 524

Pseudocholinesterase
See cholinesterase

Pyruvate

Venous	0.03-0.08 mmol/L

Pyruvate Kinase

Newborn-2 yr	1.2-2.1 IU/ml RBC
> 2 yr	1-1.4

Renin

Plasma renin activity
(Normal salt intake; 9 AM;
supine; after 1-12 hr rest)

< 3 mo	< 14 ng/L/sec	50 ng/ml/hr
3 mo-1 yr	< 4.20	< 15
1 yr-4 yr	< 2.80	< 10
4 yr-15 yr	< 1.70	< 6
Adult		
Supine after 1-12 hr rest	< 0.56	< 2.0
At 1200 hr, ambulant	< 1.11	< 4.0

Delayed separation of serum from RBCs and hemolysis both elevate result

Normal values vary with method, sodium intake, time of day, posture, and age; antihypertensive medication may alter results; if possible, medication should be discontinued
1-3 wk before test; higher in premature infant

Serum Glutamic Oxaloacetic Transaminase (SGOT)
See aspartate amino-
transferase (AST)

Continued.

Blood—cont'd

	Reference values		Notes
Agent or test	SI units	Traditional units	
Serum Glutamic Pyruvate Transaminase (SGPT)			
See alanine aminotransferase (ALT)			
Sodium			
Premature infant	132-140 mmol/L	mEq/L	
Term infant	133-142		
Child	135-143		
Adult	135-145		
Testosterone			
Male			During puberty, levels correlate with pubertal stage or bone age rather than chronologic age and progressively increase to adult values
1-15 days	< 6.6 nmol/L	< 190 ng/dl	
1-3 mo	< 12.1	< 350	
3-5 mo	< 6.9	< 200	
5-7 mo	< 2.1	< 60	
7 mo-onset of puberty	< 1.0	< 30	
Adult	12.0-38.0	350-1100	
Female			Levels during luteal phase higher on average than follicular phase; levels may rise to 3.3 nmol (95 ng/dl) during estrogen or progesterone therapy; levels higher in girls experiencing anovulatory cycles but still within normal range
Birth-onset of puberty	< 1.0 nmol/L	< 30 ng/dl	
Puberty-levels increase to adult values			
Adult	0.7-2.4	20-70	

Testosterone-free

Male

Prepuberty	1-2 pmol/L	0.03-0.06 ng/dl
Puberty-19 yr	36-90	1.04-2.6

Female

Prepuberty	1-2	0.03-0.06
Puberty-19 yr	2-11	0.06-0.32

Thyroid-stimulating Hormone (TSH)

Cord blood	< 30 mU/L	µU/ml
Rises shortly after birth to peak	< 50	
Child > 4 days of age and adult	0.5-5	

Thyroxine (T₄)

Levels rise shortly after birth to peak at 24 hr, then fall at 3 days to	115-280 nmol/L	9-22 µg/dl	Premature infants have much lower values—the more premature, the lower the value; in persons with normal thyroid function, T₄ low values may occur with absent or low levels of thyroxine-binding globulin (TBG), hypoproteinemia, drugs (e.g., phenytoin), or severe hemolysis; in persons with normal thyroid function, high T₄ values may occur with high levels of TBG, as during pregnancy or while on contraceptive or estrogen therapy; check free T₄
	100-250	8-19	
4 days-3 wk	90-200	7-16	
3 wk-2 mo	65-180	5-14	
2 mo-1 yr	65-165	5-13	
1 yr-childhood	50-155	4-12	
Adult			

Thyroxine (Free), Free T₄

0-2 days	20-45 pmol/L	1.6-3.5 ng/dl	Measure T4 not bound to protein; approximates hormonally active T4; values may be lower with phenytoin therapy
3-30 days	18-35	1.4-2.7	
30 days-adult	10-23	0.8-1.8	

Continued.

Blood—cont'd

	Reference values		
Agent or test	SI units	Traditional units	Notes
Thyroxine-binding Globulin Capacity (TBGC)			
Cord	180-1209 nmol/L		
1-4 wk	129-1158		
1-12 mo	257-978		
1-5 yr	373-695		
5-10 yr	321-643		
10-15 yr	270-592		
Adult	150-360		
Total Protein			
0-6 mo	45-75 g/L	4.5-7.5 g/dl	
6 mo-2 yr	54-75	5.4-7.5	
Child and adult	53-85	5.3-8.5	
Transferrin			
0-5 days	16-50 μmol/L		
1-9 yr	23-41		
10-19 yr	24-48		
Triglycerides			
2-17 yr	0.4-1.3 mmol/L	35-115 mg/dl	Take after 12-hr fast; before feeding in neonates and infants
> 18 yr	0.6-2.3	53-204	

Triiodothyronine (T_3)

Birth	< 1.0 nmol/L	< 70 ng/dl
Rises rapidly after birth to value at 3 days of	0.8-5.4	50-350
6 days-1 yr	1.4-4.6	90-300
1 yr-childhood	1.4-4.1	90-270
Adult	1.4-3.4	90-220

T_3 assay has low sensitivity for diagnosing hypothyroidism

Do not confuse with T_3RU

Triiodohyronine (Free), Free T_3

Adult	5-8 pmol/L

Triiodothyronine Resin Uptake Test (T_3RU)

Do not confuse with T_3	0.25-0.35	25%-35%

Synthetic resin and patient's TBG (thyroxine-binding globulin) compete for radioactive T_3; T_3RU > 0.35 (> 35%) indicates fewer available binding sites in serum, as in hyperthyroidism (sites occupied by T_4) or absence or deficiency of TBG; T_3RU < 0.25 (< 25%) indicates more available binding sites, as in hypothyroidism (little T_4 available to occupy sites) or increased TBG (e.g., during estrogen therapy or pregnancy)

Urate (Formerly Uric Acid)

Child or adult female	120-360 µmol/L	2-6 mg/dl, as uric acid
Adult male	180-420	3-7

Urea (Formerly Blood Urea Nitrogen, BUN)

Newborn	2.9-10 mmol/L	8-28 mg/dl as urea nitrogen
1-2 yr	1.8-5.4	5-15
2-16 yr	2.9-7.1	8-20

Continued.

LAB REF VALUES

Blood—cont'd

Agent or test	Reference values		Notes
	SI units	Traditional units	
Uric acid			
See urate			
Vitamin A	0.7-2.10 µmol/L	20-60 µg/dl	
Vitamin B₁₂	150-670 pmol/L	200-900 pg/ml	
Vitamin D			
See 25-hydroxyvitamin D, p. 528			
1,25-dihydroxyvitamin D, p. 522			
Vitamin E	12-46 µmol/L	0.5-2.0 mg/dl	
Zinc			
0-1 yr	11.5-22.2 µmol/L	75-145 µg/dl	
2-10 yr	10.7-20	70-130	
11-18 yr	10-19	65-124	
Adult	9.2-18.4	60-120	

URINE

Urine

	Reference values		
Agent or test	SI units	Traditional units	Notes
Acyl Carnitines			For investigation of fatty acid oxidation defects; measure after carnitine load
Acylglycine			
Hexanoylglycine	< 1.7 mmol/mmol creatinine		Elevation of both hexanoylglycine and phenylpropionylglycine strongly suggests medium- chain Acyl-CoA dehydrogenase (MCAD) deficiency
Phenylpropionylglycine	< 1		
Suberylglycine	< 7		
Amino Acids, Screen			Consists of:
			1. Two-dimensional amino acid chromatography: aminoaciduria
			2. Cyanide nitroprusside test: cystinuria, homocystinuria, glutathion-emia, certain defects of tubular transport
			3. DNPH test; detects ketoacids in PKU, MSUD, methionine malabsorp-tion, tyrosinemia
Bilirubin			Normally absent
Calcium			
Related to creatinine			
0-7 mo	< 0.1 mmol/kg body wt/day	< 4 mg/kg body wt/day	
	< 2.4 mol/mol creat-inine		
7-18 mo	< 1.7		
18 mo-6 yr	< 1.2		
Adult	< 0.6		

Continued.

Urine—cont'd

Agent or test	Reference values		Notes
	SI units	Traditional units	
Catecholamines			Values represent 95th percentile (100th percentile in parentheses); drugs such as methyl-dopa, apresoline, quinidine, epinephrine, or norepinephrine-related drugs (e.g., L-dopa) and renal function test dyes may interfere with catecholamine excretion and affect results
Norepinephrine			
0–2 yr	280 (375) μmol/mol creatinine	420 (558) μg/g creatinine	
2–4 yr	80 (150)	120 (224)	
5–9 yr	60 (90)	90 (135)	
10–19 yr	55 (60)	82 (92)	
Adult	76 (90)	114 (135)	
Epinephrine			
0–2 yr	45 (150) μmol/mol creatinine	75 (246) μg/g creatinine	
2–4 yr	35 (60)	57 (97)	
5–9 yr	20 (40)	35 (66)	
10–19 yr	20 (70)	34 (110)	
Adult	14 (50)	23 (81)	
Dopamine			
0–2 yr	2220 (3480) μmol/mol creatinine	3000 (4708) μg/g creatinine	
2–4 yr	1130 (2230)	1533 (3020)	
5–9 yr	770 (990)	1048 (1342)	
10–19 yr	400 (510)	545 (692)	
Adult	400 (580)	535 (781)	
Copper			
Normal	< 0.6 μmol/day	< 40 μg/day	

Coproporphyrin
See porphyrins

Cortisol (Urine "Free" Cortisol)

4 mo-10 yr	< 74 nmol/day	< 27 µg/day
11-20 yr	< 152	< 55
Adult	50-220	18-80
Alternatively		
4-12 yr	12-34 µmol/mol creatinine	
2-17 yr	0-190 nmol/m²	

Creatinine Clearance
Age-related reference ranges for creatinine clearance corrected for body surface area are shown in Fig. IV-1; note that SI units are printed in blue

Timed urine collection, blood taken during urine collection, patient's height and weight are required for this test; See also blood creatinine, p. 521

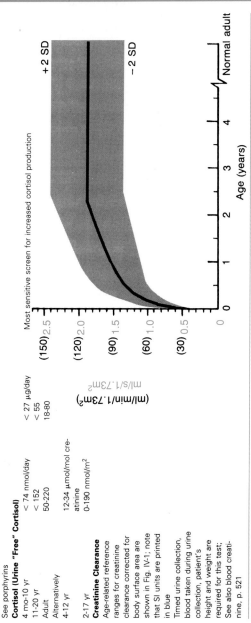

Most sensitive screen for increased cortisol production

$(ml/min/1.73m^2)$
$(ml/s/1.73m^2)$

Age (years)

+ 2 SD

− 2 SD

Normal adult

Continued.

Urine—cont'd

	Reference values		
Agent or test	SI units	Traditional units	Notes
Dinitrophenylhydrazine (DNPH) Test			
See amino acid, screen			
Glycosaminoglycuronoglycans			
See mucopolysaccharide screen			
Hemoglobin			Normally absent; may be positive after exercise and during infectious or febrile states; myoglobinuria may give false-positive result
Homovanillic Acid (HVA)			Values represent 95th percentile (100th percentile in parentheses)
0-1 yr	20 (48) mmol/mol creatinine	32 (77) mg/g creatinine	
2-4 yr	14 (37)	23 (60)	
5-9 yr	9 (21)	14 (34)	
10-19 yr	8 (27)	13 (43)	
Adult	5 (6)	8 (10)	
5 Hydroxyindoleacetic Acid (5HIAA)			
Adult	< 50 μmol/day	< 9.6 mg/day	
Ketones			Normally absent, but may be positive in febrile or toxic states, during fasting periods, diabetic ketoacidosis, and certain genetic metabolic diseases
Mercury			
Random specimen	< 5 μmol/mol creatinine	0.08	
Dental fillings may elevate value to this level			

Metabolic Study

See amino acid screen, p. 541

Metanephrines (metanephrine and normetanephrine)

< 2 yr	< 2.8 mmol/mol creatinine	< 4.6 mg/g creatinine
2-10 yr	< 1.9	< 3
10-15 yr	< 1.2	< 2
Adult	< 0.6	< 1

Medications such as hydrocortisone and phenobarbital may cause false-positive results, whereas propranolol and theophyllines may cause false-negative results with certain laboratory techniques

Mucopolysaccharide Screen (glycosaminoglycuronoglycans)

Myoglobin

Normally not detectable; normal result does not rule out all mucopolysaccharidoses

Nitroprusside Test

See amino acid screen, p. 541

Normally not detectable; reacts like hemoglobin by dipstick; confirmatory tests are available

Organic Acids

Gas chromatography; mass spectrometry results need to be interpreted by a specialist in metabolic diseases; most diagnostic if urine collected when person ill

Osmolality

Infant	50-600 mmol/kg water	mosm/kg water
Child and adult: Maximum (dehydration)	800-1400	
Child and adult: Minimum (water diuresis)	40-80	

Values should be interpreted in conjunction with serum osmolality and clinical state of patient

Continued.

LAB REF VALUES

Urine—cont'd

Agent or test	Reference values		Notes
	SI units	Traditional units	
Oxalate			
Adult	< 150-450 µmol/day		
Alternatively,			
< 1 mo	75-190 mmol/mol creatinine		
1-2.5 yr	30-140		
2.5-4 yr	20-120		
4-6 yr	20-90		
6-13 yr	20-80		
Porphobilinogen Screen			
See porphyrins			
Porphyrins			
Child: Ranges poorly defined			Screening tests are of value only during acute attack; urine porphobilinogen may be increased between and during attacks of acute intermittent porphyria; porphyrinuria may also occur in lead poisioning, liver disease, and conditions of increased erythropoiesis
Adult			
Coproporphyrin	0-380 nmol/day	0-250 µg/day	
Protoporphyrin	Not detected		
Uroporphyrin	0-35 nmol/day	< 30 µg/day	
Porphobilinogen	0-15 µmol/day	< 3 mg/day	

Potassium — Varies widely, depending on intake

Protein (Quantitative)

1 yr — < 0.1 g/m^2/day

Protoporphyrin

See porphyrins

Reducing Substances — Qualitative test (Clinitest tablet), detecting reducing substances such as glucose, galactose, fructose, lactose, pentoses, and homogentisic acid; only glucose is detected by glucose-specific dipsticks (Clinistix)

Sodium

Infant — 6-10 mmol/m^2 of body surface/day (~0.3-3.5 mmol/day) — mEq/m^2/day — Urinary sodium should be interpreted in relation to serum sodium

Child — 40-180 mmol/day — mEq/day

Adult — 80-200 mmol/day

Specific Gravity

Child > 6 mo and adult — > 1.02 (early morning sample)

Urate — 2000-4000 µmol/day or < 60 µmol/kg body wt/day — < 10 mg/kg body wt/day, as uric acid — Diet dependent

Uroporphyrin

See porphyrins

Continued.

Urine—cont'd

Agent or test	Reference values		Notes
	SI units	Traditional units	
Vanillylmandelic Acid (VMA)			
24-hr collection			Values represent 95th percentile (100th in parentheses); nonspecific elevations occur in fever, asthma, chronic anemia, or after surgery
0-1 yr	12 (16) μmol/day	2.3 (3.1) mg/day	
2-4 yr	15 (20)	3 (4)	
5-9 yr	18 (44)	3.5 (8.7)	
10-19 yr	30 (39)	6 (7.7)	
Adult	34 (41)	6.8 (8.1)	
"Spot VMA"			Less satisfactory than 24-hr collection
0-1 yr	11 (34) mmol/mol creatinine	19 (59) mg/g creatinine	
2-4 yr	6.5 (12)	11 (21)	
5-9 yr	5 (5.5)	8 (9)	
10-19 yr	5 (8)	8 (14)	
Adult	3.5 (5)	6 (8)	

FECES

Feces

Agent or test	Reference values		Notes
	SI units	Traditional units	
α₁-Antitrypsin **Clearance**	< 22 ml/day		Falsely low values where lesion(s) in esophagus, stomach, or upper small bowel because low pH environment degrades α₁-antitrypsin; collection must be free of urine; serum α₁ antitrypsin required during collection
Chymotrypsin 37° C ATEE substrate	30-750 U/g		
Coproporphyrin See porphyrins			
Fat			
Fecal fat (fraction of intake)			3- or 5-day stool collection required; accurate account of dietary fat necessary during period of stool collection; regular fat study measures only amount of long-chain fatty acids in stool
Premature infant	< 0.2		
Term infant	< 0.15		
> 3 mo	< 0.1		
Occult Blood			Qualitative study; detected when there is 4 ml whole blood/100 g feces (i.e., 6 mg Hb/g feces)
Porphyrins Adult values (values poorly defined in children)			Fecal porphyrin may be elevated after GI bleeding
Coproporphyrin	0-10 μmol/kg wet weight of stool	0-655 μg/100 g wet weight of stool	Fecal porphyrin may be elevated after GI bleeding; fecal porphyrins useful in porphyria variegata (protocoproporphyria) or hereditary coproporphyria
Protoporphyrin	0-25 μmol/kg wet weight of stool	0-1407 μg/100 g wet weight of stool	Normal values in acute intermittent porphyria or cutaneous hepatic porphyria (cutanea tarda)
Protoporphyrin See porphyrins			

LAB REF VALUES

CEREBROSPINAL FLUID (CSF)

Cerebrospinal Fluid (CSF)

Agent or test	Reference values		Notes
	SI units	Traditional units	
Glucose			
When blood glucose normal	2.1-3.6 mmol/L	38-65 mg/dl	CSF glucose should be roughly ⅔ of blood glucose
Lactate	< 2.5 mmol/L		Used in detection of inherited causes of lactic acidemia
Proteins			
CSF total protein	0.15-1.3 g/L	15-130 mg/dl	Exxessively high protein concentrations (> 5 g/L) can occur if spinal canal is blocked
Premature	0.4-1.2	40-120	
Term	0.2-0.7	20-70	
< 1 mo	0.15-0.4	15-40	
> 1 mo			
CSF IgG			
Normal	< 0.1 of CSF total protein		
Pyruvate	0.03-0.08 mmol/L		Used in detection of inherited causes of lactic acidemia

SWEAT

Sweat

Agent or test	Reference values		Notes
	SI units	Traditional units	
Sweat Chloride (Gibson Cook method)			
3 days-20 yr	< 60 mmol/L		May be erroneously elevated in malnutrition, edema, diabetes insipidus, glucose-6-phosphatase deficiency, adrenal insufficiency, ectodermal dysplasia, and hypothyroidism; may be falsely lowered by cloxacillin; test results unreliable in the first few days of life

BREATH

Breath

Agent or test	Reference values		Notes
	SI units	Traditional units	
Breath Hydrogen (Hydrogen production assessed after administration of lactose, sucrose, or lactulose)			Measurement in nonbasal samples should not exceed basal sample by more than 20 ppm in normals; false-negative test may be obtained with antibiotic usage during 2 wk before test

TOXICOLOGY

- For general screen, do urine toxicology screen by HPLC (see the following)
- When ordering, indicate patient's syndrome of toxicity at presentation
- Indicate any substances likely to be present, including medications
- If testing for barbiturates, blood is better sample
- If testing for antidepressants, urine is better sample
- Urine immunoassays better for "drugs of abuse" (cocaine, opiates, cannabinoids)

BLOOD (DRUG SCREEN)

- Tests are performed as screen for following groups:
  - Volatiles (ethanol, methanol, isopropanol)
  - Barbiturates and other sedatives
  - Benzodiazepines
  - Antidepressants
  - Ethylene glycol
- Salicylate
- Acetominophen

URINE (DRUG SCREEN)

- Broad-spectrum drug screen by high performance liquid chromatography (HPLC)
  - Does not detect barbiturates, benzodiazepines, or cannabinoids
  - Very comprehensive screen for about 500 drugs and their metabolites
  - Major classes detected include:
    - Narcotic analgesics (e.g., heroin, morphine, codeine)
    - Antidepressants (amitriptyline, fluoxetine, imipramine, doxepin)
    - Antipsychotic drugs (chlorpromazine)
    - Stimulants (cocaine, amphetamines)
    - Hallucinogens (phencyclidine)
    - Anticough/cold medication and antihistamines (pseudoephedrine, dextromethorphan, diphenhydramine, phenylpropanolamine, terfenadine)
    - Antiulcer drugs (e.g., ranitidine)
    - Cardiac drugs (diltiazem, verapamil)
- Benzodiazepine screen by immunoassay
- Barbiturate screen by immunoassay
- Cannabinoid screen by immunoassay

VIRAL AND OTHER ANTIBODY TITRES

- Note: Only changes in titer (fourfold increase or decrease over time) or detection of virus-specific IgM antibody are diagnostic of recent infection or reactivation

- Adenovirus*: complement fixation < 1:2 negative; ≥ 1:64 high positve
- Antihyaluronidase ≥ 1:300 suggestive of recent streptococcal infection
- Antistreptolysin O (ASO) ≥ 500 Todd units suggestive of recent streptococcal infection
- *Chlamydia trachomatis*: immunofluorescence < 1:8 negative; ≥ 1:64 high positive
- Cytomegalovirus (CMV)*†: latex agglutination < 1:2 negative; ≥ 1:32 high positive
- Epstein-Barr virus (EBV)
  - Heterophile antibody: agglutination of horse erythrocytes after absorption (monospot test) suggestive of recent or active infection
  - Anti-VCA (IgG) < 1:40, anti-EA negative, anti-ENBA negative: no history of infection by EBV
  - Anti-VCA (IgG) > 1:40, Anti-EA positive, anti-EBNA negative; acute or recent EBV infection, often heterophile antibody positive
  - Anti-VCA (IgG) > 1:40, anti-EA negative, anti-EBNA positive: past history of EBV infection, late convalescent stage of infection, heterophile antibody negative
  - Anti-VCA (IgG) > 1:40, anti-EA positive, anti-EBNA positive: recent EBV infection or reactivation
- Hepatitis A virus (HAV): Presence of IgM antibody consistent with recent or ongoing infection; presence of antibody in absence of IgM consistent with past infection or positive immune status (see also Table 13-3)
- Hepatits B virus (HBV) (see also Table 13-3):
  1. Presence of HBsAg consistent with active or chronic infection
  2. Presence of Anti-HBs consistent with resolution from infection or positive immune status
  3. Presence of Anti-HBc consistent with past or ongoing infection with HBV
  4. Presence of HBeAg consistent with active virus replication and presence of virus in blood
  5. Presence of Anti-HBe consistent with resolution of infection
  6. Presence of HBV DNA consistent with active virus replication and presence of virus in blood
- Hepatitis C virus (HCV) (see also Table 13-3):
  1. Presence of antibody to HCV consistent with past, ongoing, or chronic infection with HCV
  2. Presence of HCV RNA consistent with active or chronic HCV infection
- Herpes simplex*†‡: complement fixation < 1:2 negative; ≥ 1:64 high positive
- Influenza* A and B: complement fixation < 1:2 negative; ≥ 1:64 high positive

---

*Negative: no previous exposure; high postive; suggestive of recent infection or re-activation; titers in between suggestive of previous exposure.

†Neonates may have titers equal to, or one dilution higher than, maternal titers; serum titers in neonates suspected of having congenital infection must be interpreted in conjunction with maternal antibody titers.

‡In absence of CSF infection, antibody levels in serum are 200 or more times greater than in CSF.

- Measles*: immunofluorescence < 1:8 negative; ≥ 1:64 high positive
- Mumps*: immunofluorescence < 1:8 negative; ≥ 1:64 high positive
- *Mycoplasma pneumoniae:* presence of IgM antibody consistent with recent or ongoing infection; complement fixation ≥1:32 suggestive of recent infection
- Parainfluenza*: complement fixation < 1:2 negative; ≥ 1:64 high positive
- Parvovirus B19: Presence of IgM antibody consistent with recent or ongoing infection; presence of IgG antibody consistent with past infection and positive immune status
- Respiratory syncytial virus*: complement fixation < 1:2 negative; ≥ 1:64 high positive
- Rubella†: latex agglutination < 1:2 negative; ≥ 1:64 possibility of recent infection; ≥ 1:10 considered rubella immune
- Toxoplasmosis†: latex agglutination < 1:16 negative; immunofluorescence ≥ 1:256 suggestive of exposure
- Varicella zoster: immunofluorescence ≥ 1:8 considered immune to VZ

---

*Negative: no previous exposure; high postive; suggestive of recent infection or reactivation; titers in between suggestive of previous exposure.
†Neonates may have titers equal to, or one dilution higher than, maternal titers; serum titers in neonates suspected of having congenital infection must be interpreted in conjunction with maternal antibody titers.

Barbara L. Marinac and Joanne L. Smith

TABLE OF CONTENTS

Text continued p. 624.

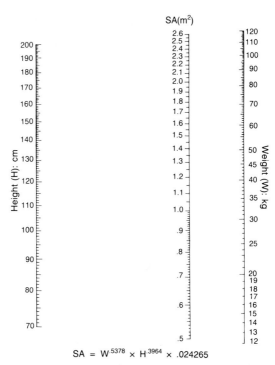

SA(m²)

$$SA = W^{.5378} \times H^{.3964} \times .024265$$

To use the nomogram, a ruler is aligned with the height and weight on the two lateral axes. The point at which the center line is intersected gives the corresponding value for surface area.

Fig.V-1   Body surface area nomogram for children and adults. (From Haycock GB, Schwartz GJ, Wisotsky DH. *J Pediatr* 1978; 93:62-66.) For simplified formula to calculate BSA, see p. 314.

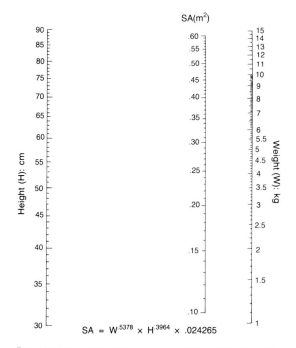

To use the nomogram, a ruler is aligned with the height and weight on the two lateral axes.
The point at which the center line is intersected gives the corresponding value for surface area.

Fig.V-2 Body surface area nomogram for infants. (From Haycock GB, Schwartz GJ, Wisotsky DH. *J Pediatr,* 1978; 93:62-66.) For simplified formula to calculate BSA, see p. 314.

Table V-1 Drug Dosage Guidelines for Infants and Children

Drug	Dose	Dose/Limit	Comments
Acetaminophen	40-60 mg/kg/day ÷ q4-6h PO/PR	65 mg/kg/day or 4 g/day	Optimal single antipyretic dose: 10-15 mg/kg
Acetylcysteine (Mucomyst)	Acetaminophen overdose: see p. 444		
Acetylsalicylic acid, ASA (aspirin)	JA, pericarditis, rheumatic fever: 60-100 mg/kg/day PO ÷ qid	Maximum initial dose: 5.4 g/day	Monitoring of serum concentrations recommended for patients with JA, pericarditis, rheumatic fever; ASA not recommended for antipyresis during viral illness; give with food; do not give enteric-coated tablets with milk, dairy products; do not give enteric-coated tablets with milk, dairy products, or antacids; use with extreme caution in hepatic impairment
	Kawasaki disease: 100 mg/kg/day PO ÷ q6h until defervescence × 24 hr then 3-5 mg/kg/day PO qam	150 mg/kg/day	
ACTH	Infantile spasms: 40-80 IU/day IM/SC 1x/day or ÷ bid		Close clinical monitoring for dose-related and idiosyncratic adverse effects recommended
Activated charcoal	Initial dose: 1 g/kg PO/NG Subsequent dose: 0.5 g/kg PO/NG q4-6h PRN		Give dose of sorbitol 70% with initial dose of activated charcoal
Acyclovir (Zovirax)	Ointment: apply 4-6 ×/day Herpes simplex encephalitis: 45 mg/kg/day IV ÷ q8h × 14 days Other herpes simplex: Treatment: 15-30 mg/kg/day IV ÷ q8h Adults and adolescents: 200 mg qid PO Prophylaxis in immunocompromised hosts: 50 mg/kg/day PO ÷ qid Varicella or zoster in immunocompromised hosts: <1 yr: 30 mg/kg/day IV ÷ q8h ≥1 yr: 1500 mg/m²/day IV ÷ q8h	1 g/day PO	Maintain fluid intake; may be given PO with food Dose interval adjustment in renal impairment: moderate, q12h; severe, q24-48h

	PO dosing (following IV therapy): 80 mg/kg/day PO ÷ qid	800 mg/dose PO 3.2 g/day PO	
	Cytomegalovirus prophylaxis: 50-80 mg/kg/day PO ÷ qid		
Adenosine	Supraventricular tachycardia: 0.05 mg/kg/dose IV; may repeat PRN in following doses q2min: 0.1 mg/kg, 0.15 mg/kg, 0.2 mg/kg, 0.25 mg/kg	12 mg/dose 30 mg total dose	Administer by rapid IV bolus
Adrenaline	See Epinephrine		
Albumin	0.5-1 g/kg dose IV	6 g/kg/day	
Albuterol	See Salbutamol		
Aldactazide	See Novospirozine		
Allopurinol	400 mg/m²/day PO ÷ tid-qid	600 mg/day	Decrease daily dose to 67% in mild and 50% in moderate renal impairment; in severe renal impairment give 3 mg/kg q2-3days
Alphacalcidol	0.01-0.02 µg/kg/day PO as single daily dose		Adjust dose according to plasma calcium concentration
Aluminum hydroxide (aluminum and magnesium hydroxides)	Infant: 2.5-5 ml PO q1-2h Child: 5-15 ml PO pc and qhs Adult: 15-45 ml PO pc and qhs		
Amantadine	Influenza A prophylaxis and treatment: 5-8 mg/kg/day PO ÷ 12h	200 mg/day	Continue prophylactic therapy for at least 10 days following exposure or throughout epidemic; active treatment should continue for 5 days after disappearance of symptoms; avoid alcohol; dose interval adjustment in renal impairment: mild, q12-24h; moderate, q2-3 days; severe, q7 days

Continued.

FORMULARY

Table V-1 Drug Dosage Guidelines for Infants and Children—cont'd

Drug	Dose	Dose/Limit	Comments
Amikacin	15-30 mg/kg/day IV/IM ÷ q8h		Monitoring of serum concentrations recommended; dose interval adjustment in renal impairment: mild-moderate, q12h; severe, q24-48h
Aminocaproic acid (Amicar)	Hemophilia before dental extraction: 200 mg/kg/day PO ÷ q6h × 7-10 days after procedure Hemophilia, acute hemorrhage: 400 mg/kg/day PO/IV ÷ q6h	30 g/day	Decrease dose to 50 mg/kg once daily in severe renal impairment
Aminophylline	See Theophylline		Contains 80% theophylline
5-Aminosalicylic acid	See Mesalamine		
Amiodarone	Loading dose (LD): 5 mg/kg IV over 1 hr followed by infusion of 5-15 µg/kg/min; or 10 mg/kg/day PO as single daily dose or ÷ bid × 7-10 days Maintenance dose: 5 mg/kg/day PO as single dose	Usual adult loading dose: 800-1600 mg/day PO Usual adult maintenance dose: 200-400 mg/day PO	Dose may require reduction in patients with liver impairment; reduce digoxin dose by 50% during concurrent therapy; reduce warfarin dose by 33%-50% during concurrent therapy; will increase phenytoin concentrations: Monitor for toxicity; monitor thyroid, liver, lung, and eye function; nausea and vomiting occur frequently with loading dose
Amlodipine	Initial dose: 0.1-0.2 mg/kg/day PO as single daily dose Maintenance dose: 0.1-0.3 mg/kg/day PO as single daily dose	15 mg/day	Reduce initial dose in patients with hepatic impairment, and titrate to effect; because of long half-life of drug, dosage adjustments should not be made more frequently than q3-5 days; doses less than 5 mg may be administered via dissolve-and-dose system; contact pharmacy for more information

Drug	Dose	Max	Remarks
Amoxicillin	20-50 mg/kg/day PO ÷ q8h Prophylaxis in asplenic patients 2-5 yrs: 20 mg/kg/day PO ÷ bid *H. pylori* eradication: Adolescents: 500 mg PO tid × 14 days	4 g/day	May be given with food
Amphotericin B	Initial: 0.25-0.5 mg/kg/day IV as single dose; increase by 0.25 mg/kg/day up to 0.5 mg/kg/day for *Candida* or 1 mg/kg/day for *Aspergillus* IV once daily or q2days	70 mg/day or 1 mg/kg/dose, whichever is less	Infuse at concentration of ≤ 0.1 mg/ml in 5% dextrose over 4-6 hr; monitor serum potassium; consider premedication with meperidine-diphenhydramine-hydrocortisone; in fluid-restricted patients, infusion of more concentrated solutions may be possible via CVL; contact pharmacy for more information
Ampicillin	Meningitis: 200-300 mg/kg/day IV ÷ q6h Other: 50-100 mg/kg/day ÷ q6h	10 g/day	Dose interval adjustment in renal failure: severe, q12-16h
Aminone	Loading dose: 0.75-3 mg/kg/dose IV over 5 min Maintenance dose: 5-20 µg/kg/min via continuous IV infusion	Loading dose: 3 mg/kg Maintenance dose: 10 mg/kg/day	Incompatible with dextrose; monitor liver function; dose may require reduction in liver impairment
Astemizole	<6 yr: 0.2 mg/kg/day PO as a single dose 6-12 yr: 5 mg PO as a single daily dose >12 yr: 10 mg PO as a single daily dose		Give on empty stomach (1 hr ac or 2 hr pc); concurrent use with drugs that inhibit hepatic metabolism (e.g., ketoconazole, erythromycin) has resulted in life-threatening cardiac arrhythmias
Atropine	Resuscitation: see inside front cover Preop: 0.01-0.02 mg/kg/dose IM/PO 30-60 min preop Minimum: 0.1 mg/dose Cholinergic crisis: 0.05 mg/kg IV q5min until secretions dry	0.6 mg/dose 2 mg/dose	

Continued.

Table V-1   Drug Dosage Guidelines for Infants and Children—cont'd

Drug	Dose	Dose/Limit	Comments
Azithromycin	Chlamydial urethritis, cervicitis in patients ≥ 16 yr: 1 g PO stat		Use with caution in severe renal impairment; give on empty stomach, at least 1 hr before or 2 hr after meal; restricted drug; for other indications, consider erythromycin or clarithromycin
Beclomethasone	Initial dose: 400 μg/day by oral inhalation ÷ bid-qid; reduce dose to minimum required for maintenance	1600 μg/day	Monitor for signs of systemic corticosteroid toxicity
Belladonna and opium	Ureteral spasm: ≥8 kg <16 kg: ¼ suppository PR q4-6h prn ≥16 kg <32 kg: ½ suppository PR q4-6h prn ≥32 kg: 1 suppository pr q4-6h prn		Minimum dose: ¼ suppository
Bisacodyl	0.3 mg/kg/dose PO 6-12 hr before desired effect < 6 yr: 5-10 mg suppository or 2.5 ml microenema PR 15-60 min before desired effect > 6 yr: 10 mg suppository or 5 ml microenema PR 15-60 min before desired effect	15mg PO	Do not divide or chew tablets; do not administer PO with milk or antacid
Bismuth subsalicylate (Pepto-Bismol)	H. pylori eradication: Adolescents: 524 mg PO qid × 14 days		Avoid in patients with renal failure; contraindicated in patients with influenza or chicken pox because of risk of Reye's syndrome; may cause grayish-black stools, darkened tongue
Budesonide	Severe acute asthma: Children: 0.5-1 mg bid via nebulizer Adults: 1-2 mg bid via nebulizer Maintenance: Children: 0.25-0.5 mg via nebulizer Adults: 0.5-1 mg bid via nebulizer		

Bupivacaine	Epidural: Bolus: 2-3 mg/kg epidurally Infusion: 0.2-0.4 mg/kg/hr epidurally	May be given epidurally with or without epinephrine or fentanyl
Calcitriol (1,25-dihydroxycholecalciferol)	Hypoparathyroidism, vitamin D resistant rickets, dialysis: Initial: 0.015-0.025 µg/kg/day PO ÷ bid Maintenance: increase prn gradually to 0.5-1 µg/day PO	Adjust dose according to serum calcium concentration
Calcium carbonate	Calcium deficiency and hyperphosphatemia prophylaxis in renal patients: Infants: 125 mg elemental Ca/dose PO tid Children: 250 mg elemental Ca/dose PO tid	Titrate dose according to serum PO_4; oral suspension 200 mg/ml contains 80 mg elemental Ca/ml; tablet 625 mg contains 250 mg elemental Ca
Calcium	Resuscitation: see inside front cover Hypocalcemia: 0.1-0.2 mmol Ca/kg/hr IV Adjust IV rate q4h according to plasma Ca concentration	For IV administration, dilute to 0.05 mmol/ml or less; avoid extravasation; cardiac monitoring recommended 100 mg calcium chloride = 28 mg elemental Ca = 0.68 mmol Ca 100 mg calcium gluconate = 9.6 mg elemental Ca = 0.23 mmol Ca
Calcium polystyrene sulfonate (Resonium Calcium)	Initial: 1 g/kg/day PO/pr in divided doses Maintenance: 0.5 g/kg/day PO/pr in divided doses	Contains 8% w/w calcium (1.6-2.4 mmol/g); use for patients with hyperkalemia and restricted sodium intake
Captopril	Hypertension: Initial dose: 0.3-0.9 mg/kg/day PO ÷ tid Maintenance dose: 0.3-4 mg/kg/day PO ÷ tid CHF: Initial dose: 0.1 mg/kg/**dose** PO tid Maintenance dose: 1.5-6 mg/kg/day PO ÷ bid-tid	6 mg/kg/day Reduce dose to 50% in severe renal impairment

Continued.

Table V-1 Drug Dosage Guidelines for Infants and Children—cont'd

Drug	Dose	Dose/Limit	Comments
Carbamazepine	Initial dose: 10 mg/kg/day PO ÷ 1-2 ×/day Maintenance dose: up to 20-30 mg/kg/day PO ÷ q8h; increase dose gradually over 2-4 wk		Chewable tablets must be thoroughly chewed and not swallowed whole; controlled-release tablets may be split; give with food or milk; dose may require reduction in liver impairment; monitoring of serum drug concentrations recommended
Cefaclor	20-40 mg/kg/day PO ÷ q8h	1.5 g/day	May be given with food; dose adjustment in renal impairment: moderate, 50%-100%; severe, 33%; consider use of cefuroxime axetil in older children
Cefazolin	Mild to moderate infections: 25-50 mg/kg/day IV/IM ÷ q8h	2 g/day	Dose interval adjustment in renal impairment: moderate, q12h; severe, q24-48h
	Severe infections: 50-150 mg/kg/day IV/IM ÷ q8h	6 g/day	
	Cardiac surgery prophylaxis: 40 mg/kg/dose IV/IM q8h × 6 doses	750 mg/dose	
Cefixime	8 mg/kg/day PO as a single daily dose Gonorrhea: 8 mg/kg PO × 1 dose	400 mg/day	Inactive against staphylococci; dose adjustment in renal impairment: moderate, 75%; severe, 50%
Cefotaxime	Mild to moderate infections: 75-100 mg/kg/day IV/IM ÷ q6-8h	6 g/day	Dose interval adjustment in renal impairment: moderate, q8-12h; severe, q12-24h
	Severe infections: 150-200 mg/kg/day IV/IM ÷ q6-8h	8 g/day	
	Meningitis in infants 1-3 mo of age: 200 mg/kg/day IV/IM ÷ q6h	8 g/day	

Drug	Dose	Max	Comments
Cefoxitin	Mild to moderate infections: 80-100 mg/kg/day IV/IM ÷ q6-8h Severe infections: 80-160 mg/kg/day IV/IM ÷ q4-6h	4 g/day 12 g/day	Dose interval adjustment in renal impairment: moderate, q8-12h; severe, q24-48h
Ceftazidime	Mild to moderate infections: 75-100 mg/kg/day IV/IM ÷ q8h Severe infections: 125-150 mg/kg/day IV/IM ÷ q8h CF Patients: 200 mg/kg/day IV/IM ÷ q6h	3 g/day 6 g/day 6 g/day	Dose interval adjustment in renal impairment: mild, q8-12h; moderate, q24-48h; severe, q48-72h
Ceftriaxone	Meningitis in children > 3 mo of age: 80 mg/kg/dose IV at 0, 12, and 24h followed by 80 mg/kg/day IV q24h Other infections: 80 mg/kg/day IV/IM q24h Uncomplicated gonorrhea: < 45 kg: 125 mg/dose IM as single dose ≥ 45 kg: 250 mg/dose IM as single dose	4 g/day	Treat uncomplicated gonorrhea in children ≥ 45 kg with tetracycline/doxycycline or azithromycin as well
Cefuroxime	75 mg/kg/day IV/IM ÷ q8h	4.5 g/day	Dose interval adjustment in renal impairment: moderate, q8-12h; severe, q24h; not to be used for treatment of meningitis
Cefuroxime axetil (Tablets)	≥ 12 yr: Mild-moderate infection: 125-250 mg PO bid Moderate-severe infection: 250-500 mg PO bid < 12 yr: Pharyngitis, tonsillitis: 125 mg PO bid	1 g/day	Administration with food may decrease GI adverse effects; do not crush tablets; taste is very bitter
Cephalexin	25-50 mg/kg/day PO ÷ qid	4 g/day	May be given with food; Dose interval adjustment in renal impairment: severe, q8-12h

Continued.

Table V-1 Drug Dosage Guidelines for Infants and Children—cont'd

Drug	Dose	Dose/Limit	Comments
Charcoal, activated	see Activated Charcoal		
Chloral hydrate	Hypnotic: 50 mg/kg/dose PO/PR 20-45 min preexam Sedative: 25 mg/kg/dose PO/PR qhs PRN	1 g/dose	Reduce dose in patients with CNS impairment; dose may require reduction in liver impairment; capsules may be given rectally
	Conscious sedation: 50-80 mg/kg/dose PO 20-45 min preprocedure; may repeat 25-40 mg/kg/dose in 1 hr prn	1 g/initial dose 500 mg/ supplemental dose	
Chloramphenicol	Meningitis: 75-100 mg/kg/day IV/PO ÷ q6h Other: 50-75 mg/kg/day IV/PO ÷ q6h	4 g/day	Avoid in liver impairment; do not use chloramphenicol palmitate in infants < 1 yr or in patients with cystic fibrosis; give PO on empty stomach (1 hr ac or 2 hr pc); monitoring of serum drug concentrations recommended
Chloroquine	Malaria prophylaxis: < 1 yr: 37.5 mg base/dose 1-3 yr: 75 mg base/dose 4-6 yr: 100 mg base/dose 7-10 yr: 150 mg base/dose 11-16 yr: 225 mg base/dose > 16 yr: 300 mg base/dose Dosed once weekly, beginning 1-2 wk before entering malaria zone and continuing for 4 wk after leaving malaria area	300 mg base/dose	250 mg chloroquine phosphate = 150 mg chloroquine base; give PO with food or milk; PO drug extremely bitter; chloroquine widely available as syrup in malaria-endemic countries; tablets may be crushed and mixed with cereal or jam; parenteral drug available on emergency release

	Malaria: 10 mg base/kg/dose PO × 1 dose 5 mg base/kg/dose PO 6 hr later Then 5 mg base/kg/day PO as single daily dose × 2 days or 3.5 mg base/kg/dose IM/SC Repeat × 1 in 6 hr PRN	First dose: 600 mg base Subsequent doses: 300 mg base PO	
Chlorpheniramine (nonformulary)	0.35 mg/kg/day PO ÷ q6-12h	Usual adult dose: 4 mg PO q4-6h prn or 8 mg PO q12h prn (sustained-release tablets)	Give with food or milk; may cause drowsiness or CNS stimulation
Chlorpromazine	Afterload reduction: 0.025-0.05 mg/kg/dose IV Nausea and vomiting: 2 mg/kg/day PO/IM/IV ÷ q4-6h 4 mg/kg/day PR ÷ q6-8h Sedation: 0.5mg/kg/**dose** PO/IV	< 5 yr: 40 mg/day 5-12 yr: 75 mg/day	Monitor blood pressure after IV therapy; give PO with food or milk
Cholestyramine	0.24-1.1 g/kg/day PO ÷ bid/tid		May alter absorption of other drugs
Cimetidine (Nonformulary)	20 mg/kg/day PO/IV ÷ q6h or ÷ tid with meals and qhs	2400 mg/day	Dose adjustment in renal impairment: moderate, 75%; severe, 50%; monitor gastric pH in patients requiring IV therapy; coadministration of cimetidine and propranolol may decrease effect of propranolol; coadministration of cimetidine and either theophylline, phenytoin, or procainamide may produce toxicity because of latter drug

Continued.

Table V-1 Drug Dosage Guidelines for Infants and Children—cont'd

Drug	Dose	Dose/Limit	Comments
Cisapride	0.6-1 mg/kg/day PO ÷ tid ac or ÷ tid ac and qhs	40 mg/day	Dose may require reduction in renal or liver impairment; may alter absorption of other drugs; concurrent use with drugs that inhibit hepatic metabolism (e.g., ketoconazole, erythromycin) may cause life-threatening cardiac arrhythmias
Clarithromycin	*Mycobacterium avium* complex: 15-30 mg/kg/day PO ÷ q12h Other infections: 15 mg/kg/day PO ÷ q12h	1 g/day	Dose reduction in renal impairment: moderate, 75%; severe; 50%-75%, give 1 or 2 doses/day

Clindamycin	Mild to moderate infections:
	  15-25 mg/kg/day IM/IV ÷ q6-8h
	  10-30 mg/kg/day PO ÷ q6h
	Severe infections:
	  25-40 mg/kg/day IM/IV ÷ q6-8h
	Chloroquine-resistant *falciparum* malaria:
	  9-21 mg base/kg/day PO ÷ tid
	  10 mg base/kg IV loading dose followed by 5 mg base/kg/dose IV q8h until blood clear of asexual parasites
		1.8 g/day IV/IM
		2 g/day PO
		
		2.7 g/day IV/IM
		
		1.8 g/day PO
			Do not use palmitate in infants < 1 yr or in patients with CF; give capsule PO with food or full glass of water to avoid esophageal ulceration; use with quinine/quinidine for chloroquine-resistant malaria only if patient unable to take doxycycline, tetracycline, or Fansidar

Clobazam	Initial dose: 0.25 mg/kg/day PO as single daily dose hs or ÷ bid Increase gradually to 0.5 mg/kg/day PO ÷ bid-tid	Initial: 10 mg/dose Maintenance: 1 mg/kg/day or 80 mg/day	

Clonazepam	≤ 30 kg: Initial dose: 0.05 mg/kg/day PO ÷ bid or tid increasing by 0.05 mg/kg/day every 3 days PRN up to 0.2 mg/kg/day > 30 kg: Initial dose: 1.5 mg/kg/day PO ÷ tid increasing by 0.5-1 mg/day every 3 days up to 20 mg/day PO ÷ tid	20 mg/day	Dose may require reduction in liver impairment
Clonidine	Growth hormone stimulation test: SA ≤ 0.39 m²: 0.05 mg/dose 0.4-0.7 m²: 0.1 mg/dose 0.71-1.1 m²: 0.15 mg/dose > 1.1 m²: 0.2 mg/dose	0.2 mg/dose	
Cloxacillin	Mild-moderate infections: 50-100 mg/kg/day PO/IV/IM ÷ q6h Severe infections: 150-200 mg/kg/day IV/IM ÷ q6h Febrile neutropenia: 160 mg/kg/day IV/IM ÷ q6h 100 mg/kg/day PO ÷ q6h	4 g/day PO/IV/IM 12 g/day IV/IM 4 g/day PO	Give PO on empty stomach (1 hr ac or 2 hr pc); oral suspension extremely bitter; consider flucloxacillin or cephalexin if oral liquid required
Codeine	Analgesic: 3-6 mg/kg/day PO/IM ÷ q4-6h prn Antitussive: 0.8-1.2 mg/kg/day PO ÷ q4-6h	1.5 mg/kg/dose	Max dose should not be given for > 24 hr; avoid IM route if possible
Cortisone acetate	Hypoadrenalism: 25 mg/m²/day PO ÷ tid		Give with food or milk; to discontinue in patients receiving therapy for ≥ 10 days, reduce dose by 50% q10-14 days

Continued.

Table V-1 Drug Dosage Guidelines for Infants and Children—cont'd

Drug	Dose	Dose/Limit	Comments
Cotrimoxazole	Bacterial infection: 5-10 mg trimethoprim/kg/day PO/IV ÷ q12h (includes 25-50 mg/kg/day sulfamethoxazole) *Pneumocystis carinii:* Treatment: 20 mg trimethoprim/kg/day IV or PO ÷ q6h (includes 100 mg/kg/day sulfamethoxazole) Prophylaxis: HIV infected/exposed children: 5 mg trimethoprim/kg/day 3 or 7 days per week PO ÷ bid Prophylaxis: Other immunocompromised children: 2.5-5 mg trimethoprim/kg/day PO q2day or 3 × weekly as single daily dose Prophylaxis: Otitis media and urinary tract infection: 2-5 mg trimethoprim/kg/day PO Prophylaxis: asplenia (≤ 6 mo): 5 mg trimethoprim/kg/day PO 1 × day		Maintain fluid intake; may be given PO with food; dose interval adjustment in renal impairment: moderate, q18h; severe, 24h For prophylaxis in asplenic patients > 6 mo, penicillin (all ages) or amoxicillin (2-5yr) recommended
Cromoglycate sodium	1% inhalation solution: 20-mg (2-ml) dose bid-qid via nebulizer Metered-dose aerosol: 2 mg (2 puffs) qid via inhalation Spincap: 60-80 mg/day via inhalation ÷ tid/qid Nasal: 1-2 squeezes into each nostril, up to 6 ×/day		Use of Aerochamber or Aerochamber with mask recommended with metered dose inhaler

Cyclosporine	Bone marrow transplant: Initial dose: 3 mg/kg/day IV ÷ q12h Liver transplant: Initial dose: 3 mg/kg/day IV as continuous infusion Renal transplant: 5-10 mg/kg/day PO ÷ q12h Cardiac transplant: Initial dose: 1 mg/kg/day IV as continuous infusion		Dose may require reduction in liver impairment; give PO on empty stomach (1 hr ac or 2-3 hr pc); many other drugs may increase or decrease the effects of cyclosporine; monitoring of level recommended
Dapsone (Non-formulary)	PCP prophylaxis: 1-2 mg/kg/day PO as single daily dose	100 mg/day	Use with caution in patients with G6PD deficiency, hypersensitivity to sulfonamides; may cause photosensitivity; do not administer with antacids
Deferoxamine mesylate (Desferal)	Acute iron intoxication: See p. 448 Chronic iron overload: 50 mg/kg/day as 8-12 hr SC infusion	4 g/day	Titrate dose according to serum ferritin
Desmopressin (DDAVP)	*Diabetes insipidus:* 5-20 µg/day intranasally 1 ×/day or ÷ bid Coagulopathy: 0.3 µg/kg/dose IV/SC Enuresis: Initial dose: 20 µg (10 µg in each nostril) qhs × 7 days; may increase dose q7 days in 10 µg increments up to 30-40 µg qhs	25 µg/dose 40 µg/day	For enuresis, maintain lowest effective dosage × 4 wk, then taper by decreasing dose by 10 µg/night each mo, if possible

Continued.

Table V-1 Drug Dosage Guidelines for Infants and Children—cont'd

Drug	Dose	Dose/Limit	Comments
Dexamethasone	Extubation (if previous difficulties with extubation): 1-2 mg/kg/day PO/IV/IM ÷ q6h beginning 24 hr before extubation and continuing 4-6 hr afterward Increased ICP: Initial dose: 0.2-0.4 mg/kg IV Subsequent dose: 0.3 mg/kg/day IV/IM ÷ q6h; may be useful in cerebral tumors and malaria, but not in head injury Croup: 0.6 mg/kg IV × 1 Meningitis: 0.6 mg/kg/day IV ÷ q6h × 4 days Antiemetic: 10mg/m²/dose IV prechemo and q12h afterward 0.2 mg/kg/dose PO prechemo and q6h afterward	Initial dose: 10 mg Max 20 mg/dose IV Max 4 mg/dose PO	Give PO with food or milk; to discontinue in patients receiving therapy for ≥ 10 days, reduce dose by 50% q48h until 0.3 ± 0.1 mg/m²/day achieved; then reduce dose by 50% q10-14days In meningitis, administer first dose before giving antibiotics; avoid in children with peptic ulcer disease
Dextromethorphan	1 mg/kg/day PO ÷ q6-8h	1 mg/kg/day Usual adult dose: 10-20 mg PO q4h prn	
Dextrose	Resuscitation: see inside front cover		
Diazepam	Status epilepticus: 0.1-0.3 mg/kg/dose IV q10min × 3 or 0.3-0.5 mg/kg/dose PR × 1 Preop: 0.1-0.5 mg/kg/dose PO 30-90 min before surgery Conscious sedation: 0.1 mg/kg/dose IV 0.2 mg/kg/dose PO 45-60 min before procedure	< 5 yr: 5 mg/dose ≥ 5 yr: 10 mg/dose 20 mg/dose PO 20 mg/dose IV/PO	May cause hypotension and apnea when given IV; dose may require reduction in liver impairment

	Anxiolytic: 0.1-0.8 mg/kg/day PO ÷ q6h	Usual adult dose (anxiolytic): 2-10 mg/dose bid-qid PO
Diazoxide	Acute hypertension: 1-3 mg/kg/dose IV q5-15min prn	Max total dose: 8 mg/kg or 4 doses	Give IV undiluted over 30 sec
Didanosine (Videx, ddI) (Non-formulary)	180 mg/m²/day PO ÷ bid-tid	Tablets: 250 mg/day Powder: 334 mg/day	Dose interval in renal impairment: Severe, q48h; moderate, q24h; use with caution in hepatic impairment; adult strengths contain sodium: 264.5mg/buffered tablet, 1380mg/powder packet; tablets should be chewed, crushed, or dispersed in water; do not mix tablets or powder with fruit juice or other acidic liquids; may cause pancreatitis, peripheral neuropathy, headache, diarrhea

Digoxin	Digitalization dose: (3 doses: 1st stat, 2nd in 6 hr, 3rd in another 6 hr)
	≥ 37 weeks postconceptual age (PCA) -2 year:
	  17 µg/kg/**dose** PO
	  12 µg/kg/**dose** IV
	> 2 yr: 13µg/kg/**dose** PO
	  10 µg/kg/**dose** IV
	Maintenance dose:
	≥ 37 wk PCA-2 yr old:
	  10 µg/kg/day PO ÷ bid or as single daily dose
	> 2 yr:
	  8 µg/kg/day PO ÷ bid or as single daily dose
		Total digitalization dose: 1mg
		
		Maintenance dose: 250 µg/day
			Calculate dose according to ideal body weight, reduce dose by 50% during concurrent administration of amiodarone, propafenone, or quinidine; digitalizing dose adjustment in renal impairment: severe, 50%-65%; maintenance dose adjustment in renal impairment: moderate, 25%-75%; severe, 10%-25%; once daily dosing may be satisfactory, especially in patients > 2 yr; monitoring of serum drug concentrations recommended; Digoxin antibody (Digibind) available to treat potentially life-threatening digoxin toxicity; contact the poison center for more information

Continued.

Table V-1 Drug Dosage Guidelines for Infants and Children—cont'd

Drug	Dose	Dose/Limit	Comments
Dimenhydrinate	5 mg/kg/day PO/IV/IM/pr ÷ q6h	300 mg/day	
Dimercaprol (BAL in oil)	Severe lead poisoning (blood lead > 70 µg/dl or 3.35 µmol/L): 300 mg/m²/day IM ÷ q4h × 3-5 days		Give by deep IM injection; start calcium disodium edetate with 2nd dose of dimercaprol; ensure adequate urine output; discontinue when blood lead < 50 µg/dl (2.4 µmol/L); turnaround time for results of blood lead analysis may be 2-3 days
Diphenhydramine	Antihistamine: 5 mg/kg/day PO/IV/IM ÷ q6h Anaphylaxis: 1-2 mg/kg/dose IV	300 mg/day 50 mg/dose	
Dipyridamole	5 mg/kg/day PO ÷ tid	400 mg/day	Given on empty stomach (1 hr ac or 2 hr pc)
Dobutamine	2-30 µg/kg/min IV	40 µg/kg/min	Avoid extravasation; administer via central line whenever possible
Docusate sodium	5 mg/kg/day PO ÷ q6-8h or as single daily dose	Usual adult dose: 100-200 mg/day	Dilute liquid in milk or juice; onset of action = 24-72 hr
Domperidone (nonformulary)	1.2-2.4 mg/kg/day PO ÷ tid-qid; give 15-30 min ac ÷ qhs	80 mg/day Usual adult dose: 10 mg tid-qid	
Dopamine	5-30 µg/kg/min via continuous IV infusion	30 µg/kg/min	Avoid extravasation; administer via central venous line whenever possible

Doxycycline	5 mg/kg/day PO ÷ q12h	200 mg/day	May be given PO with food; not recommended for children ≤ 8 yr; for treatment of malaria, use in combination with quinidine/quinine for 7 days
	Chloroquine-resistant *Falciparum* malaria: 4 mg/kg/day PO ÷ bid		
Edetate cal-cium disodium	Lead poisoning: 1000 mg/m^2/day by continuous IV infusion or ÷ q12h		Begin therapy with second dose of dimercaprol; ensure good urine output; allow at least 2 days' interval before re-peating course of treatment
Edrophonium	Supraventricular tachycardia:	10 mg/dose	Have atropine ready
	0.2 mg/kg/dose IV over 3 min		
Epinephrine	Resuscitation: see inside front cover		Incompatible with sodium bicarbonate; administer IV via cen-tral venous line whenever possible
	0.01 mg/kg/dose (0.01 ml of 1:1000 solution/kg/dose) sc q10-20 min prn; minimum 0.1 mg (0.1 ml)/dose		To prepare infusion:
	0.1-1 µg/kg/min via continuous IV infusion		0.3 × weight (kg) = dose (mg) added to IV fluid to make
	0.1 mg + 0.01 mg/kg IV/ETT, q5min prn (1 ml + 0.1 ml/kg/dose of 1:10,000 solution)		50 ml; then 1 ml/hr = 0.1 µg/kg/min
Epinephrine (Racemic) for inhalation	0.5 ml/dose in 3 ml NS via nebulizer prn up to max q1h	0.5 ml/dose	
Erythromycin	Base: 40 mg/kg/day PO ÷ q6h	2 g/day PO	Use base for CF patients; give PO on empty stomach (1 hr ac or 2 hr pc) unless GI upset occurs; dose interval adjust-ment in renal impairment: severe, 50%-75%; multiple drug interactions, including astemizole, terfenadine, cyclosporine, carbamazepine, cisapride, and warfarin; consult pharmacy for details
	Stearate and estolate:		
	20-40 mg/kg/day PO ÷ q6-12h		
	Ethylsuccinate:		
	40 mg/kg/day PO ÷ q6h		
	Glucoptate and lactobionate:	4 g/day IV	
	20-50 mg/kg/day IV ÷ q6h		

Continued.

Table V-1 Drug Dosage Guidelines for Infants and Children—cont'd

Drug	Dose	Dose/Limit	Comments
Erythromycin—cont'd	Inflammatory acne: 500-1000 mg/day PO ÷ q6-8h May be decreased to 250 mg/day PO as single daily dose for maintenance		
Erythropoietin	Anemia of chronic renal failure: Initial dose: 50 U/kg/day IV/SC 3 × weekly		Titrate dose according to hemoglobin
Esmolol	Loading dose: 100-500 µg/kg IV over 1 min Maintenance: 100-300 µg/kg/min IV infusion		Use with caution in patients with impaired renal function
Ethambutol	Initial dose: 15-25 mg/kg/day PO as single daily dose or 50 mg/kg/dose PO 2×/wk Retreatment: 25 mg/kg/day PO as single daily dose	2.5 g/day	Bacteriostatic; give with food if GI upset occurs; dose interval adjustment in renal impairment: Moderate, q24-36h; severe, q48h
Ethosuximide	Initial dose: 15 mg/kg/day PO as single dose or ÷ bid: increase gradually q3days prn to maximum dose	1.5 g/day or 40 mg/kg/day, whichever is less	Dose may require reduction in liver impairment; monitoring of serum drug concentrations recommended
Fansidar	Chloroquinine-resistant *Falciparum* malaria: 2-11 mo: ¼ tablet PO × 1 1-3 yr: ½ table PO × 1 4-8 yr: 1 tablet PO × 1 9-14 yr: 2 tablets PO × 1 > 14 yr: 3 tablets PO × 1		Each tablet contains 25 mg pyrimethamine, and 500 mg sulfadoxine; Fansidar may cause Stevens-Johnson syndrome and toxic epidermal necrolysis
Fentanyl injection	Epidural Bolus: 1-3 µg/kg epidurally Infusion: 0.4-0.8 µg/kg/hr epidurally		

Ferrous fumerate, ferrous sulfate	Treatment: 6 mg elemental Fe/kg/day PO ÷ tid Prophylaxis: 0.5-2 mg elemental Fe/kg/day PO as single daily dose or ÷ bid-tid		Dilute drops, syrup, or suspension before administration in glass of water or juice and mix thoroughly; administer tablets with ½ to 1 glass of water or juice; administer 1 hr before or 2 hr after dairy products, eggs, coffee, tea, or whole-grain bread or cereal
Flucloxacillin	25-100 mg/kg/day PO ÷ q6h	2 g/day	Give on empty stomach (1 hr ac or 2 hr pc); consider cephalexin if oral liquid required; dose may require reduction in renal impairment
Fluconazole	3-12 mg/kg/day PO/IV as single daily dose Oropharyngeal candidiasis: 3 mg/kg/day PO as single daily dose Esophageal candidiasis: 3-6 mg/kg/day PO as single daily dose Secondary prophylaxis of candidiasis in HIV-infected patients: 3-5 mg/kg/day PO as single daily dose BMT prophylaxis: 5 mg/kg/day PO/IV as single daily dose beginning day -7 and continuing until ANC ≥ 0.5 (usually day +14 to +21)	400 mg/day Dropharyngeal candidiasis: 200mg/day PO	Use with caution in patients with liver impairment; dose interval adjustment in renal impairment: moderate, q48h; severe, q72h or adjust dose (not interval): moderate, 50%; severe, 25%
Fludrocortisone	Salt-losing hypoadrenalism: 0.05-0.2 mg/day, PO ÷ q12h		Give with food or milk
Flumazenil	10 μg/kg IV over 15 sec; wait 1-3 min; if necessary, dose may be repeated up to 4 × at 1-3 min intervals to total dose of 50 μg/kg; if resedation occurs, doses may be repeated every 20 min, or effective dose may be given as hrly infusion	200 μg/dose 1000 μg total dose	Dose adjustment may be required in liver impairment

Continued.

Table V-1 Drug Dosage Guidelines for Infants and Children—cont'd

Drug	Dose	Dose/Limit	Comments
Fluoxetine	≥ 6 yr: Depression: 10-20 mg/day OCD, bulimia: Initial dose 1-20 mg/day; increase dose every few weeks to desired effect or maximum of 80 mg/day	80 mg/day	Dose adjustment may be required in liver impairment
Furazolidone	Giardiasis: 5-8 mg/kg/day PO ÷ qid × 7-10 days		Emergency release drug
Furosemide	1-2 mg/kg/day PO ÷ q6-12h prn; may increase to 3-8 mg/kg/day PO ÷ q6-8 hr prn 0.5-2 mg/kg/dose IV/IM q6-8h prn	6 mg/kg/dose	Give IV over 5-10 min no faster than 20 mg/min; IV doses have been given as often as q2h for acute pulmonary edema
Ganciclovir	CMV infection: Treatment: 10 mg/kg/day IV ÷ q12h Allogeneic bone marrow transplant prophylaxis: Day −5 to day 0: 10 mg/kg/day IV ÷ q12h Posttransplant when ANC ≥ 1:5 mg/kg/day IV as single daily dose, until day 100 or patient able to tolerate PO acyclovir		Handle as biohazard; dose and interval adjustment in renal impairment: CrCl Dose (ml/1.73m²/min) 50-79 2.5 mg/kg/dose IV q12h 25-49 2.5 mg/kg/dose IV q24h < 25 1.25 mg/kg/dose IV q24h Discontinue ganciclovir in bone marrow transplant patients if absolute neutrophil count (ANC) < 0.5
Gelusil (extra strength)	See Aluminum and magnesium hydroxides		
Gentamicin	7.5 mg/kg/day IV/IM ÷ q8h Cardiac surgery prophylaxis: 2 mg/kg/dose IV 1 hr preop and 8 hr postop	120 mg/dose before serum concentration determination 120 mg/dose	Calculate dose according to effective body weight; monitoring of serum drug concentrations recommended; dose interval adjustment in renal impairment: mild-moderate, q12hr; severe, q24-48h

Glucagon	Hypoglycemia in *diabetes mellitus*: < 5 yr: 0.5 mg/dose SC > 5 yr: 1 mg/dose SC May repeat in 5-20 min	
GoLytely	See PEG-electrolyte liquid	
Growth hor- mone	0.06 mg/kg/dose IM or SC 3 × week	
Heparin	Loading dose: 75 U/kg IV over 10 min Initial maintenance dose: ≤ 1 yr: 28 U/kg/hr > 1 yr: 20 U/kg/hr	Adjust heparin to maintain APTT at 60-85 sec; usual dilution is 80 U/ml in children ≤ 10 kg and 40 U/ml in children > 10 kg; avoid concurrent use of ASA or other antiplatelet drugs. Antidote: Protamine sulfate
Hydralazine	Initial dose: 0.15-0.8 mg/kg/dose IV q4-6h or 1.5 µg/kg/min IV Maintenance dose: 0.75-7 mg/kg/day PO ÷ q6h 25 mg/dose IV 200 mg/day or 7 mg/kg/day, whichever is less	Associated with development of drug-induced lupus
Hydrochlo- rothiazide	2-4 mg/kg/day PO ÷ q12h Usual adult dose: 25-100 mg/dose PO as single daily dose, bid or q2days	For hydrochlorothiazide in combination with spironolactone, see Novospirozine; ineffective when GFR < 30 ml/min

Continued.

Table V-1 Drug Dosage Guidelines for Infants and Children—cont'd

Drug	Dose	Dose/Limit	Comments

Hydrocortisone	Acute asthma: 4-6 mg/kg/dose IV q4-6h
	Anaphylaxis: 5-10 mg/kg IV
	Hypoadrenalism
	  Normal endogenous production: 10 ± 3 mg/m²/day
	  Maintenance dose: 20 mg/m²/day PO ÷ tid or 12 mg/m²/day IV ÷ q6h
	Precp 100 mg/m² IV × 1 preop, then 100 mg/m²/day IV ÷ q6h
	Acute adrenal crisis: 100 mg/m² IV stat, then 100 mg/m²/day IV ÷ q6h
			Bioavailability of PO hydrocortisone: 50%; triple maintenance dose during concurrent illness or stress; in CAH, administer ½ daily dose at bedtime to suppress AM surge of ACTH; give PO with food or milk; to discontinue in patients receiving therapy for ≥ 10 days, reduce dose by 50% q48h until 10 ± 3 mg/m²/day achieved; then reduce dose by 50% q10-14 days

Hydroxychloroquine	Juvenile arthritis: ≤ 6 mg/kg/day PO as single daily dose	400 mg/day	Give with food or milk; avoid alcohol; monitor visual acuity
Hydroxyzine	2 mg/kg/day PO ÷ tid or qid Chronic urticaria: 2-4 mg/kg/day PO ÷ tid or qid	400 mg/day	
Imipenem-cilastatin	60-100 mg/kg/day IV/IM ÷ q6h	4g/day	Dose interval adjustment in renal impairment: Mild, q6-8h; moderate, q8-12h; severe q12h (max, 1 g/day); avoid use in patients with CrCl < 5 ml/min/1.73 m² who are not being dialyzed; high doses have been associated with neurotoxicity, including seizures
Immune globulin (human, IV)	Hypogammaglobulinemia: 600 mg/kg/dose IV 1 ×/mo Bone-marrow transplant: 200-500 mg/kg/dose IV 1 ×/mo Idiopathic thrombocytopenia purpura: 1 g/kg/dose IV as single daily dose × 1 or 2 days		Supplied as Gamimune except for Kawasaki disease (use Iveegam) and study patients

	Kawasaki disease: 2 g/kg IV as single dose Polymyositis/dermatomyositis: 1 g/kg/dose IV 1 ×/day for 2 days/mo Guillain-Barré syndrome: 1 g/kg/day IV 1 ×/day × 2 days JRA: 1.5 g/kg/dose IV 1 ×/mo Perinatal HIV: 400 mg/kg IV 1×/mo Bone-marrow transplant, SCIDS: 5-20 ml PO bid	70 g
Indomethacin	1.5-3 mg/kg/day PO ÷ tid with meals	200 mg/day	Give with food or milk; sustained-release capsules may be dosed bid
Iodine	see Potassium iodide		
Iodoquinol	Intestinal amoebiasis: 30-40 mg/kg/day PO ÷ tid pc × 20 days	1.95 g/day	
Ipecac	9-12 mo: 10 ml PO 1-10 yr: 15 ml PO > 10 yr: 30 ml PO	≤ 1 yr: 1 single dose > 1 yr: can repeat once after 20 min	Contact Poison Center for treatment of patients < 9 mo old
Ipratropium	Metered dose aerosol: 1-2 puffs (20-40 µg) tid-qid	12 puffs/day (240 µg)	

Continued.

Table V-1 Drug Dosage Guidelines for Infants and Children—cont'd

Drug	Dose	Dose/Limit	Comments
Ipratropium—cont'd	Inhalation solution: 250 µg/dose Give each dose in 3 ml NS via nebulizer tid-qid prn; in severe acute asthma, may be given q20min	Usual adult dose: 250-500 µg/dose in 3 ml NS via nebulizer q4-6h prn	
Iron	See Ferrous fumarate		
Isoniazid	10-20 mg/kg/day PO as single daily dose or ÷ q12 or 10-20 mg/kg/dose PO twice weekly	CNS disease: 500 mg/day 2×/wk regimen: 900 mg/day Other: 300 mg/day	Dosage reduction may be required in liver impairment; give on empty stomach (1 hr ac or 2 hr pc), unless GI upset occurs; pyridoxine supplementation should be considered in patients at risk of pyridoxine deficiency (e.g., malnourished; breast-feeding infant)
Isoproterenol	0.05-1 µg/kg/min IV as a continuous infusion		To prepare infusion: 0.3 × weight (kg) = dose (mg) added to IV solution to make 5 ml; 1 ml/hour = 0.1 µg/hg/min
Isotretinoin (Accutane)	Cystic scarring acne: Initial dose: 0.5-2 mg/kg/day PO ÷ bid; reduce dose to low-est effective dose after ≥ 2 wk		Must avoid pregnancy for 1 mo before, during, and 1 mo following therapy; give with food; usual duration of course of treatment is 15-20 wk; repeat course may be required after interval of ≥ 8 wk
Itraconazole	Oropharyngeal candidiasis treatment or secondary prophy-laxis: 2-5 mg/kg/day PO as single daily dose	400 mg/day	Dose adjustment may be required in liver impairment; give with food; caution regarding drug interactions, especially with terfenadine, cyclosporine; may cause hepatic dysfunc-tion; oral liquid is emergency release drug

Kayexalate	See Sodium polystyrene sulfonate		
Ketoconazole	5-10 mg/kg/day PO as single daily dose or ÷ q12h	400 mg/day	Give with food
Ketotifen	6 mo-3 yr: Initial dose: 0.05 mg/kg/day PO ÷ bid or qhs Maintenance dose: 0.1 mg/kg/day PO ÷ bid > 3 yr: Initial dose: 0.5 mg PO qhs or 0.25 mg PO bid Maintenance dose: 1 mg PO bid		Give with food
Labetalol	Acute hypertension: 1-3 mg/kg IV Hypertension: 1 mg/kg/hr by continuous IV infusion	3 mg/kg/hr	Dose may require reduction in liver impairment
Lactulose	Constipation: Initial dose: 5-10 ml/day PO 1 ×/day Double daily dose until stool produced	Usual adult dose: 15-60 ml/day (constipation)	
	Hepatic encephalopathy: < 1 yr: 2.5 ml PO bid Older children and adolescents: 10-30 ml PO tid	< 1 yr: 2.5 ml PO qid	For hepatic encephalopathy: Decrease/discontinue if severe diarrhea develops; treatment is effective if stool is soft with pH < 5.5; hypernatremia or hypokalemia may occur
Lamivudine (3TC) (Nonformulary)	HIV-infected children, usually in combination with zidovudine: 8 mg/kg/day PO ÷ bid	300 mg/day	May cause pancreatitis, peripheral neuropathy; oral solution contains sugar
Lamotrigine	**Children 2-12 yr:** not taking valproic acid Initial dose: 2 mg/kg/day PO ÷ for 2 wk then increase to 5 mg/kg/day PO ÷ bid for 2 wk, then titrate dose Usual maintenance dose 5-15 mg/kg/day PO ÷ bid		Use with caution in patients with impaired renal or liver function

Continued.

Table V-1 Drug Dosage Guidelines for Infants and Children—cont'd

Drug	Dose	Dose/Limit	Comments
Lamotrigine—cont'd	**Children 2-12 yr:** taking valproic acid as only other anticonvulsant		
	Initial dose:		
	0.25 mg/kg/day PO as single daily dose for 6 wk, then increase to 0.5 mg/kg/day PO as single daily dose for 6 wk, then titrate dose		
	Usual maintenance dose:		
	1-5 mg/kg/day PO as single daily dose or ÷ bid		
	Children > 12 yr: taking enzyme-inducing agents but not valproic acid		
	Initial dose:		
	25 mg PO bid for 2 wk, then increase to 50 mg PO bid for 2 wk, then titrate dose		
	Usual maintenance dose:	400 mg/day	
	200 mg PO bid		
	Children > 12 yr: taking enzyme-inducing agents with valproic acid		
	Initial dose:		
	25 mg PO as single daily dose for 2 wk, then increase dose by 50 mg/day every 2 wk according to response, to maximum of 400 mg/day	400 mg/day	
	Children > 12 yr: taking valproic acid but not enzyme-inducing agents		
	Initial dose:		
	25 mg PO as single dose every other day for 2 wk, then increase to 25 mg PO as single daily dose for 2 wk, then titrate dose		
	Usual maintenance dose:	200 mg/day	
	100 mg PO as single daily dose		

Levocarnitine	Metabolic crisis: Give loading dose 50-300 mg/kg IV, then give same dose over next 24 hr ÷ q4h IV Maintenance: 50-100 mg/kg/day PO/IV ÷ q4-6h	Usual adult dose: 4g/day PO ÷ bid-tid	
Levothyroxine	1-6 mo: 7-12 µg/kg/day PO 1 ×/day 6-12 mo: 6-8 µg/kg/day PO 1 ×/day 1-5 yr: 4-6 µg/kg/day PO 1 ×/day 5-10 yr: 3-5 µg/kg/day PO 1 ×/day 10-20 yr: 2-3 µg/kg/day PO 1 ×/day		Adjust dose according to clinical status and thyroid function tests; give on empty stomach (1 hr ac or 2 hr pc)
Lidocaine	Resuscitation: See inside front cover		
Lindane (Kwellada)	Scabies: Apply cream or lotion in thin layer to skin below neck and leave on overnight; bathe in 8-12 hr		In children < 2 yr consider use of alternative scabicide because of possible CNS toxicity
Loperamide	0.08-0.24 mg/kg/day PO ÷ bid or tid	16 mg/day 2 mg/dose	Following first treatment day, give 0.1 mg/kg/dose only after loose stool
Loratidine	< 30 kg: 5 mg PO 1 ×/day ≥ 30 kg: 10 mg PO 1 ×/day		
Lorazepam	Preop: 0.05 mg/kg/dose SL Status epilepticus: 0.05 mg/kg/dose IV/PR May repeat 1 × PRN	SL: 4 mg IV/PR 4 mg/dose 8 mg/12 hr or 0.1 mg/kg/12 hr, whichever is less	Dose may require reduction in liver impairment; for PR administration, dilute injection according to IV instructions
Magnesium citrate	Cathartic: 4 ml/kg/dose PO	296 ml/dose	Use with caution in renal failure

Continued.

Table V-1 Drug Dosage Guidelines for Infants and Children—cont'd

Drug	Dose	Dose/Limit	Comments
Magnesium glucoheptonate	Hypomagnesemia: 20-40 mg elemental magnesium/kg/day PO ÷ tid		Large doses may cause diarrhea; use with caution in renal failure
Magnesium hydroxide	Cathartic: 0.5 ml/kg/dose PO	Usual adult dose: 30-60 ml	Use with caution in renal failure
Magnesium sulfate	Hypomagnesemia Initial dose: 0.21-0.42 mmol/kg/dose IV (5-10 mg/kg/dose elemental magnesium) Maintenance: Continuous infusion: 0.12 mmol/kg/day IV (2.9 mg/kg/day elemental magnesium)	40 mmol (1000 mg elemental magnesium) per dose	Must be diluted before administration; use with caution in renal failure; 500 mg magnesium sulfate = 50 mg elemental magnesium = 2 mmol magnesium = 4 mEq magnesium
Mannitol	Test for oliguria: 0.2 g/kg/dose IV over 10 min × 1 dose Diuresis, reduction of intracranial pressure, reduction of intraocular pressure: 0.2-2 g/kg/dose IV push or as IV infusion over up to 6 hr	Test dose: 12.5 g	Contraindicated in patients with anuria or impaired renal function who do not respond to test dose with adequate urine output; monitor fluid and electrolyte balance
Mebendazole	Pinworm: 100 mg PO × 1 dose; repeat in 2 wk Other nematodes: 200 mg/day PO ÷ bid × 3 days		Do not use for children < 2 yr; tablets may be chewed or swallowed whole or crushed and mixed with food
Mefloquine	Prophylaxis (start prophylaxis 1 wk before traveling, continue 1 ×/wk during travel and for 4 wk after leaving area): Weight < 15kg: 5 mg/kg PO 1 ×/wk 15-19 kg: 62.5 mg (¼ tab) PO 1 ×/wk		Use in children < 15 kg not recommended by manufacturer; however, should be considered for children at high risk Semiimmune patients defined as those who have resided in malaria-endemic areas and who have previous history of malarial infection with same species of parasites

20-30 kg: 125 mg (½ tab) PO 1 ×/wk
31-45 kg: 187.5 mg (¾ tab) PO 1 ×/wk
> 45 kg: 250 mg (1 tab) PO 1 ×/wk
Treatment:
Weight
≤ 45 kg: 25 mg/kg PO (irrespective of immune status) as single dose
46-60 kg: Nonimmune patients: 750 mg PO followed by 500 mg PO after 6-8 hr
46-60 kg: Semiimmune patients: 750 mg PO as single dose
> 60 kg: Nonimmune patients: 750 mg PO followed by 500 mg PO in 6-8 hr and 250 mg PO after additional 6-8 hr
> 60 kg: Semiimmune patients: 750 mg PO followed by 250 mg PO in 6-8 hr

| Meperidine | Analgesic: 1-1.5 mg/kg/dose IV/SC/IM/PO q3-4h prn
Preop: 1-2 mg/kg/dose IM/SC/PO 60 min preop | IV/IM/SC:
2 mg/kg/dose
or 100 mg/
dose, which-
ever is less
PO:
4 mg/kg/dose
or 150 mg/
dose, which-
ever is less | Dose reduction in renal impairment: Severe, 50%-75%; dose may require reduction in liver impairment; may cause constipation, respiratory, or CNS depression; dose is cumulative; metabolite may cause seizures; for patients being converted from parenteral to oral therapy, IM:PO dose ratio = 1:4; avoid IM route, if possible; skin reactions and itching often respond to antihistamines and usually do not imply allergy |

Continued.

Table V-1 Drug Dosage Guidelines for Infants and Children—cont'd

Drug	Dose	Dose/Limit	Comments
Mesalamine (5-ASA)	Ulcerative colitis, Crohn's disease: Children: 30-50 mg/kg/day PO ÷ bid-qid Adolescents, adults: 2400-4800 mg/day PO ÷ tid-qid, then reduce to lowest possible maintenance dose; rectal suspension: 1-4g PR qhs × 3-6 wk, then reduce to lowest possible dose and frequency for maintenance; rectal suppositories: 500 mg PR bid-tid or 1 g qhs, then reduce to lowest possible dose and frequency for maintenance	4.8 g/day PO 4 g/day PR	Retain rectal suspension or suppository for as long as possible for best results
Methotrexate	Juvenile arthritis: 5-10 mg/m²/dose PO 1 ×/wk; may double dose prn after 6-8 wk		Give on empty stomach (1 hr ac or 2 hr pc); monitor liver function
Methylprednisolone	Pulse therapy (rheumatology, immunology): 10-30 mg/kg/dose IV over 1 hr Acute asthma: 2-4 mg/kg/day IV ÷ q6h	1 g/dose	
Metoclopramide	Small bowel intubation: 0.1 mg/kg/dose PO/IM or IV Delayed gastric emptying: < 5 yr: 0.5 mg/kg/day PO ÷ tid with meals 5-14 yr: 2.5-5 mg PO tid before meals > 14 yr: 5-10 mg PO tid before meals Antineoplastic-induced emesis prophylaxis 1.5-2 mg/kg/dose IV prechemo and q2-3h × 3 doses and prn thereafter	50 mg/dose or 300 mg/day	May alter absorption of other drugs; when used as antiemetic, concomitant diphenhydramine 1.25 mg/kg IV (max 50 mg/dose, 300 mg/day) recommended

Metoprolol	1-5 mg/kg/day PO ÷ bid	400 mg/day	Dose may require reduction in severe liver impairment
Metronidazole	Anaerobes, including *Clostridium difficile*:		Give PO with food or milk; avoid alcohol; in *Trichomonas vaginalis* partner must also be treated; dose reduction required in severe liver impairment; dose adjustment in renal impairment: severe, 50%
	15-30 mg/kg/day PO ÷ tid	2 g/day PO	
	30 mg/kg/day IV ÷ q6-8h	4 g/day IV	
	Giardiasis: 15 mg/kg/day PO ÷ tid × 5 days or single daily dose as follows:	750 mg/day	
	< 25 kg: 35 mg/kg/day PO × 3 days		
	25-40 kg: 50 mg/kg/day PO × 3 days		
	> 40 kg: 2 g/day PO × 3 days	2 g/day	
	Amoebiasis: 35-50 mg/kg/day PO ÷ tid × 5-10 days	2.25 g/day	
	Trichomonas vaginalis		
	>13 yr: 2 g PO stat		
	H. pylori eradication:		
	Adolescents: 250 mg PO qid × 14 days	1 g/day	
	Ulcerative colitis, Crohn's: 10-20 mg/kg/day PO ÷ tid pc	1 g/day	
	Gut sterilization: 10 mg/kg/dose PO given at 1 PM, 2 PM, and 11 PM on day before surgery		
Mexilitene	Loading dose: 6-8 mg/kg PO	1200 mg/day	Give with caution in patients with hepatic or renal impairment, CHF, pulmonary disease; adjust doses of both drugs when used in combination with other CNS depressants; concomitant use of cimetidine or erythromycin may increase effects of midazolam; do not discontinue abruptly in patients on prolonged midazolam infusions
	Maintenance dose: 6-16mg/kg/day PO ÷ tid-qid	Usual adult dose: 600 mg/day PO ÷ qid	
Midazolam	Weight < 20 kg: 0.5-0.75 mg/kg/dose PO	20 mg/dose PO except when ordered by anesthesia for preop	Use with caution in patients with hepatic or renal impairment, CHF, pulmonary disease; adjust doses of both drugs when used in combination with other CNS depressants; concomitant use of cimetidine or erythromycin may increase effects of midazolam; do not discontinue abruptly in patients on prolonged midazolam infusions
	Weight ≥ 20 kg: 0.3-0.5 mg/kg/dose PO administered 20-45 min before procedure or surgery		
	0.05 mg/kg/dose IV for conscious sedation, repeat × 1 prn		
	0.1-0.2 mg/kg/dose IV preop		

Continued.

Table V-1 Drug Dosage Guidelines for Infants and Children—cont'd

Drug	Dose	Dose/Limit	Comments
Mineral oil (heavy)	1 ml/kg/dose PO qhs	Usual adult dose: 15-45 ml PO as single dose	Avoid in children < 1 yr
Minocycline	Inflammatory acne: 50-100 mg/day PO ÷ bid	200 mg/day	May be taken with food or milk; contraindicated in children < 8 yr
Minoxidil	0.1-1 mg/kg/day PO ÷ bid		
Morphine	Conscious sedation: 0.05-0.1 mg/kg IV may repeat × 1 in 15 min prn 0.3 mg/kg PO, 30-60 min before procedure Preop sedation: 0.05-0.2 mg/kg/dose IM 30-60 min preop Analgesia: Intermittent dosing: 0.15-0.3 mg/kg/dose PO/PR q4h or 0.05-0.1 mg/kg/dose IV/SC q2-4h Continuous infusion: 0.1-0.2 mg/kg IV loading dose 0.01-0.04 mg/kg/hr IV/SC infusion 0.02-0.05 mg/kg/dose IV/SC q4h prn for breakthrough pain Increase infusion rate q8h prn in increments ≤ 25% of previous infusion rate Epidural: 0.05-0.1 mg/kg bolus	Analgesia: IV/IM/SC: 15 mg/dose; no dose limit for palliative care	Dose adjustment may be required in liver impairment; dosage adjustment in renal impairment: moderate, give 75% of standard dose; severe, give 50% of standard dose For patients being converted from parenteral to oral therapy, IM:PO dose ratio = 1:3 Capsules may be opened, and contents sprinkled on soft food; pellets should not be chewed Continuous IV/SC infusion is preferred to intermittent dosing for management of prolonged pain requiring frequent or high-dose morphine administration; do not adjust maintenance infusion dose until current dose has been running for at least 8 hr; if maintenance dose of > 0.1 mg/kg/hr or additional boluses seem to be required, contact pain service or clinical pharmacology

	Vasoocclusive crisis in sickle cell disease: Loading dose: 0.15 mg/kg IV over 5 min Maintenance dose: 0.04 mg/kg/hr IV Increase dose q8h prn in increments of 0.02 mg/kg/hr up to max of 0.1 mg/kg/hr	Vasoocclusive crisis: Loading dose: 7.5 mg Maintenance dose: 0.1 mg/ kg/hr	Consider pain service or clinical pharmacology consult for difficulties with pain management (see p. 424) Epidural morphine use restricted to anesthesia/pain service
Nadolol	Hypertension: 1 mg/kg/day PO 1 ×/day Increase daily dose by 1 mg/kg/day q3-4days prn	4 mg/kg/day or 320 mg/day, whichever is less	Dose reduction in renal impairment: Moderate, 50%; severe, 25%
Naloxone	< 5 yr or < 20kg: 0.1 mg/kg/dose IV/ETT, repeat prn ≥ 5yr or ≥ 20 kg: 2mg/dose IV/ETT, repeat prn		
Naproxen	10-20 mg/kg/day PO ÷ bid ≥ 50 kg: 500 mg/dose PR 25-49 kg: 250 mg/dose PR	1g/day	Dose may require reduction in hepatic impairment Use with caution in patients with hepatic impairment
Neomycin	Hepatic encephalopathy: 20-30 mg/kg/day PO ÷ q6h Gut sterilization: 25 mg/kg/dose PO given at 1 PM, 2 PM, and 11 PM on day before surgery	Encephalopathy: 2 g/day Sterilization: 1 g/dose	
Neostigmine	Supraventricular tachycardia: 0.01-0.04 mg/kg/dose IV Curare antagonism: 0.02-0.08 mg/kg/dose IV	2.5 mg/dose	Have atropine on hand

Continued.

Table V-1 Drug Dosage Guidelines for Infants and Children—cont'd

Drug	Dose	Dose/Limit	Comments
Nifedipine	Hypertension: Initial dose: 0.5 mg/kg/day PO ÷ q8h Increase gradually prn 1-1.5 mg/kg/day PO	Usual adult dose: 10-30 mg/dose	Prolonged action tablets may be dosed q12h; do not crush or split prolonged-action tablets; for more rapid action, direct patient to bite and swallow capsule
Nitrazepam	Initial dose: 0.25 mg/kg/day PO 1 x/day or ÷ tid; increase gradually prn to 1.2 mg/kg/day PO		Give with food or milk; dose reduction may be required in liver impairment
Nitrofurantoin	5-7 mg/kg/day PO ÷ q6h	600 mg/day or 10 mg/kg/day	Give with food or milk; do not give to infants < 1 mo; do not give if creatinine clearance is < 40 ml/min; may discolor urine rust-yellow to brown
Nitroglycerin	0.5-1C μg/kg/min via continuous IV infusion		
Nitroprusside	0.5-8 μg/kg/min via continuous IV infusion	2.5 mg/kg/day cumulative dose	Caution regarding cyanide toxicity
Norepinephrine	0.02-0.1 μg/kg/min via continuous IV infusion		Avoid extravasation; administer via central line whenever possible
Novospirozine	2-4 mg of each component/kg/day PO ÷ bid	Usual adult dose: 2-4 tablets/day	Give with food or milk; contains spironolactone and hydrochlorothiazide in equal amounts; ineffective when GFR < 30 ml/min
Nystatin	400,000-2,400,000 U/day PO ÷ q4-6h		
Ondansetron	3-5 mg/m² IV 15 min prechemo then PO q8h as follows: < 0.3 m²: 1 mg/dose 0.3-0.6 m²: 2 mg/dose > 0.6-1 m²: 3 mg/dose > 1 m²: 4-8 mg/dose		Consider switching to alternative regimen after 48 hr of ondansetron therapy because of tachyphylaxis

Orciprenaline	0.9-2 mg/kg/day PO ÷ tid-qid 0.01-0.03 ml of inhalation solution/kg/dose in 3 ml NS q4-6h via nebulizer	20 mg/dose PO Inhalation: 1 ml/ dose	
Oxybutynin	Neurogenic bladder: < 5 yr: 0.5 mg/kg/day PO ÷ qid ≥ 5 yr: 10-15 mg/day PO ÷ bid-tid		Use with caution in children < 5 yr
Pancrelipase (Cotazym)	Infants: 1 regular capsule/120 ml formula Children and adults Regular capsules: 6/meal; 2/snack Enteric-coated (EC) capsules: 3/meal; 1/snack		Do not chew or crush capsule contents; titrate dose to stool fat content; cotazym capsules contain lipase, 8,000 IU; amylase, 30,000 CIU; and protease, 30,000 IU; powder is irritating to skin
Pancuronium	Muscle paralysis for mechanical ventilation: 0.1 mg/kg/dose IV q30min prn Prevention of fasciculation associated with succinylcholine: 0.006-0.01 mg/kg/dose IV		If succinylcholine used for intubation, decrease initial pancuronium dose by 33%; dose adjustment in renal impairment: Mild-moderate, 50%; severe, do not use
Paraldehyde	200-400 mg/kg/dose (0.2-0.4 ml of undiluted paraldehyde/kg/dose) PR q4-8h; give PR as 30%-50% solution in oil or NaCl 0.9% 100-150 mg/kg/dose (2-3 ml of 5% solution/kg/dose) IV over 15-20 min, then 20 mg/kg/hr (0.4 ml of 5% solution/kg/hr) as continuous IV infusion	PR: 10 g/dose	Dose reduction may be required in renal or liver impairment; undiluted paraldehyde contains 1 g/ml; do not administer in polyvinyl chloride plastic
Pediazole	Otitis media: 40 mg erythromycin/kg/day PO ÷ qid (includes 120 mg/kg/day sulfamethoxazole)	1600 mg erythromycin/day	Maintain fluid intake; dose interval adjustment in renal impairment: Moderate, q8-12h; severe, q12-24h

Continued.

Table V-1 Drug Dosage Guidelines for Infants and Children—cont'd

Drug	Dose	Dose/Limit	Comments
Penicillamine	Juvenile arthritis: Initial dose: 5 mg/kg/day PO as single daily dose; increase dose in increments of 5 mg/kg/day at 2-3 mo intervals up to 15 mg/kg/day PO ÷ bid-qid	Initial dose: 250 mg/dose Final dose: 1.5 g/day	Give on empty stomach (1 hr ac or 2 hr pc)
PEG-electrolyte liquid	See Polyethylene glycol-electrolyte solution		
Penicillin G	Mild to moderate infections: 25,000-50,000 U/kg/day IM/IV ÷ q6h Severe infections: 100,000-400,000 U/kg/day IM/IV ÷ q4-6h Meningitis: 250,000 U/kg/day IM/IV ÷ q4-6h	20 MIU/day	Dose interval adjustment in renal impairment: Moderate, q8-12h; severe, q12-16h 600 mg = 1 million U Contains 1.7 mmol Na^+ or K^+ per 1 million U
Penicillin G benzathine (Bi-cillin 1200 LA)	Rheumatic heart disease prophylaxis: 1.2 MU IM 1 ×/mo Streptococcal pharyngitis/rheumatic fever: < 27 kg: 600,000 U IM × 1 ≥ 27 kg: 1.2 MU IM × 1		
Penicillin VK	Infection: Streptococcal: 25-30 mg/kg/day PO ÷ bid Other: 50-100 mg/kg/day PO ÷ q6-8h Rheumatic fever: 125-250 mg PO tid-qid × 10 days Rheumatic fever prophylaxis: > 5 yr: 125-300 mg PO bid Prophylaxis in asplenics: 6 mo-5 yr: 125 mg PO bid > 5 yr: 250 mg PO bid	3 g/day	May be given with food; dose reduction in renal impairment: Moderate, 75%; severe, 25%-50%; 250 mg ∼ 400,000 U; prophylaxis for asplenic patients: cotrimoxazole recommended for patients < 6 mo; amoxicillin is alternate agent for patients 2-5 yr

Pentamidine	*Pneumocystis carinii:*		Use Respirgard II jet nebulizer to administer inhalation. Dose interval adjustment for IM/IV therapy in renal impairment as follows: moderate, q24-36h; severe, q48h
	Treatment:		
	4 mg/kg/day IM/IV as single daily dose for 12-21 days		
	Prophylaxis:		
	4 mg/kg/dose IV q2 or 4 wk		
	300 mg/dose by inhalation monthly		
Pentobarbital (Nembutal)	Pre x-ray:	200 mg/dose	Rapid IV administration may cause respiratory depression, apnea, laryngospasm, and hypotension; dose reduction in liver impairment may be required
	< 15 kg: 6 mg/kg/dose IM/PR		
	≥ 15 kg: 5 mg/kg/dose IM/PR 20-30 min pre x-ray		
	or 2.5 mg/kg (max 50 mg) IV over 1 min; wait 1 min; then 1.25 mg/kg (max 25 mg) IV over 30 sec; wait 1 min; then 1.25 mg/kg (max 25 mg) IV over 30 sec; wait 1 min; if required, additional dose of 1 mg/kg (max 20 mg) IV may be given, to a total dose of 4-5 mg/kg IV	100 mg/dose	
	Preop sedative:		
	< 8 yr: 3-4 mg/kg/dose PR		
	≥ 8 yr: 2-4 mg/kg/dose PO		
	20-60 min preop		
Permethrin (Nix)	*Pediculosis capitis:*		Removal of nits may improve efficacy; presence of live lice 24-48h after treatment is indication to use alternative agent
	Shampoo, rinse, and towel dry hair as usual; saturate hair and scalp with cream rinse and leave on hair for 10 min; repeat in 7 days prn × 1		

Continued.

Table V-1 Drug Dosage Guidelines for Infants and Children—cont'd

Drug	Dose	Dose/Limit	Comments
Phenobarbital	Status epilepticus: 20 mg/kg IV × 1 Maintenance dose: < 3 mo: 5-6 mg/kg/day PO 1 ×/day or ÷ bid ≥ 3 mo: 3-5 mg/kg/day PO 1 ×/day or ÷ bid Adolescents: 2-4 mg/kg/day PO 1 ×/day or ÷ bid	800 mg/dose Maintenance dose: 200 mg/ day	Calculate loading dose according to total body weight; calculate maintenance dose according to ideal body weight; dose reduction in liver impairment may be required; monitoring of serum drug concentrations recommended; coadministration of phenobarbital and valproic acid may lead to phenobarbital toxicity; administer IV at rate not to exceed 60 mg/min or 1 mg/kg/min, whichever is less
Phenoxybenza-mine	Loading dose: 1 mg/kg IV over 1 hr Maintenance dose: 0.5-2 mg/kg/day IV/PO ÷ q6-12h		Emergency release drug
Phentolamine	Acute hypertension: 0.1-0.2 mg/kg dose IV Treatment of extravasation of vasoactive drug (e.g., dopamine): Prepare solution of 5 mg in 10 ml NS, and use SC to infiltrate area of extravasation	Usual adult dose: 5 mg	
Phenylephrine	Supraventricular tachycardia: Initial dose: 0.01-mg/kg/dose IV Increase in 0.01-mg/kg increments up to 0.1 mg/kg/total dose Tetralogy of Fallot spell: 5 μg/kg IV followed by continuous infusion of 0.1-4 μg/kg/min IV		For SVT and hypercyanotic spells, the final dose should be based on a successful result or a 50% increase in blood pressure over baseline

Phenytoin	Status epilepticus: 20 mg/kg IV Maintenance dose: 0.5-3 yr: 7-9 mg/kg/day PO ÷ q8-12h 4-6 yr: 6.5 mg/kg/day PO ÷ q8-12h 7-9 yr: 6 mg/kg/day PO ÷ q8-12h 10-16 yr: 3-5 mg/kg/day PO ÷ q8-12h Arrhythmia: Loading dose: 15 mg/kg/dose IV over 1 hr Simultaneously give 3 mg/kg/dose PO × 1; then 6 hr later give 2 mg/kg/dose PO × 1 Start maintenance 6 hr later or 5 mg/kg/dose PO q6h × 4 doses Then 2.5 mg/kg/dose PO q6h × 4 doses Maintenance: 5-6 mg/kg/day PO ÷ q12h	Loading dose: 1 g	Calculate loading dose according to total body weight; calculate maintenance dose according to ideal body weight; administer IV at rate not to exceed 1 mg/kg/min or 50 mg/min, whichever is less; dose reduction may be required in severe liver disease; monitoring of serum drug concentrations recommended; may interact with many other medications; consult pharmacy for details
Phosphate (Phosphate Sandoz)	Hypophosphatemia (moderate): Oral therapy: 1-2 mmol/kg/day PO ÷ bid-qid Hypophosphatemic rickets: 1-3 mmol/kg/day PO ÷ qid Hypophosphatemia (moderate-severe) IV therapy: 1-2 mmol phosphate/kg/day IV or 0.042-0.083 mmol phosphate/kg/hr IV as continuous infusion	Monitor serum phosphate Maximum rate of infusion 0.125 mmol/kg/hr	For peripheral IV administration, use sodium phosphate and dilute 1:10 with IV fluids to concentration of 0.3 mmol phosphate/ml; monitor serum phosphate q6h and adjust infusion accordingly; for central venous line administration, use sodium or potassium phosphate and dilute to concentration of 15 mmol phosphate/50 ml of IV fluids; monitor serum potassium q3h (for potassium phosphate) and phosphate q6h and adjust infusion accordingly

Continued.

Table V-1 Drug Dosage Guidelines for Infants and Children—cont'd

Drug	Dose	Dose/Limit	Comments

Phytonadione (vitamin K₁)	Warfarin antidote:
	No bleeding, future need for warfarin:
	  0.5-2 mg/dose SC
	No bleeding, no future need for warfarin:
	  2-5 mg/dose SC/IV
	Significant bleeding:
	  5 mg/dose IV over 10-20 min
	Acute hepatic failure:
	Infants: 1-2 mg/dose IM/SC/IV
	Children: 5-10 mg/dose IM/SC/IV
	Malabsorption: 2.5-5 mg/dose PO given 1-7 days/wk (titrate to effective maintenance dose); 1-2 mg/dose IM/IV
		25 mg/dose PO	Injection may be given by mouth, undiluted; oral tablets (5 mg) are available by emergency release for long-term patients; severe anaphylactoid reactions have occurred with IV administration; give IV in emergency situations only
			
			Administer IV at rate not to exceed 1 mg/min

Piperacillin	200-300 mg/kg/day IV/IM ÷ q6h CF patients: 300 mg/kg/day IV/IM ÷ q6h Febrile neutropenia: 200 mg/kg/day IV/IM ÷ q6h	24 g/day	Dose interval adjustment in renal impairment: moderate, q6-8h; severe, q8h
Piperazine	Roundworm: 75 mg/kg/day PO ÷ bid-tid × 2 days	3.5 g	

Pivampicillin (nonformulary)	Mild-moderate infections:
	  20-50 mg/kg/day PO ÷ bid
	Otitis media:
	  40-50 mg/kg/day PO ÷ bid
	Serious infections:
	  40-100 mg/kg/day PO ÷ q8h
		1 g/dose	May be given with food; dose interval adjustment in renal impairment: Severe, q12-16h

Polyethylene glycol-electrolyte solution (e.g., Golytely, Peg-Lyte)	25 ml/kg/hr PO/NG until rectal effluent is clear Adolescents: 240 ml PO q10min until rectal effluent is clear	2L/hr, 4L total 2L/hr, 4L total	Use with caution in patients with renal insufficiency; for PO administration, product is more palatable when chilled
Potassium chloride	Maintenance requirement: 30-40 mmol/m²/day Hypokalemia: 3 mmol/kg/day + maintenance requirement IV as continuous infusion or PO in divided doses		Give PO with food; dilute oral solution in water or juice; capsules may be opened and contents sprinkled on soft food for administration (pellets should not be chewed); for peripheral IV administration, dilute to at least 0.04 mmol/ml and infuse at rate not to exceed 10 mmol/hr or 0.2 mmol/kg/hr
Potassium iodide	Radiation protection: 30 mg iodine/day PO as single daily dose	100 mg iodine daily	Dilute in 1 glassful of water, juice, or milk; give with food or milk; Lugol's solutions = 126 elemental iodine/ml; duration of treatment depends on type of radiation exposure
Prazosin	Test dose: 5 μg/kg PO Maintenance: 0.05-0.1 mg/kg/day PO ÷ bid-qid; increase dose gradually to effect or to maximum of 0.4 mg/kg/day	Maximum daily dose: 20 mg Usual initial adult dose: 0.5 mg/dose Usual adult maintenance dose: 2-20 mg/day ÷ bid-tid	Dose reduction may be required in renal impairment; first dose may cause excessive postural hypotension and syncope

Continued.

Table V-1 Drug Dosage Guidelines for Infants and Children—cont'd

Drug	Dose	Dose/Limit	Comments
Prednisone	Asthma: 1-2 mg/kg/day PO as single daily dose × 5 days Nephrotic syndrome: Initial dose: 60 mg/m^2/day PO as single daily dose or in divided doses JRA, IBD, etc: Initial dose: 2 mg/kg/day PO as single daily dose or in divided doses	80 mg/day	Individualize dose according to response; give with food or milk; to discontinue in patients receiving therapy for ≥ 10 days, reduce dose by 50% q48h until 2.5 ± 0.8 mg/m^2/day achieved; then reduce dose by 50% q10-14days
Primaquine	Malaria: 0.3 mg base/kg/day PO as single daily dose × 14 days	15 mg base/day	Rule out G6PD deficiency before therapy; give with food or milk; 26.3 mg primaquine phosphate = 15 mg primaquine base
Primidone	0-8 yr: Starting dose: 125 mg PO qhs Increase on day 7 to: 125 mg PO bid Increase on day 14 to: 125 mg PO tid Increase on day 21 to: 10-25 mg/kg/day PO ÷ tid/qid	> 8 yr: 250 mg PO qhs 250 mg PO bid 250 mg PO tid 750-1500 mg/day PO ÷ tid/qid	Monitoring of serum concentrations of primidone and phenobarbital recommended; dose interval adjustment in renal impairment: Moderate, q8-12h; severe, q12-24h; use with caution in patients with hepatic impairment; may interact with many other medications; contact pharmacy for details
Procainamide	Loading dose: 12-15 mg/kg/hr IV for no longer than 75 min Maintenance dose: 20-80 μg/kg/min by continuous IV infusion 15-60 mg/kg/day PO ÷ q4-6h	 2 g/day IV 500 mg/dose PO	Dose may require reduction in severe CHF; dose reduction in renal impairment: Moderate, q6-12h; severe, q8-24h; monitoring of serum procainamide and NAPA concentrations recommended; may be associated with SLE; IV loading dose should be switched to maintenance infusion rate before 75 min if arrhythmia reverts or if QRS is prolonged 50% over baseline; give PO on empty stomach (1 hr ac or 2 hr pc) unless GI upset occurs

Propafenone	200-600 mg/m^2/day PO ÷ tid-qid	900 mg/day Usual adult dose: 450-600 mg/day PO ÷ q8-12h	Give with food or milk; reduce digoxin dose by 50% when initiating concurrent propafenone therapy; dose reduction in renal impairment may be required; reduce dose in hepatic impairment
Propranolol	Arrhythmia: 0.01-0.15 mg/kg/dose IV q6-8h prn Wolff-Parkinson-White syndrome: 2-10 mg/kg/day PO ÷ tid-qid Antihypertensive: 0.5-4 mg/kg/day PO ÷ tid or qid Tetralogy spell: 0.05-0.10 mg/kg/dose IV over 2-10 min Maintenance dose: 1-6 mg/kg/day PO ÷ tid-qid	3 mg/dose IV	Give IV propranolol only under ECG monitoring over 2-10 min at rate not to exceed 1 mg/min; reduce dose in hepatic impairment
Propylthiouracil	Initial dose: 150 mg/m^2/day PO ÷ q8h or 10 mg/kg/day PO ÷ q8h Maintenance: Usually ⅓-½ of initial dose once patient is euthyroid	Initial dose: 6-10 yr: 150 mg/day > 10 yr: 300 mg/day However, higher doses may be required in some patients	Give at same time in relation to meals each day; may rarely cause agranulocytosis, exfoliative dermatitis, hepatitis
Protamine	1 mg IV for every 100 U of heparin administered in previous 3-4 hr at rate not to exceed 5 mg/min	50 mg/dose	Actual protamine neutralization factor for each heparin lot listed on manufacturer's label

Continued.

FORMULARY

Table V-1   Drug Dosage Guidelines for Infants and Children—cont'd

Drug	Dose	Dose/Limit	Comments
Pseudoephed-rine	4 mg/kg/day PO ÷ q6h prn	Usual adult dose: 60 mg/dose PO q4-6h prn	Use with caution in hypertensive patients < 2 yr; dose combination products (e.g., Sudafed DM) according to pseudoephedrine content
Pyrantel pamoate	Roundworm, pinworm: 11 mg of base/kg/dose PO × 1 dose only Hookworm: 11 mg of base/kg/day PO as single daily dose × 3 days	1 g of base/dose	For pinworm, repeat dose after 2 wk; may be given with food or on empty stomach
Pyrazinamide	15-30 mg/kg/day PO ÷ q6-8h or 50-70 mg/kg/dose PO 2 ×/wk	2 g/day; 4 g/dose for 2 ×/wk regimens	Dose reduction may be required in hepatic impairment
Pyrimethamine (nonformulary)	Toxoplasmosis prophylaxis: 1-2 mg/kg/day PO as single daily dose	50 mg/day	Use with caution in patients with impaired renal or hepatic function, and patients with possible folate deficiency; may cause photosensitivity, blood dyscrasias; administration with food may decrease gastrointestinal irritation
Quinacrine (emergency release)	Giardiasis: 6 mg/kg/day PO ÷ tid pc × 5-7 days	300 mg/day	Give with full glass of water or juice

Quinidine	Dysrhythmia: 15-60 mg of base/kg/day PO ÷ q4-6h Chloroquine-resistant *Falciparum* malaria: Severe infection or patient unable to take PO medications: 6.2 mg (base)/kg IV over 1-2 hr, then 0.0125 mg (base)/kg/ min by continuous IV infusion × 72 hr or until patient can swallow or 15 mg (base)/kg IV over 4 hr, then beginning 8 hr after end of loading infusion, 7.5 mg (base)/kg IV q8h	500 mg/dose	Dose may require reduction in severe CHF; reduce dose to 30% in severe liver impairment; digoxin maintenance dose requires reduction during concurrent quinidine therapy; moni- toring of serum drug concentrations recommended; do not break or chew controlled-release tablets Quinidine bisulfate = 66% base Quinidine sulfate = 83% base Treatment of malaria: Loading dose should not be used if patient received quinine, quinidine, or mefloquine within pre- ceding 12-24 hr, switch from IV quinidine to oral quinine as soon as possible, in patients requiring more than 48 hr of IV therapy, reduce quinidine maintenance dose by ⅓ to ½
Quinine sulfate	Uncomplicated *Falciparum* or sequential oral therapy: 22.5 mg (base)/kg/day PO ÷ tid × 3-7 days	1.5 g (base)/day	Give with food or milk; chloroquine-resistant strains generally require total of 7 days' treatment with quinine or quinidine and second drug
Ranitidine	2-6 mg/kg/day IV ÷ q6-12h Peptic ulcer, gastro-esophageal reflux: Treatment: 5-8 mg/kg/day PO ÷ q12h × 8 wk Maintenance: 2.5-5 mg/kg/day PO 1 ×/day	300 mg/day ex- cept in Zollinger- Ellison syndrome Usual adult PO dose: 300 mg/ day as single HS dose or ÷ q12h	Monitor gastric pH in patients requiring IV therapy; dose re- duction in renal impairment: Moderate, 75%; severe, 50%
Ribavirin	6 g/day; 20 mg/ml solution via inhalation over 12-18 hr/day for 3-7 days		Use small-particle aerosol generator (SPAG-2) for administra- tion; do not wear contact lenses when exposed to ribavirin aerosol

Continued.

Table V-1 Drug Dosage Guidelines for Infants and Children—cont'd

Drug	Dose	Dose/Limit	Comments
Rifampin	Tuberculosis: 10-20 mg/kg/day PO 1 ×/day or ÷ q12h or 10-20 mg/kg/dose PO 2 ×/wk	600 mg/day	Reduce dose in liver impairment; may discolor urine, sweat, saliva, and tears; give on empty stomach (1 hr ac or 2 hr pc) unless GI upset occurs; concurrent use may decrease efficacy of oral contraceptives; may interact with many other medications also; consult pharmacy for details
	Meningococcal prophylaxis: 20 mg/kg/day PO ÷ q12h × 2 days	1200 mg/day	
	H. influenzae prophylaxis: 20 mg/kg/day PO 1 ×/day × 4 days	600 mg/day	
Salbutamol	Acute Asthma: Inhalation solution: 0.01-0.03 ml/kg/dose in 3 ml NS via nebulizer q½-4h prn; in severe cases give initial dose of 0.03 ml/kg/dose (max 1 ml/dose) q20min via nebulizer Metered dose inhaler (mild to moderate asthma): Weight: ≤ 12 kg: 4 puffs (400 μg) q½-4h 12-' 6 kg: 5 puffs (500 μg) q½-4h 16-25 kg: 6 puffs (600 μg) q½-4h 25-35 kg: 8 puffs (800 μg) q½-4h ≥ 35 kg: 10 puffs (1000 μg) q½-4h Infusion: Initial rate: 1 μg/kg/min IV; increase by 1 μg/kg/min q15min prn up to a maximum of 10 μg/kg/min Maintenance therapy for asthma: 100-200 μg tid via metered dose aerosol/diskhaler/rotahaler, 0.3 mg/kg/day PO ÷ tid or qid Hyperkalemia: 4 μg/kg IV over 20 min	PO: 16 mg/day Inhalation solution: 1 ml/dose	Limit nebulized salbutamol to 4 ×/day for outpatients; may cause hypokalemia Metered aerosol: 100 μg/puff Diskhaler: 200 μg or 400 μg/blister Rotahaler: 200 μg or 400 μg/capsule Inhalation solution: 5 mg/ml
Sodium bicarbonate	Resuscitation: See inside front cover		

Sodium polystyrene sulfonate (Kayexalate)	1 g/kg/dose PO q6h prn 1 g/kg/dose PR q2-6h prn	Exchanges approximately 1 mmol/kg; administer rectally in appropriate volume of tap water, 10% dextrose, or equal parts tap water and 2% methylcellulose; moisten resin with honey or jam for PO use
Sorbitol	Cathartic: 1.5-2 ml/kg PO 150 ml/dose	
Sotalol	Arrhythmias: 2-5 mg/kg/day PO ÷ bid 480 mg/day Usual adult dose: 320 mg/day PO ÷ bid	Dose reduction in renal impairment: Moderate, 30%; severe, 15%-30%; dose may require reduction in liver impairment
Spironolactone	1-4 mg/kg/day PO ÷ into 1, 2, 3, or 4 daily doses Usual adult dose: 25-200 mg/day PO	For spironolactone in combination with hydrochlorothiazide, see Novospirozine; avoid when creatinine clearance < 10 ml/min
Streptokinase	Loading dose: 4000 IU/kg IV over 10 min Maintenance dose: 2000 IU/kg/hr × 6hr as continuous IV infusion	Do not use streptokinase in patients who have previously been treated with this drug or in patients < 3 mo; use with heparin
Succinylcholine	1-2 mg/kg/dose IV One dose only; no repeats	
Sucralfate (Sulcrate)	Adolescents and adults: 4 g/day PO ÷ qid (1 hour ac + qhs)	
Sulfadiazine (nonformulary)	Toxoplasmosis prophylaxis: 25-100 mg/kg/day PO as single daily dose 2 g/day	Use with caution in patients with impaired renal or hepatic function, G6PD deficiency, or blood dyscrasias; may cause severe hypersensitivity reactions; ensure adequate urine output; give on empty stomach

Continued.

Table V-1 Drug Dosage Guidelines for Infants and Children—cont'd

Drug	Dose	Dose/Limit	Comments
Sulfasalazine	JA: 40-60 mg/kg/day PO ÷ bid-qid Ulcerative colitis: Acute management: 40-70 mg/kg/day PO ÷ tid-qid pc Maintenance: 20-50 mg/kg/day PO ÷ bid-qid	6g/day 2g/day	Begin with ⅓ recommended dose and increase q2days to maximum required dose; maintain fluid intake; give with food; use with caution in patients with renal impairment; may discolor skin, tears, urine orange-yellow; monitor for blood dyscrasias; caution in patients with hypersensitivity to salicylates, sulfonamides, G6PD deficiency
Terfenadine	3-6 yr: 30 mg/day PO ÷ bid 7-12 yr: 60 mg/day PO ÷ bid > 12 yr: 120 mg/day PO ÷ bid		Give with food or milk; concurrent use with drug that inhibit hepatic metabolism (e.g., ketotifen, erythromycin) has re-sulted in life-threatening cardiac arrhythmias
Tetracycline capsule: 250 mg	Inflammatory acne: 1 g/day PO ÷ qid × 1 wk Then, 500 mg/day PO ÷ bid *H. pylori* eradication Adolescents: 500 mg PO qid × 14 days		Dose interval adjustment in renal impairment: Moderate, q12-24h; avoid in severe renal impairment; use with caution in patients with hepatic insufficiency; do not use in children < 8 yr; may cause permanent discoloration of teeth, enamel hypoplasia, and (usually reversible) retardation of skeletal development; give on empty stomach; do not administer with dairy products, milk formulas, antacids, bismuth, or iron products; enhances effects of warfarin; may cause photo-sensitivity reaction

Theophylline	For patients not currently receiving aminophylline or theophylline: Loading dose: 6 mg/kg IV Initial maintenance dose: 2-6 mo: 0.4 mg/kg/hr IV 6-11 mo: 0.7 mg/kg/hr IV 1-12 yr: 0.8 mg/kg/hr IV 12-16 yr: 0.7 mg/kg/hr IV > 16 yr (nonsmoker): 0.6 mg/kg/hr IV Cardiac decompensation, cor pulmonale, liver dysfunction: 0.2 mg/kg/hr IV Maximum maintenance dose before TDM: 6-52 wk: [0.2 × (age in wk) + 5] mg/kg/day PO ÷ q6-8h 1-12 yr: 20 mg/kg/day PO ÷ q8-12h 12-16 yr: 18 mg/kg/day PO ÷ q12h > 16 yr: 14 mg/kg/day PO ÷ q12h or 900 mg/day, whichever is less	Calculate loading dose according to effective body weight and maintenance dose according to ideal body weight; dose reduction required in liver impairment; administer IV at rate not to exceed 20 mg/min; IV doses are conservative; titrate dose according to serum concentration; oral doses apply to sustained-release products, which are preferred for chronic dosing; maximum oral doses should be attained stepwise to prevent intolerance in patients not being converted from IV therapy; begin at 50% of recommended doses; give PO on empty stomach (1 hr ac or 2 hr pc) unless GI upset occurs; coadministration of theophylline and nonselective β-blockers may decrease effects of theophylline; coadministration of theophylline and cimetidine or erythromycin may produce theophylline toxicity; coadministration of theophylline and phenytoin may decrease effects of both drugs.
Ticarcillin	200-300 mg/kg/day IM/IV ÷ q4-6h CF patients: 300 mg/kg/day IM/IV ÷ q4-6h	24 g/day	Dose interval adjustment in renal impairment: Moderate, q6-8h; severe, q8h
Tobramycin	7.5 mg/kg/day IV/IM ÷ q8h CF patients: 10 mg/kg/day IV/IM ÷ q8h 80 mg TID via nebulizer	120 mg/dose before serum concentration determination No maximum single dose	Calculate dose according to effective body weight; dose interval adjustment in renal impairment: Mild-moderate, q12h; severe, q24-48h; monitoring of serum drug concentrations recommended

Continued.

Table V-1   Drug Dosage Guidelines for Infants and Children—cont'd

Drug	Dose	Dose/Limit	Comments
Tolmetin	20-40 mg/kg/day PO ÷ tid or qid	1.6 g/day	Dose adjustment may be required in hepatic impairment
Trimethoprim	4 mg/kg/day PO ÷ q12h	200 mg/day	Dose interval adjustment in renal impairment: Moderate, q18h; severe, q24h; Give on empty stomach (1 hr ac or 2 hr pc) unless GI upset occurs
Urokinase	For blocked central venous catheters: Instill 2 ml of 5000 U/ml solution into each lumen of catheter (3 ml into subcutaneous port) and leave for 2-4 hr: withdraw drug, and if possible, flush with NS; may repeat 1 × in 24 hr Low-dose infusion for blocked CVL: 150 U/kg/hr through each lumen of catheter × 24 hr Systemic thrombolytic therapy: 4000 U/kg IV loading dose over 10 min, followed by 4000 U/kg/hr IV infusion × 6 hr		Use with heparin for systemic thrombolytic therapy
Ursodiol	15 mg/kg/day PO ÷ tid		
Valproic acid	Initial dose: 15 mg/kg/day PO 1 ×/day or ÷ q8-12h; increase dose weekly prn by 5-10 mg/kg/day up to 30-60 mg/kg/day PO ÷ tid or qid	60 mg/kg/day	Reduce dose in liver impairment; monitoring of serum drug concentration recommended; coadministration of valproic acid and either phenobarbital or primidone may result in toxicity because of latter drug; coadministration of valproic acid and phenytoin may decrease effects of both drugs
Vancomycin	Mild to moderate infections: 40 mg/kg/day IV ÷ q6h Severe infections: 40-60 mg/kg/day IV ÷ q6h Patients with neutropenia: 60 mg/kg/day IV ÷ q6h Meningitis: 60 mg/kg/day IV ÷ q6h	2 g/day 4 g/day 4 g/day 4 g/day	Calculate doses according to effective body weight; dose interval adjustment in renal impairment: Mild, q8-18h; moderate, q18-72h; severe, q3-7days, monitoring of serum drug concentrations recommended; injection or oral dosing may be used; restrict use of drug to prevent emergence of resistant organisms

	Pseudomembranous colitis: 50 mg/kg/day PO ÷ q6h Cardiac surgery prophylaxis: 20 mg/kg/dose IV q12h × 2 doses	500 mg/day 1 g/dose	
Varicella zoster immune globulin	125 U/10 kg/dose IM minimum: 125 U/dose	625 U	Do not administer part vials; round dose up to next number of whole vials; approximately 125 U/vial
Verapamil (Isoptin)	0-2 yr: 0.1-0.2 mg/kg/dose IV 2-15 yr: 0.1-0.3 mg/kg/dose IV May repeat × 1 in 30 min PRN Maintenance dose: 4-10 mg/kg/day PO ÷ tid/qid	10 mg/dose IV Usual adult dose: 240-480 mg/day PO	Administer IV under ECG monitoring; avoid use in early post-cardiosurgical period, in severe CHF, or in presence of β-blockers
Vigabatrin	Initial dose: 30 mg/kg/day PO as single daily dose or ÷ bid; increase gradually Usual maintenance dose: 60 mg/kg/day PO as single daily dose or ÷ bid.	Initial: 1 g/day Maintenance dose: 100 mg/kg/day or 4 g/day	Reduce initial dose in renal impairment; and monitor for adverse effects such as sedation, confusion; may be given with food; concurrent use of vigabatrin may decrease serum phenytoin levels
Vitamin K$_1$	See Phytonadione		

Continued.

Table V-1 Drug Dosage Guidelines for Infants and Children—cont'd

Drug	Dose	Dose/Limit	Comments
Warfarin (Coumadin)	Loading dose Day 1: 0.2 mg/kg PO as single daily dose Reduce to 0.1 mg/kg/dose in patients with liver impairment or Fontan Days 2-5: Adjust based on INR: INR Adjustment 1.1-1.3 repeat initial LD 1.4-1.9 50% of initial LD 2-3 50% of initial LD 3.1-3.5 25% of initial LD > 3.5 Hold until INR < 3.5 then restart at 50% less than previous dose If INR ≤ 1.5 on day 4, dosing must be individualized Maintenance dose adjustments: INR Adjustment 1.1-1.4 increase dose by 20% 1.5-1.9 increase dose by 10% 2-3* no change 3.1-3.5 decrease dose by 10% > 3.5 hold until INR < 3.5, then restart at 20% less than previous dose *For patients with mechanical valves, maintain INR between 2.5-3.5.	Loading dose: 10 mg/dose (5 mg in patients with liver impairment or Fontan)	Start warfarin on day 1 or 2 of heparin therapy (except for treatment of extensive DVT; then start warfarin on day 5 of heparin); loading period is approximately 3-5 days for most patients; heparin should be continued for minimum of 5 days and until INR > 2 for 2 consecutive days; adjust dose to maintain INR between 2 and 3 (children with mechanical valves require INR between 2.5 and 3.5) Discontinue vitamin K in TPN when warfarin started; use formula with low Vitamin K content (e.g., Pediasure); warfarin may interact with many medications; consider consulting pharmacist regarding patient on multiple medications Monitor INR: Daily during loading doses; within 3 days of discharge from hospital on maintenance dose; 5-7 days after changing maintenance dose; and minimum of 1 ×/mo on stable maintenance dose

Zalcitabine (Hivid, ddC) (nonformulary)	0.015-0.03 mg/kg/day PO ÷ tid	2.25 mg/day	Dose interval adjustment in renal impairment: CrCl (ml/min) Interval 40-55 no change: monitor for ADRs 10-40 q12h < 10 q24h Use with caution in patients with hepatic dysfunction; concurrent use with pentamidine not recommended; other drugs may also increase risk of adverse effects; may cause pancreatitis, peripheral neuropathy; give on empty stomach, if possible
Zidovudine (AZT)	Infants: 360-720 mg/m²/day PO ÷ qid Older children: 100-150 mg PO qid Perinatal HIV exposure: 8 mg/kg/day PO ÷ q6h starting 6-8 hr after birth and continuing for 6 wk	600 mg/day	
Zinc	Supplementation: 0.5-1 mg elemental zinc/kg/day PO ÷ bid-tid Acrodermatitis enteropathica: 1-2 mg elemental zinc/kg/day PO ÷ bid-tid	15 mg elemental zinc/day 45 mg elemental zinc/day	Give with food to reduce GI irritation

Table V-2 Neonatal Drug Dosage Guidelines*

Drug	Dose	Comments
Acetaminophen (Tempra, Tylenol)	10-15 mg/kg/dose PO or per rectum q4-6h	Max: 60 mg/kg/day; for doses ≤ 80 mg, oral drops may be administered rectally
Acyclovir (Zovirax)	Herpes simplex infections: < 34 wk PCA: 20 mg/kg/day IV ÷ q12h ≥ 34 wk PCA: 30 mg/kg/day IV ÷ q8h	Reduce dose in renal impairment; higher doses may be required in herpes zoster infections
Albumin	0.5-1 g/kg/dose (10-20 ml of 5% solution/kg) IV	Dilute 25% albumin to 5% strength (e.g., 4 ml 25% albumin + 16 ml 5% dextrose), or give 5% undiluted
Alprostadil	0.05-0.1 µg/kg/min IV as continuous infusion	May cause apnea; formula for dilution: 500 µg in 80 ml at 1 ml/kg/hr = 0.1 µg/kg/min
Amikacin	< 2 kg: 0-7 days: 15 mg/kg/day IV or IM ÷ q12h > 7 days: 20 mg/kg/day IV or IM ÷ q8h ≥ 2 kg: 0-7 days: 20 mg/kg/day IV or IM ÷ q12h > 7 days: 30 mg/kg/day IV or IM ÷ q8h	Reduce dose in renal impairment; monitoring of serum drug concentrations is recommended; indicated for organisms resistant to gentamicin
Amphotericin B	0.25 mg/kg/day IV as single daily dose Increase by 0.25 mg/kg/day up to 1 mg/kg/day IV as tolerated	Infuse in a concentration of ≤ 0.1 mg/ml in 5% dextrose over 4-6 hr; contact pharmacy for administration to fluid restricted patients; may be given on alternate days; consider therapy at 0.5 mg/kg/day if clinical situation warrants and/or if flucytosine given concurrently; *Aspergillus* infections require treatment at 1 mg/kg/day; monitor serum potassium

Ampicillin	< 2 kg: 0-7 days:	Reduce dose in severe renal impairment
	Meningitis: 100 mg/kg/day IV ÷ q12h	
	Other: 50 mg/kg/day IV ÷ q12h	
	> 7 days:	
	Meningitis: 150 mg/kg/day IV ÷ q8h	
	Other: 75 mg/kg/day IV ÷ q8h	
	≥ 2 kg: 0-7 days:	
	Meningitis: 150 mg/kg/day IV ÷ q8h	
	Other: 75 mg/kg/day IV ÷ q8h	
	> 7 days:	
	Meningitis: 200 mg/kg/day IV ÷ q6h	
	Other: 100 mg/kg/day IV ÷ q6h	
Atropine	Resuscitation: see inside front cover	
Caffeine	Loading: 10 mg/kg PO or IV	Monitoring of serum drug concentrations recommended; dose expressed as caffeine base; 2 mg caffeine citrate = 1 mg caffeine base
	Maintenance: 2.5 mg/kg/dose PO or IV 1 ×/day	
Calcium gluconate	Resuscitation: 1.5 ml/kg/dose of 2% solution = 30 mg/dose IV q10-20 min prn	Avoid extravasation; preferable to use central line when giving 10% solution; administer at rate not to exceed 10 mg/min
	Maintenance: 200-400 mg/kg/day (2-4 ml of 10% solution/kg/day) IV	10% solution: 1 ml = 100 mg of calcium gluconate = 9.3 mg elemental calcium = 0.23 mmol of calcium
Cefazolin	< 2 kg regardless of age and ≥ 2 kg age 0-7 days: 40 mg/kg/day IV or IM ÷ q12h	Reduce dose in renal impairment
	≥ 2 kg age > 7 days: 60 mg/kg/day IV or IM ÷ q8h	
	Cardiac surgery prophylaxis:	
	0-7 days: 40 mg/kg/dose IV or IM q12h × 4 doses	
	> 7 days: 40 mg/kg/dose IV or IM q8h × 6 doses	

Continued.

*These dosage guidelines apply to all neonates until postconceptional age (PCA) of > 38 wk and postnatal age of > 4 wk have been achieved.

Table V-2 Neonatal Drug Dosage Guidelines*—cont'd

Drug	Dose	Comments
Cefotaxime	0-7 days: 100 mg/kg/day IV ÷ q12h > 7 days: 150 mg/kg/day IV ÷ q8h	Reduce dose in renal impairment
Ceftazidime	< 2 kg: 0-7 days: 100 mg/kg/day IV or IM ÷ q12h > 7 days: 150 mg/kg/day IV or IM ÷ q8h ≥ 2 kg: 0-7 days: 100 mg/kg/day IV or IM ÷ q8h > 7 days: 150 mg/kg/day IV or IM ÷ q8h	Reduce dose in renal impairment
Chloral hydrate	10-50 mg/kg/dose PO or PR 3 or 4 ×/day Sedation preprocedure: 25-50 mg/kg/dose PO or PR	Reduce dose in patients with CNS impairment; dose may require reduction in liver impairment
Chloramphenicol	< 2 kg: 25 mg/kg/day IV as single daily dose ≥ 2 kg: 0-7 days: 25 mg/kg/day IV as single daily dose > 7 days: 50 mg/kg/day IV ÷ q12h	Monitoring of serum drug concentrations recommended; avoid in liver impairment; do not administer chloramphenicol palmitate PO
Clindamycin	< 2 kg: 0-7 days: 10 mg/kg/day IV ÷ q12h > 7 days: 15 mg/kg/day IV or PO ÷ q8h ≥ 2 kg: 0-7 days: 15 mg/kg/day IV ÷ q8h > 7 days: 20 mg/kg/day IV or PO ÷ q6h	Do not administer PO to infants < 7 days; do not administer clindamycin palmitate PO; use clindamycin phosphate in neonates ≥ 7 days
Cloxacillin	< 2 kg: 0-7 days: Meningitis: 100 mg/kg/day IV ÷ q12h Other: 50 mg/kg/day PO or IV ÷ q12h > 7 days: Meningitis: 150 mg/kg/day IV ÷ q8h Other: 75 mg/kg/day PO or IV ÷ q8h	

≥ 2 kg: 0-7 days:
    Meningitis: 150 mg/kg/day IV ÷ q8h
    Other: 75 mg/kg/day PO or IV ÷ q8h
  > 7 days:
    Meningitis: 200 mg/kg/day IV ÷ q6h
    Other: 100 mg/kg/day PO or IV ÷ q6h

Dexamethasone (Decadron)	Short course:	0.3-0.6 mg/kg/day ÷ bid × 3 days
	Intermediate course:	0.3-0.6 mg/kg/day ÷ bid × 3 days
		0.15-0.3 mg/kg/day ÷ bid × 3 days
		0.075-0.15 mg/kg/day ÷ bid × 3 days
	Long course–18 days:	0.5 mg/kg/day ÷ bid × 3 days
		0.25 mg/kg/day ÷ bid × 3 days
		0.125 mg/kg/day ÷ bid × 3 days
		0.06 mg/kg/day as single daily dose × 3 days
		0.06 mg/kg/dose every other day × 7 days
	Long course–42 days:	0.5 mg/kg/day ÷ bid × 3 days
		0.25 mg/kg/day ÷ bid × 3 days
		Reduce dose by 10% every 3 days until day 34, then 0.1 mg/kg/day × 3 days, then 0.1 mg/kg/dose every other day × 7 days
	Subglottic edema:	1 mg/kg/dose tid × 2 days, then reassess

May be given IV or PO

Continued.

Table V-2 Neonatal Drug Dosage Guidelines*—cont'd

Drug	Dose	Comments
Dextrose	Transient hypoglycemia: 5-7 mg/kg/min IV Acute hypoglycemia: Loading dose: 0.1-0.2 g/kg IV Maintenance dose: 5-7 mg/kg/min IV	Dilute 50% solution before administration
Diazepam (Valium)	Seizure: 0.1-0.2 mg/kg/dose IV	Administer at rate not to exceed 0.05 mg/kg/min
Digoxin	Digitalization dose: (3 doses: 1st stat, 2nd in 6 hr, 3rd in another 6 hr) < 37 wk postconceptional age (PCA): 7 µg/kg/dose PO 5 µg/kg/dose IV ≥ 37 wk PCA: 17 µg/kg/dose PO 12 µg/kg/dose IV Maintenance dose: < 37 wk PCA: 4 µg/kg/day PO ÷ q12h 3 µg/kg/day IV ÷ q12h ≥ 37 wk PCA: 10 µg/kg/day PO ÷ q12h 7 µg/kg/day IV ÷ q12h	Do not administer IM; reduce dose by 50% during concurrent indomethacin therapy; when digitalizing to terminate tachycardia, total digitalization dose is divided ½, ¼, ¼; decrease maintenance dose in renal impairment; monitoring of serum drug concentrations recommended
Dobutamine	5-25 µg/kg/min IV	Formula for dilution: (body weight [kg] × 15) mg in 50 ml 5% dextrose at 1 ml/hr = 5 µg/kg/min
Dopamine	Renal: 2-5 µg/kg/min IV Inotropic: 5-20 µg/kg/min IV Vasoconstrictive: > 20 µg/kg/min IV	Neonates may be less sensitive to dopamine Formula for dilution: (body weight [kg] × 15) mg in 50 ml 5% dextrose at 1 ml/hr = 5 µg/kg/min
Doxapram	0.5 mg/kg/hr IV; may increase gradually up to 2.5 mg/kg/hr IV	Nonformulary; caffeine or theophylline should be given concurrently; monitor abdominal girth, blood pressure, and blood glucose

Epinephrine	Resuscitation: see inside front cover Minimum dose: Premature neonate: 0.5ml (0.05mg) Full-term neonate: 1 ml (0.1 mg) 0.05-1 µg/kg/min IV	1:10,000 = 0.1 mg/ml Verify concentration of solution before use; formula for dilution: (body weight [kg] × 0.3) mg in 50 ml IV fluid at 1 ml/hr = 0.1 µg/kg/min
Epinephrine (racemic)	0.05 ml/kg/dose in 3 ml NS via nebulizer prn to maximum q1h	

Erythromycin estolate	< 2 kg: 0-7 days: 20 mg/kg/day PO ÷ q12h
	       > 7 days: 30 mg/kg/day PO ÷ q8h
	≥ 2 kg: 0-7 days: 20 mg/kg/day PO ÷ q12h
	       > 7 days: 30-40 mg/kg/day PO ÷ q8h	

Erythromycin gluceptate or lactobionate	20-40 mg/kg/day IV ÷ q6h	
Furosemide	1-2 mg/kg/dose IV or PO 1 ×/day or 2 ×/day	

Gentamicin	≤ 1 kg: 0-7 days: 2.5 mg/kg/dose IV daily
	       > 7 days: 3.5 mg/kg/dose IV daily
	> 1 kg: 0-7 days: 2.5 mg/kg/dose IV q18h
	       > 7 days: < 37 weeks gestational age (GA) 2.5 mg/kg/dose IV q12h
	       ≥ 37 weeks GA 2.5 mg/kg/dose IV q8h
		Reduce dose in renal impairment; monitoring of serum drug concentrations recommended

Glucagon	1-1.5 mg/day IV as continuous infusion	Dilute in 5% or 10% dextrose
Heparin	Thrombosis: Loading dose: 50-100 U/kg IV Maintenance dose: 20-30 U/kg/hr IV via continuous infusion	Monitor PTT and titrate infusion rate accordingly Maintenance of indwelling lines: Mix weight in units per ml of IV solution and run at 0.5 ml/hr (e.g., 2 kg patients: 2 U heparin in 1 ml IV solution; run at 0.5 ml/hr)

Continued.

Table V-2 Neonatal Drug Dosage Guidelines*—cont'd

Drug	Dose	Comments
Hydralazine	1.7-3.5 mg/kg/day IV ÷ q4-6h	

Indomethacin	Patent ductus arteriosus:
	0.1 mg/kg/dose IV q24h × 5 doses or age at 1st dose:
	  < 48 hr: 0.2 mg/kg/dose IV followed 12 hrs later by 0.1 mg/kg/
	    dose q12h IV × 2 doses
	  > 48 hr: 0.2 mg/kg/dose IV q12h × 3 doses
		Reduce doses of aminoglycosides and digoxin to ½ until good urine output returns; infuse over 20 min

Insulin	0.01-0.02 U/kg/hr IV as continuous infusion	Titrate infusion rate according to blood glucose; use regular insulin only
Iron	Supplementation (prematurity, long-term PN): Birth weight ≥ 1000 g: 2-3 mg/kg/day PO as single daily dose Birth weight < 1000 g: 3-4 mg/kg/day PO as single daily dose	Supplementation for premature infants usually begins at 6-8 wk postnatal age; iron-fortified formula (instead of iron drops/syrup) recommended for bottle-fed infants; patients on long-term parenteral nutrition (PN) may require iron supplementation
Isoproterenol	0.05-1 μg/kg/min IV as continuous infusion	Stop or slow infusion if heart rate > 200/min
Lorazepam	Seizures: 0.05 mg/kg/dose IV or PR May repeat once prn	For PR administration, dilute injection according to IV instructions
Mannitol	1 g/kg/dose IV (5 ml of 20% solution/kg/dose)	
Metoclopramide	Initial dose: 0.1 mg/kg/day PO or IV ÷ q8h Max: 0.5 mg/kg/day	Extrapyramidal side effects may be reversed with diphenhydramine, 1 mg/kg/dose IV
Metronidazole	Weight (g) Age (days) Dose < 1200 7.5 mg/kg/dose IV q48h 1200-2000 ≤ 7 7.5 mg/kg/dose IV q24h > 2000 ≤ 7 7.5 mg/kg/dose IV q12h 1200-2000 > 7 7.5 mg/kg/dose IV q12h > 2000 > 7 15 mg/kg/dose IV q12h	Reduce dosage in patients with severe liver impairment; may discolor urine dark or reddish brown

Morphine	Pain: Loading dose: 0.05-0.1 mg/kg IV Maintenance dose: 0.005-0.01 mg/kg/hr IV as continuous infusion	
Naloxone	0.1 mg/kg/dose IV/ETT; repeat prn	Contact poison control in cases of narcotic overdose
Novospirozine	2-4 mg of each component/kg/day PO ÷ q12h	Contains equal amounts of hydrochlorothiazide and spironolactone
Pancuronium (Pavulon)	0.05-0.1 mg/kg/dose IV prn	
Paraldehyde	150 mg/kg/hr (3 ml of 5% solution/kg/hr) IV over 2 hr 1 ×/day 300 mg/kg (0.3 ml of undiluted paraldehyde/kg) × 1 per rectum diluted in oil or normal saline to make 30%-50% solution	Use with caution in patients with liver impairment; make 5% solution by adding 1.75 ml of paraldehyde to 5% dextrose to make total volume of 35 ml in syringe; undiluted paraldehyde contains 1 g/ml
Penicillin G (Benzylpenicillin)	< 2 kg: 0-7 days: Meningitis: 100,000 U/kg/day IV ÷ q12h Other: 50,000 U/kg/day IV ÷ q12h > 7 days Meningitis: 150,000 U/kg/day IV ÷ q8h Other: 75,000 U/kg/day IV ÷ q8h ≥ 2 kg: 0-7 days: Meningitis: 150,000 U/kg/day IV ÷ q8h Other: 50,000 U/kg/day IV ÷ q8h > 7 days: Meningitis: 200,000 U/kg/day IV ÷ q6h Other: 100,000 U/kg/day IV ÷ q6h	Reduce dose in severe renal impairment
Phenobarbital	Loading dose: < 37 wk PCA: 10-20 mg/kg IV; may repeat dose of 5-10 mg/kg IV up to max total dose of 25 mg/kg ≥ 37 wk PCA: 10-20 mg/kg IV; may repeat dose of 10 mg/kg IV up to max total dose of 30 mg/kg Maintenance dose: 4-6 mg/kg/day IV or PO 1 ×/day	Reduce dose in liver impairment; administer undiluted at rate not to exceed 1 mg/kg/min; monitoring of serum drug concentrations recommended

Continued.

FORMULARY

Table V-2 Neonatal Drug Dosage Guidelines*—cont'd

Drug	Dose	Comments
Phenytoin	Loading dose: 20 mg/kg IV Maintenance dose: 4-8 mg/kg/day PO or IV 1 ×/day or ÷ bid	Reduce dose in liver impairment; monitor for hypotension during infusion; administer undiluted at rate not to exceed 1 mg/kg/min; poorly absorbed orally in infant; monitoring of serum drug concentrations recommended
Piperacillin	< 2 kg: 0-7 days: 150 mg/kg/day IV ÷ q12h > 7 days: 225 mg/kg/day IV ÷ q8h > 2 kg: 0-7 days: 225 mg/kg/day IV ÷ q8h > 7 days: 300 mg/kg/day IV ÷ q6h	Reduce dose in severe renal impairment
Propranolol	Resuscitation: 0.01-0.10 mg/kg/dose IV Other: 0.5-1 mg/kg/day PO ÷ q6h	
Prostaglandin E$_1$	see alprostadil	
Pyridoxine (vitamin B$_6$)	50-100 mg/dose IV	Monitor EEG concurrently
Ranitidine	1.25-1.9 mg/kg/day IV ÷ q6-12h 2.5-3.8 mg/kg/day PO ÷ q12h	Reduce dose in renal impairment
Rifampin	20 mg/kg/day PO ÷ q12h	Use with caution in patients with liver impairment
Sodium bicarbonate	IV dose (mmol) = wt (kg) × 0.3 × base deficit 1-3 mmol/kg IV over 5 min in mild asphyxia 3-5 mmol/kg IV over 5 min in severe asphyxia	4.2% = 0.5 mmol/ml 8.4% = 1 mmol/ml Dilute 8.4% 1:1 with sterile water or 5% dextrose or use 4.2% undiluted
Sodium polystyrene sulfonate (Kayexalate)	1 g/kg/dose PO or per rectum	Mix in water or 5% dextrose; exchanges ~ 1 mmol K$^+$/g
Spironolactone	2-4 mg/kg/day PO ÷ q12h	For spironolactone in combination with hydrochlorothiazide, see Novospirozine

Theophylline	For patients not currently receiving aminophylline or theophylline: Loading dose: 5 mg/kg IV or PO Maintenance dose: 2 mg/kg/day IV or PO ÷ q12h	Monitoring serum theophylline and caffeine concentrations recommended; administer at rate not to exceed 0.4 mg/kg/min
Ticarcillin	< 2 kg: 0-7 days: 150 mg/kg/day IV ÷ q12h > 7 days: 225 mg/kg/day IV ÷ q8h ≥ 2 kg: 0-7 days: 225 mg/kg/day IV ÷ q8h > 7 days: 300 mg/kg/day IV ÷ q6h	Reduce dose in severe renal impairment
Tobramycin	≤ 1 kg: 0-7 days: 2.5 mg/kg/dose IV daily > 7 days: 3.5 mg/kg/dose IV daily > 1 kg: 0-7 days: 2.5 mg/kg/dose IV q18h > 7 days < 37 weeks GA 2.5 mg/kg/dose IV q12h ≥ 37 weeks GA 2.5 mg/kg/dose IV q8h	Reduce dose in renal impairment; monitoring serum drug concentrations recommended
Tolazoline (Priscoline)	Loading dose: 1-2 mg/kg IV Maintenance dose: 0.5-2mg/kg/hr IV via continuous infusion	Monitor blood pressure; emergency-r ease or investigational agent; should be used in critical care areas only
Trimethoprim	UTI prophylaxis: 2 mg/kg/day PO ÷ bid or as single daily dose	Reduce dose in renal impairment; monitoring serum drug concentrations recommended
Vancomycin	Post- conceptional Weight (g) Age (wks) Dosage < 800 or < 27 27 mg/kg/dose IV q36h 800-1200 or 27-30 24 mg/kg/dose IV q24h 1201-2000 or 31-36 18 mg/kg/dose IV q12h or 27 mg/kg/dose IV q18h > 2000 or > 37 22.5 mg/kg/dose IV q12h	
Vitamin K₁ (phytonadione)	Hemorrhagic disease of newborn: Prophylaxis: 0.5-1 mg IM or SC at birth Treatment: 1 mg/dose IM or IV	Administer IV at rate not to exceed 1 mg/min

THERAPEUTIC DRUG MONITORING (TDM)

TDM CONCEPTS FOR PEDIATRICIANS IN PRACTICE (Table V-3)

- Elimination half-life of drug defined as time taken for serum concentration to decrease to half its original value; this parameter is a useful index of dose requirements, dosage interval, and time to steady state, but "normal" listed values are subject to interindividual variability
- Routine drug levels should not be measured before attainment of steady-state conditions (normally equivalent to duration of constant therapy involving 5 elimination half-lives), unless failure of therapeutic response or onset of toxicity suspected
- If individualization of therapy critical factor in acute phase of patient care, two blood samples drawn approximately one half-life apart (in first dosage interval or during constant rate infusion) can provide useful information about maintenance dose requirements
- Adequacy of oral therapy can be most reliably assessed by steady-state trough level analysis
- Time of sampling less critical for patients receiving long-term therapy if drug has long elimination half-life and given by regular intermittent dosing or if constant rate infusions are used
- If lack of efficacy or suspicion of toxicity transient and occurs at regular point in dosage interval, TDM samples should be collected at these times
- To facilitate TDM interpretation, all TDM serum samples should have accurately recorded on requisition and on patient's permanent record:
  1. Time that sample was drawn
  2. Actual time that previous dose was given

OPTIMAL SAMPLING GUIDELINES FOR TDM (Table V-4)

- *Earliest time for first TDM* refers to first routine opportunity for sampling after new order or order change; normally represents attainment of steady state
- *Ideal sampling time* permits direct comparison with normal therapeutic range
- Results of tests conducted on samples collected at other than ideal times must be interpreted cautiously
- Under certain circumstances, may be necessary to collect samples for monitoring at times that do not coincide with normal "peak" and "trough" assessment; such samples are referred to as "special" concentrations; special drug concentrations may have to be obtained when:
  1. Patients receiving peritoneal dialysis, hemodialysis, or CVVH
  2. Patients have unstable or poor renal function
  3. Therapy has been stopped after previous high drug concentration
- Except where indicated, minimum of 0.5 ml blood (either heparinized or clotted) required for each drug assayed; cyclosporine samples must be sent in EDTA vial

GUIDELINES FOR OBTAINING AMINOGLYCOSIDE CONCENTRATIONS

- All patients prescribed aminoglycosides (i.e., gentamicin) have concentrations ordered day 4 (if therapy to continue), except for following patients:
  1. Patients with renal impairment
  2. Premature infants
  3. Term infants < 7 days
  4. Documented infections when therapy continues beyond 72 hr
  5. Patients with fever and neutropenia
  6. Therapy beyond 7 days
  7. Patients on concurrent nephrotoxic drugs (i.e., amphotericin, cyclosporin)
  8. Patients with severe burns
- Above exceptions should have preaminoglycoside (trough) and post aminoglycoside (peak) concentrations ordered with third or fourth dose
- Continued monitoring should be at suggestion of pharmacy; however, in stable patients, creatinine and preconcentrations usually obtained approximately every 5 days; clinical status and renal function dictate degree of monitoring
- Consult pharmacy regarding aminoglycoside monitoring in dialysis patients

GUIDELINES FOR OBTAINING VANCOMYCIN CONCENTRATION

- Following guidelines reflect the maximal amount of routine investigation required:
  - Initial preconcentration (trough) before 4th or 5th dose
  - Initial preconcentration (trough) and postconcentrations (peak) before 4th or 5th dose:
    1. Febrile neutropenics
    2. Burn patients
  - Additional preconcentration (trough):
    1. Dosage adjustment
    2. Treatment of >10 days
    3. Additional nephrotoxic drugs
    4. Stable renal insufficiency/failure
    5. High MIC isolate
  - Additional preconcentration (trough) or postconcentration (peak):
    1. Patients not improving clinically
    2. Unstable renal function requiring full kinetic workup
  - Post concentrations (peak) of no use when drug infused over > 1 hr
  - Consult pharmacy regarding vancomycin monitoring in dialysis patients

Table V-3   Therapeutic Drug Monitoring (TDM) Concepts for Pediatricians in Practice

Drug	Time to steady state (elimination half-life)				Physician's routine inpatient orders (earliest time for initial TDM and suggested frequency with maintenance therapy)	Optional serum concentration range	Comments
	Neonates	Infants > 1 mo	Children > 1 yr				
Amikacin	24 hr* (6 hr)	24 hr (1.5 hr)	24 hr (1.5 hr)		See guidelines for obtaining aminoglycoside concentrations p. 625	Trough: 2.5-10 mg/L Peak: 20-35 mg/L	Half-life may be prolonged in patients with renal dysfunction; both clearance and volume of distribution may be increased in cystic fibrosis
Caffeine	14 days (3 days)	24 hr (2.5 hr)			Initial: After 1 wk therapy Maintenance: Trough: 1 ×/wk	30-100 μmol/L	Half-life of up to 100 hr in premature neonates decreases gradually throughout infancy to reach normal adult values by approximately 9 mo
Carbamazepine	30 days (12 hr)	30 days (10 hr)	30 days (8 hr)		Initial: Trough: 1 wk after initial dose, then 2 ×/wk until stable Trough: Day 3 after dose, change Maintenance: Patient specific	17-50 μmol/L Monitoring of active metabolite, carbamazepine 10, 11 epoxide not routine but may be of assistance Trough: 5-12 μmol/L	Because of enzyme autoinduction, half-life during chronic dosing may be considerably shorter than after first dose; consequently, within first 2-4 wk of therapy, dose may need to be increased to maintain therapeutic levels
Chloramphenicol	72 hr (15 hr)	48 hr (10 hr)	24 hr (5 hr)		Initial: Trough and peak on day 2 of therapy Maintenance: Trough: 2 ×/wk Peak: 2 ×/wk	Trough: 2-10 mg/L Peak: 15-25 mg/L	Pharmacokinetics in pediatric patients vary greatly and are unpredictable

Drug			Sampling Times	Optimal Concentration Range	Comments
Cyclosporine	—	36 hr (6 hr)	Initial: Trough: Day 2 of therapy Maintenance: Trough: Based on clinical picture	Optimal concentration range dependent on clinical status of patient, type and time since transplant, sample matrix, and analytic method	Monitoring considered mandatory to avoid extremely low or high levels, which may precipitate therapeutic failure or nephrotoxicity, respectively
Digoxin	7 days (1.5 days)	10 days† (2.5 days)	Initial: Trough: Neonate: Baseline, per first dose No risk factors: Day 5 Risk factors present: 48 hr postload Risk factors include clinical suspicion of toxicity, renal or hepatic impairment, poor response, drug interactions or noncompliance Maintenance: Trough: 1 ×/wk	1-2.5 μmol/L	Half-life may be prolonged in renal impairment, in infants and children, concentration-effect relationship somewhat imprecise, particularly in renal and hepatic impairment, because of cross-reactivity of standard assays with digoxin metabolites
Ethosuximide	7 days (1.5 days)	—	Initial: Trough: After 1 wk therapy Maintenance: Trough: Patient specific	280-710 μmol/L	Selected patients may tolerate and benefit from serum levels that are significantly higher than "recommended maximum limit"

Continued.

*Prolonged in premature neonates to 36 hr.
†Prolonged in premature neonates from 12-14 days.
‡Prolonged in premature neonates from 36-48 hr.
||Prolonged in patients with renal impairment; reduced in patients with cystic fibrosis.
§May be prolonged by birth asphyxia.
¶Neonates may respond to lower levels.

Table V-3 Therapeutic Drug Monitoring (TDM) Concepts for Pediatricians in Practice—cont'd

Drug	Time to steady state (elimination half-life)			Physician's routine inpatient orders (earliest time for initial TDM and suggested frequency with maintenance therapy)	Optional serum concentration range	Comments
	Neonates	Infants > 1 mo	Children > 1 yr			
Gentamicin	24 hr‡ (7 hr)	24 hr (4 hr)	24 hr (2 hr)‖	See guidelines for obtaining aminoglycoside concentrations, p. 625	Trough: 0.6-2 mg/L Peak: 5-10 mg/L	Target Peak (mg/L) Indication UTI 3-5 5-7 Pyelonephritis; cellulitis 6-8 Pneumonia, wound infection 7-9 Positive culture with neutropenia
Methotrexate	Not applicable; monitoring of high single doses only			Dependent on specific chemotherapy protocol	Calcium leucovorin therapy usually continues until methotrexate levels are < 0.08 μmol/L; however, may vary depending on protocol	Refer to individual protocol for target levels at specific points after initiation of high-dose infusion; concentrations elevated by impairment of renal filtration or secretion
Phenobarbital	14 days (5 days)§	7 days (2.5 days)	10 days (3 days)	Initial: Trough: Day 4 of therapy then 2 ×/wk during stabilization Maintenance: Trough: Patient specific	65-170 μmol/L	Specific patients tolerate and may benefit from serum levels that are significantly higher than "recommended maximum limit"

Phenytoin	7 days Half-life is concentration dependent, which makes time to steady state highly variable and unpredictable		Initial: Trough: Day 3 of therapy then 2 ×/wk until stable Maintenance: Trough: Patient specific	40-80 μmol/L¶	Simultaneous monitoring of free phenytoin levels not routine but may be of assistance Trough: 4-8 μmol/L
Primidone	No data available		Initial: Trough: Day 3 of therapy, then 2 ×/wk Maintenance: Trough: 1 ×/wk	23-55 μmol/L	Phenobarbital is major metabolite of primidone in vivo and therefore should be monitored concurrently; expected parent drug-to-metabolite ratio varies from 1:4 to 1:2
Salicylate (ASA)	7 days 7 days Approximate values only (half-life is concentration dependent)		Initial: Trough: Day 3 Maintenance: Trough: 1 ×/wk Overdose: See p. 442	JRA: 1.1-2.2 mmol/L Kawasaki disease, pericarditis: < 2.2 mmol/L	Nonlinear relationship may exist between dose and concentration because of "capacity-limited" protein binding and hepatic metabolism
Tobramycin	Refer to gentamicin guidelines				
Valproic acid	10 days 72 hr 36 hr (2 days) (15 hr) (8 hr)		Initial: Trough: Day 3 Maintenance: Trough: 2 ×/wk	350-700 μmol/L	Half-life may be prolonged in patients with hepatic disease and may be shortened in patients receiving other anticonvulsant drugs
Vancomycin	36 hr 24 hr 24 hr (7.5 hr) (4.0 hr) (2.5 hr)		See guidelines for obtaining vancomycin concentrations	Trough: 5-12 mg/L Peak: 25-40 mg/L	Half-life may be prolonged in premature low-birth weight neonates and in patients with renal impairment; peak concentrations are of no utility when drug is infused over > 1 hr

Table V-4 Optimal Sampling Guidelines for Therapeutic Drug Monitoring (TDM)

Drug	Earliest time for first TDM	Ideal sampling time	Comments
Acetaminophen		4 or more hr after ingestion	Toxicology only see nomogram p. 444
Amikacin	See guidelines for obtaining aminoglyco-		
Trough	side concentrations	0-30 min before dose	
Peak		IV: 30-60 min after finish of drug flush	
		IM: 60 min postflush	
Caffeine	1 wk	Trough: 0-4 hr before dose	
Carbamazepine			
Initial dose	1 wk	Trough: 0-1 hr before dose	
Dose change	Day 3		
Chloramphenicol			
Trough	Day 2	0-30 min before dose	If bacteriologic assay used, identify concur-
Peak	Day 2	60-90 min after finish of PO dose or drug	rent antibiotics
		flush	
Cyclosporine			Sampling protocol dependent on sample
Constant infusion	Day 2	No restrictions	matrix, analytic method, clinical indication,
Intermittent	Day 2	Trough: 0-60 min before dose	and time since transplantation
(IV or PO)			
Digoxin			1 ml sample volume
After loading	48 hr	Trough: 0-60 min before dose or at least 8	
Maintenance	Day 5	hr after last dose	
Ethosuximide	Day 7	Trough: 0-1 hr before dose	
Gentamicin	See guidelines for obtaining aminoglyco-		
Trough	side concentrations	0-30 min before dose	
Peak		IV: 30-60 min after finish of drug flush	
		IM: 60 min postflush	

Lithium	Trough: 12hr postdose	Must be clotted sample
Methotrexate	Sampling procedures dependent on treatment protocol	
Phenobarbital		
IV loading	At least 1 hr after load	
Maintenance	Trough: 0-2 hr before dose	
Phenytoin		
IV loading	At least 1 hr after load	
Maintenance	Trough: 0-1 hr before dose	
Primidone	Trough: 0-1 hr before dose	Take concurrent phenobarbital level
Quinidine	Trough: 0-1 hr before dose	
Salicylate		See p. 442
Toxicology	At least 6hr after acute ingestions	
Therapeutic	Trough: 0-1 hr before dose	Time to peak varies and is prolonged with enteric-coated product
Tobramycin		
Trough	0-30 min before dose	
Peak	30-60 min after finish of drug flush	
Valproic acid	Trough: 0-1hr before dose	
Vancomycin		
Trough	0-30 min before dose	
Peak	IV: 60-90 min after finish of drug flush; not routinely done	When infusion period > 60 min, peak concentrations will be lower than indicated in therapeutic range

Lithium	4-6 days
Phenobarbital	
IV loading	No restrictions
Maintenance	Day 4 (day 7 for steady state)
Phenytoin	
IV loading	No restrictions
Maintenance	Day 3 (day 7 for steady state)
Primidone	Day 3
Quinidine	Just before fifth regular dose
Salicylate	
Toxicology	No restrictions
Therapeutic	Day 3
Tobramycin	
Trough	See guidelines for obtaining aminoglycoside concentrations
Peak	
Valproic acid	Day 2
Vancomycin	See guidelines for obtaining vancomycin concentrations, p. 625

Table V-5 Equivalent Doses of Systemic Corticosteroids (Intravenous or Oral)

Drug	Equivalent dose
Cortisone	25 mg
Hydrocortisone	20 mg
Prednisone	5 mg
Prednisolone	5 mg
Methylprednisolone	4 mg
Triamcinolone	4 mg
Dexamethasone	0.75 mg

(From Schimmer BP, Parker KL: Adrenocorticotropic hormone; adrenocortical steroids and their synthetic analogs; inhibitors of the synthesis and actions of adrenocortical hormones. In: Hardman JG, Limbrid LE, eds: *Goodman and Gilman's the pharmacological basis of therapeutics*, ed 9, Toronto, 1996, McGraw Hill)

Table V-6 Maximum Volumes of Enemas to Be Administered Rectally*

Age	Volume
0-3 mo	30-100 ml
3-12 mo	100-250 ml
1-6 yr	250-500 ml
6-12 yr	500-1000 ml

*Note: Above volumes are guidelines only; in certain circumstances (e.g., encopresis), larger volumes may be recommended (see appropriate section).

Table V-7 Recommendations for Endocarditis Prophylaxis

1. Dental Procedures, Oropharyngeal Surgery, Instrumentation of Respiratory Tract, Including Children With Prosthetic Tissue or Heart Valves:

Children able to receive penicillin:	Children allergic to penicillin or on continuous penicillin prophylaxis for rheumatic fever or who have been treated with antibiotics more than once in past month:
Ampicillin 50 mg/kg (max 2 g) IV/IM 30 min before procedure, then 25 mg/kg (max 1 g) IV/IM 6 hr later; second dose may be replaced by amoxicillin 25 mg/kg (max 1.5 g) PO 6 hr later, except in neonates	Clindamycin 10 mg/kg IV (max 300 mg) 30 min before procedure, then 5 mg/kg IV/PO (max 150 mg) 6 hr later
or	or
Amoxicillin 50 mg/kg (max 3 g) PO 1 hr before procedure, then 25 mg/kg (max 1.5 g) PO 6 hr later; neonates should not receive oral prophylaxis; use IV/IM regimen above	Clindamycin 10 mg/kg PO (max 600 mg) 1 hr before procedure; no repeat dose; neonates should not receive oral prophylaxis; use IV/IM regimen above

Table V-7 Recommendations for Endocarditis Prophylaxis—cont'd

2. Gastrointestinal and Genitourinary Procedures or Instrumentation, Including Children With Prosthetic Tissue or Heart Valves

If urine is infected, antibiotic should be chosen that is active against infecting pathogen and against enterococci

Children able to receive penicillin:

Children allergic to penicillin or on continuous penicillin prophylaxis for rheumatic fever or who have been treated with antibiotics more than once in past month:

Major procedures:

Ampicillin 50 mg/kg (max 2 g) IV/IM 30 min before procedure, then 8 hr later

plus

Gentamicin* 2 mg/kg (max 100 mg) IV/IM 30 min before procedure, then 8 hr later; second doses may be replaced by pivampicillin 25 mg/kg (max 1.5 g) 6 hr after initial doses, except in neonates

Minor procedures:

Amoxicillin 50 mg/kg (max 3 g) PO 1 hr before procedure, then 25 mg/kg (max 1.5 g) PO 6 hr later; neonates should not receive oral prophylaxis; use IV/IM regimen above

Major procedures:

Vancomycin* 20 mg/kg (max 1 g) over 1 hr starting 1 hr before procedure and 8 hr later

plus

Gentamicin* 2 mg/kg (max 100 mg) IV/IM 30 min before procedure, then 8 hr later

Minor procedures:

Clindamycin 10 mg/kg (max 600 mg) PO 1 hr before procedure; no repeat dose; neonates should not receive oral prophylaxis; use IV/IM regimen above

3. Surgical Procedures on Infected and Contaminated Tissues, Including Incision and Drainage of Abscesses Where *Staphylococcus aureus* is Suspected, Including Children With Prosthetic Tissue or Heart Valves

Children able to receive penicillin:

Children allergic to penicillin or on continuous penicillin prophylaxis for rheumatic fever or who have been treated with antibiotics more than once in past mo:

Major procedures:

Cloxacillin 50 mg/kg (max 2 g) IV/IM 30-60 min before procedure and 6 hr later

plus

Gentamicin* 2 mg/kg (max 100 mg) IV/IM 30 min before procedure and 8 hr later

Minor procedures:

Flucloxacillin 25 mg/kg (max 1 g) PO 1 hr before procedure and 6 hr later

Major procedures:

Clindamycin 10 mg/kg IV (max 300 mg) 30 min before procedure; no repeat dose

plus

Gentamicin* 2 mg/kg (max 100 mg) IV/IM 30 min before procedure and 8 hr later

Minor procedures:

Clindamycin 10 mg/kg (max 600 mg) 1 hr before procedure; no repeat dose

*Reduce or omit second dose appropriately in patients with renal impairment.
Modified from Recommendations of the British Society of Antimicrobial Therapy, *Lancet* 335:88, 1990; and American Heart Association, *JAMA* 264:2919, 1990.

INDEX